Eating Disorders

Eating Disorders

A Guide to Medical Care and Complications

SECOND EDITION

PHILIP S. MEHLER, M.D., CEDS
Chief Medical Officer, Denver Health
Glassman Professor of Medicine,
University of Colorado Health Sciences Center
Denver, Colorado

and

ARNOLD E. ANDERSEN, M.D.
Professor, Department of Psychiatry
Carver College of Medicine, University of Iowa
Iowa City, Iowa

The Johns Hopkins University Press

Baltimore

© 1999, 2010 The Johns Hopkins University Press
All rights reserved. Published 2010
Printed in the United States of America on acid-free paper
9 8 7 6 5 4 3 2 1

The Johns Hopkins University Press
2715 North Charles Street
Baltimore, Maryland 21218-4363
www.press.jhu.edu

Library of Congress Cataloging-in-Publication Data

Mehler, Philip S.
    Eating disorders : a guide to medical care and complications / Philip S. Mehler
and Arnold E. Andersen. — 2nd ed.
      p. ; cm.
    Rev. ed. of: Eating disorders : a guide to medical care and complications / edited
by Philip S. Mehler and Arnold E. Andersen. 1999.
    Includes bibliographical references and index.
    ISBN-13: 978-0-8018-9368-1 (hardcover : alk. paper)
    ISBN-10: 0-8018-9368-2 (hardcover : alk. paper)
    ISBN-13: 978-0-8018-9369-8 (pbk. : alk. paper)
    ISBN-10: 0-8018-9369-0 (pbk. : alk. paper)
    1. Eating disorders—Complications. 2. Eating disorders—Treatment.
    I. Andersen, Arnold E. II. Eating disorders. III. Title.
    [DNLM: 1. Eating Disorders—therapy. 2. Eating Disorders—complications.
WM 175 M498e 2009]
    RC552.E18E28215 2009
    616.85'26—dc22   2009011816

A catalog record for this book is available from the British Library.

*Special discounts are available for bulk purchases of this book. For more information,
please contact Special Sales at 410-516-6936 or special sales*

The Johns Hopkins University Press uses environmentally friendly book materials,
including recycled text paper that is composed of at least 30 percent post-consumer
waste, whenever possible. All of our book papers are acid-free, and our jackets and
covers are printed on paper with recycled content.

To Leah, Avi, Ilana, and Benji Mehler, for their devotion and love, and to the memory of my late parents, Irving and Bernice Mehler, for their unfailing efforts and invaluable guidance.

—Philip S. Mehler

To Helen, my wife, and Allan, Karl, and Ellie, for their loving patience and encouragement.

Arnold E. Andersen

CONTENTS

The second edition of *Eating Disorders: A Guide to Medical Care and Complications* was prompted by both the success of the first edition and the substantial increase in medical information available for the care of persons with eating disorders since 2000. The intended audience is primarily clinicians with direct care responsibility for treating eating disorders, but a host of other professionals who are involved in detection, treatment, and prevention, such as coaches and teachers, as well as families, will find this book useful. The role of the primary care clinician is emphasized. Our goal is to advocate excellence in care with adequate detail but a minimum of obscure medical terminology. The approach continues to be directive and selective, based on a broad and long clinical practice in psychiatry and internal medicine as well as references from the published literature. The approach described in this book emphasizes hands-on practical methods of treatment, albeit with a reasoned explanation, while being unfailing in our commitment to being evidence-based. Individual circumstances will guide medical care in other directions where appropriate. We believe the principles and practices detailed herein will be most useful and offer substantial benefit for the reader.

The method of each chapter is to identify common questions to be answered and to offer a clinical case or two with highlights pertinent to the subject. We strive to describe the background for understanding the nature of the medical or psychiatric issue, to offer an approach to diagnosis and treatment, and finally, to recommend a list of selected up-to-date and pertinent references. The full literature is so voluminous at present, and will continue to expand, that winnowing out pertinent references is crucial.

We chose to rewrite the book between the two of us rather than continue with editing contributions from multiple authors. A number of chapter authors of the edited first edition have dispersed far and wide, making a close working relationship between an experienced psychiatrist and a widely published internist the most feasible method for updating the book. Dr. Andersen is the primary author of Chapters 1, 2, and 11–15, while Dr. Mehler wrote Chapters 3–10. An earlier version of Chapter 14 on the ethics of care of patients with anorexia nervosa appeared in *Eating Disorders Review* in 2008. The appendix outlines a pragmatic approach to the daily care of inpatients with eating disorders on a dedicated unit for those who wish not to have to rediscover the wheel regarding practical nuances of care. When there is a tree in the middle of the road, it may not matter whether you go left or right around it, but it is important to do one or the other. Likewise, some semiprotocolized approach to patient care is helpful, with periodic revisions and updates.

Because of its importance and special characteristics, gynecological endocrinology is presented in chapter 8 in association with osteoporosis, separate from general endocrinology in chapter 9. There is no chapter exclusively on obesity in this second edition because obesity by itself is not reflective of an eating disorder and because the topic is too broad to be covered in a single chapter. Where obesity affects eating disorders, as it does for the approximately 25 percent of obese patients who engage in binge eating, the interaction is described.

The first goal is to describe an approach to effective medical care, with an important but secondary concern with cost-effectiveness. Many publications support the definitive multidisciplinary care that is emphasized in this book rather than a "revolving door" approach of removing the immediate danger and then discharging the patient. This latter approach is not only less humane but also more costly in the long run. Good care involves concern with the whole person, including improving each person's psychological and medical status, ensuring minimal mortality and the lowest possible morbidity, and respecting the unique and individual humanity of each person's life journey. This approach offers realistic hope based on evidence from formal treatment trials as well as a wealth of clinical experience.

Both of us are deeply indebted to our patients for their trust and for what each one teaches us about the nature and the course of eating disorders. We could not have written this second edition without the constant guidance and encouragement of Wendy Harris, our editor at the

Johns Hopkins University Press. Thanks also to Adriana Padgett, Kelly Smith, and Claire Sabin for their superb administrative support. We, of course, are responsible for any errors in the publication.

Ambrose Pare (1519–90) summarized the role of the physician: "To cure sometimes, to relieve often, but to comfort always." We believe there is currently sufficient medical information regarding eating disorders that we can advocate "to care and comfort always, and to cure many times." We hope that in the near future the phrase will be modified as "to cure most times."

Eating Disorders

CHAPTER ONE

The Diagnosis and Treatment of Eating Disorders in Primary Care Medicine

COMMON QUESTIONS

How are eating disorders defined?

How do eating disorders present to primary care clinicians?

What simple screening questions can primary care clinicians ask patients to detect eating disorders?

What are the differences among anorexia nervosa, bulimia nervosa, binge eating disorders, and atypical or subsyndromal eating disorders?

What is the relationship between eating disorders and obesity?

Do males develop eating disorders?

Don't you need a psychiatrist to diagnose and treat eating disorders?

How is healthy weight determined for an individual?

What role do medications play in the treatment of eating disorders?

When should a primary care clinician refer a patient, and when should a primary care clinician carry out the treatment?

What are the criteria for hospitalization?

What are the most common comorbid psychiatric disorders?

Case 1

A.H., a 25-year-old female, was referred by her local psychiatrist for treatment of severe anorexia nervosa, complicated by a fractured humerus. She had developed body image distress and perception of fatness starting at age 13. She had been slightly chubby and was teased by her peers, especially about her "thunder thighs." She restricted food and lost weight from 151 pounds at 5 feet 4 inches (body mass index [BMI] of 26) to 84.9 pounds (BMI 14.6) at admission. In addition to eating fewer than 500 calories a day, she ran 6–8 miles a day and lifted weights. She limited herself to no more than 5 grams of fat a day and became vegetarian, not a family tradition. She developed fearfulness about "dangerous foods," such as cheese.

A.H. stated: "I felt cold all the time. My skin was dry. My hair started to fall out and my nails were brittle." Menses stopped at age 19. She was preoccupied with thoughts of food, weight, and shape for "80 to 90 percent of the day." She experienced a severe fear of becoming fat, even as her weight plunged. Her mood became brittle, often tearful. Family "walked on egg shells" to avoid displeasing her and provoking irritability. Her temperament was that of a self-critical, perfectionistic young woman for whom expression of emotions was a foreign experience.

Three previous residential treatments resulted in only temporary improvement, followed by relapse into her anorexic pattern of behavior and thinking. No binges or purges developed. Shortly before admission, she fell on an icy sidewalk and fractured her humerus. Bone mineral density by dual-energy X-ray absorptiometry (DEXA) scan for L1-L4 was 0.675 g/cm^3, 3.4 standard deviations below the mean for a woman her age. Left hip bone density was 0.674 g/cm^3, -2.2 standard deviations. Hemoglobin of 5.4 required four transfusions. Labs showed hyponatremia of 126 meq/L. Calcium was low, but potassium and phosphorus were within normal limits. ECG showed bradycardia of 45. Her displaced fracture was treated surgically with a rod, followed by physical therapy. A.H. had never abused alcohol or street drugs. Her two previous relationships had ended poorly, and she had a sense of distrust about future relationships.

During the inpatient portion of comprehensive treatment, A.H. restored her weight to 85 percent of her goal weight of 122–26 pounds. She accomplished the remainder of her weight restoration in partial hospital (a day program, 5 days a week), achieving 100 percent of her goal weight. Her morbid fear of fatness diminished, and she developed an acceptance of a healthy weight and body image, learning cognitive-behavioral skills in group, individual, and family therapy to challenge her overvalued beliefs. Her mood became good and stable. No psychotropic medications were needed. She made considerable progress in catching up with normal development during a year of relapse-prevention outpatient therapy after discharge.

Background

Eating disorders are disorders of eating behavior that individuals develop to deal with problems in emotional regulation, fears of development, and relationship conflicts, growing out of an overvaluation of the benefits of slimness to deal with these issues. They have almost nothing to do with food, weight, or shape, just as fear of elevators has little to do with elevators. They essentially serve as strategies, as pseudosolutions, to deal with a variety of distressed emotions and personal conflicts, especially a sense of lack of adequate control and effectiveness for life situations. Our society promotes the belief that weight loss is the way to improve low self-esteem, become respected, feel effective and in control, and avoid criticism. While often discussed as separate disorders, anorexia nervosa, bulimia nervosa, and binge eating disorder are all part of one overarching larger disorder of eating dysregulation driven by cognitive distortions, especially a shared irrational fear of fatness, a drive for thinness, and a distortion in body perception (Andersen and Yager, 2005).

Eating disorders are one of the "great pretenders" of the twentieth and twenty-first centuries, along with HIV/AIDS, presenting to primary care clinicians in many disguised forms, much like tuberculosis and syphilis in the nineteenth century. The physician may encounter them as symptoms related to almost any organ system (Table 1.1). A brief psychiatric history and mental state exam will reveal the true picture of the underlying disorder behind the medical presentation. Anorexia nervosa (AN) is a relatively "public" disorder because it produces obvious thinness, often in an otherwise energetic younger individual (Fig. 1.1). Bulimia nervosa (BN), however, is usually private, secretive, and marked by shame, and it generally involves planned or impulsive exits from functions involving food. A spouse living with someone who has bulimia may not be aware of the condition despite a decade or more of symptomatology.

Anorexia nervosa has been recognized for several centuries, but bulimia nervosa was given a diagnostic name only in 1979 (Russell, 1979). These two disorders are two sides of the same coin: they both begin by an attempt at weight loss, leading in one case to sustained low weight

TABLE 1.1   Typical ways in which eating disorders present to primary care
physicians

- Maternal concerns about medical illnesses causing loss of periods in daughter, unexplained weight loss, finding signs of vomiting without medical illness
- Physician notes decreased weight, preoccupation with dieting, or new amenorrhea in established patient compared to past visit
- Referral by coach, teacher, psychologist for evaluation of possible eating disorder
- Patient complaints compatible with disorders of specific organ systems but also compatible with eating disorders: thyroid (hyperactive, weight loss), malabsorption (diarrhea), other GI disorders such as gastroesophageal reflux disorder, ulcers, lactose intolerance (reflux, stomach pain, bloating), cancer (especially in older patients with weight loss, complaints of loss of appetite), parasites (unexplained weight loss), dermatological (loss of hair), dental (multiple new caries, loss of enamel), worsened obesity
- Positive answers to routine behavioral surveys, written or in person, for presence of an eating disorder
- Routine examinations in a patient in a high-risk sport or interest group or sexual orientation
- Failure to grow in weight (less commonly, height) appropriate for age

and in the other to the breakthrough of hunger in the form of binge eating, followed by compensatory efforts to avoid weight gain using self-induced vomiting, laxatives, diuretics, exercise, or bouts of fasting. Bulimia nervosa in many ways is a failed attempt at anorexia nervosa: a dieting effort in a person without the persevering traits of a classic anorexic, a person whose physiology and psychology do not tolerate prolonged semistarvation. Bulimia nervosa quickly evolves from being driven by hunger alone to being triggered by dysphoric mood and automatic habits of time and place, as well as probable autonomic conditioning. Binge eating disorder (BED) is defined as chronic binge eating with *no* compensation for the binges—no purging and no dietary restriction. Its definition is even more recent (Latner and Clyne, 2008). Commonly, there is migration between these subtypes, most often from anorexia to bulimic symptoms. Approximately 50 percent of patients with bulimia nervosa had had a past episode of anorexia nervosa, either full or partial syndrome.

These disorders are culture-bound: they occur only in industrialized

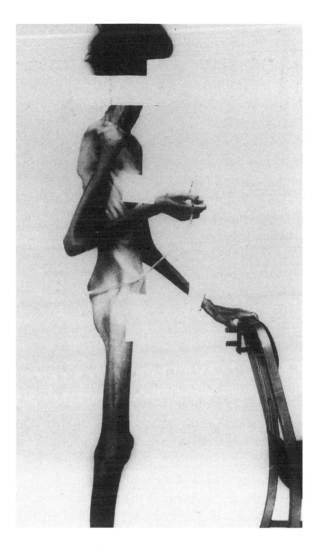

FIGURE 1.1 A typical very ill woman with anorexia nervosa. Note the extreme emaciation and lack of soft tissue.

cultures that value thinness and have sufficient availability of food that being overweight is a realistic possibility. Except in the governing or wealthy classes of developing countries, anorexia nervosa is infrequent. In cultures that value slimness (which include much of the Western hemisphere, most of Europe, Japan, and Westernized subgroups within other countries), a number of increasingly specific risk factors have been identified that predict which individuals will be more vulnerable to developing eating disorders, even though the risk for a given individual is probabilistic, not deterministic. Table 1.2 identifies several risk factors that increase the probability of developing eating disorders in proportion to their number and severity.

The natural history of eating disorders usually begins with several years of preoccupation with weight in the 8- to 12-year-old age group, with the subsequent development of attitudes valuing thinness and fearing fatness, often with unrealistic goals of an idealized thin but fashionable body size and improbable body shape (defined abs, no "stomach," slim hips). Dieting behavior usually begins later, during adolescence, when the body shape undergoes pubertal changes. The attitudes and values learned earlier drive the weight loss. Sometimes a specific precipitating factor (such as comments by friends or family, especially the mother, coaches, educators, or peers, suggesting that a particular individual is overweight, is in danger of becoming overweight, or should change the shape of a body part) may trigger a predisposed individual to develop an illness. Up to 40 percent of 9- to 10-year-olds are already worried about becoming fat, even though many fewer have any actual problem with even mild medical overweight. The increasingly alarmist leapfrogging of announcements of how many children are overweight begs the question of whether they are overfat, underfit, or simply above average.

Once dieting has started, a number of outcomes are possible. A frequent outcome is the development of the most common subsyndromic eating disorder, chronic dieting, without fulfilling strict criteria for a diagnosable eating disorder. About 1 percent of teenage girls go on to develop classical anorexia nervosa, and about 5 percent of those have a mild case. Two to four percent develop the full bulimia nervosa syndrome, whereas up to 19 percent of college women (5% of college men) experience some bulimic symptoms. Eighteen percent of high school wrestlers show partial eating disorders syndromes. Anorexia nervosa may present as a pure food-restricting subtype (ANR) or as a binge and/or purge subtype (ANB/P). A subgroup defined as purging-only subtype (Keel, 2007) is still controversial. The first binge of bulimia nervosa is usually triggered by dieting-induced hunger, provoking binge eating and

TABLE 1.2   Risk factors that increase the probability of eating disorders

Risk factor	Comments
Gender	More females than males, but not as large a discrepancy as previously thought (although 10:1 in clinical referrals, only 2–3:1 in community sample)
Age	Persons in teens and early 20s most likely, with peaks at ages 13–14 and 17–18; however, cases noted in patients from 7 to 77 years of age
Location	Highest incidence in Westernized societies valuing slimness and in upper socioeconomic classes in developing countries
Personality (typical, though not universal, features)	Anorexia nervosa: sensitive, perfectionistic, persevering, self-critical features of temperament
	Bulimia nervosa: impulsivity, emotional intensity, mood lability, dramatic features
	Binge eating disorder: high novelty seeking, high harm avoidance, low self-directedness
Family history	Increased in patients from families with history of obesity, depressive illness, anxiety disorders, eating disorders
Heritability	Estimated 50%–70% of risk factors are heritable. Concordance in monozygotic twins 3–4 times as high as in dizygotic twins
Interest groups	Dancers, body builders, models, wrestlers, sports with high performance and appearance demands, visual media professionals, actors
Critical sensitizing events	Teasing, criticism for overweight, especially by mothers, coaches, peers, significant others; involuntary weight loss for medical/surgical reasons (8% of cases); occasionally iatrogenic; demands for improved athletic performance; need for meeting military weight standards; obesity at menarche; childhood abuse
Sexual orientation	Increased in gay males (related to higher demand for perfectionistic body ideals, especially lean muscularity, not to sexuality); heterosexual females. Lesbian females may be slightly protected (controversial)

(continued)

TABLE 1.2 *(continued)*

Risk factor	Comments
Age of onset of dieting behavior	Girls starting to worry about weight by ages 9–10; by age 14, 60–70% trying to reduce weight
Racial and ethnic group	Largely independent of racial and ethnic identification, but increased with adoption of Westernization body ideals within groups; increased with higher socioeconomic status of African Americans
Medical diseases predisposing	Type I diabetes mellitus; cystic fibrosis
Psychiatric disorders predisposing	Depressive disorders, anxiety disorders, ADHD, PTSD, OCD
Location	More common in urban areas than in rural
Influence of media	Decreased self-esteem, more self-critical body image after viewing impossible-to-achieve body size/shape ideals in media

then compensatory measures to get rid of the unwanted calories eaten due to the fear of fatness. Soon, however, the binges of bulimia nervosa generalize to become a way to deal with any distressed mood, including depression, anxiety, anger, or feeling stuck or bored. Autonomic patterning helps lock in the syndrome behaviors. Finally, both eating disorders go on to give a personal identity whereby the individual cannot imagine life without either self-starving or binge/purge behavior or both.

No age, social class, or race is excluded from developing eating disorders (Striegel-Moore et al., 2003). Recently, the entity of binge eating disorder has emerged as a diagnostic relative of bulimia nervosa and is now the most common eating disorder. It is less obvious, being characterized by bingeing only (often with relentless grazing), without any purging or any other compensation to avoid weight gain. It tends to present less dramatically than bulimia nervosa, generally in patients in their 30s or 40s, and contributes to 25 percent of cases of medical obesity. It is often dismissed by patients, families, and doctors as simply a lack of willpower. A fairly rare entity, "reverse anorexia," may occur in body builders and weight lifters, who fear they are never big enough. A more recent term for this is "muscle dysmorphia."

Diagnosis and Evaluation

Table 1.3 lists five screening questions—the SCOFF Questionnaire (Morgan, Reid, and Lacey, 1999)—that primary care physicians may ask in assessing patients for the possibility of an eating disorder. It is helpful to have a brief but systematic set of questions for each behavioral disorder commonly seen in patients, such as the CAGE questionnaire for alcohol problems. The key concept in a diagnosis of eating disorder is that it is made not by ruling out all conceivable medical causation but by confidently ruling in the disorder based on a brief history and mental status examination.

The pertinent diagnostic criteria for eating disorders are summarized in Table 1.4 Anorexia nervosa is present when (1) *self-induced dieting* results in persistent substantial weight loss (or lack of normal weight gain during adolescent or preadolescent development); (2) the individual experiences the typical core psychopathology (overvaluation of the benefits of slimness or shape change associated with an intense drive for thinness and/or irrational fear of fatness, two sides of the same coin); (3) there is an abnormality of body image such that self-esteem depends disproportionately on weight or shape, often with an overestimation of size; and (4) there is abnormality of reproductive hormones or other signs and symptoms of medical starvation such as hypothermia, bradycardia,

TABLE 1.3   The SCOFF Questionnaire

---

1. Do you make yourself Sick because you feel uncomfortably full?
2. Do you worry you have lost Control over how much you eat?
3. Have you recently lost Over 14 pounds in a three-month period?
4. Do you believe yourself to be Fat when others say you are too thin?
5. Would you say that Food dominates your life?

Source: Adapted from Morgan, Reid, and Lacey, 1999, for American readers. In the original publication, item 3 reads "One stone" rather than "Over 14 pounds."
Note: Ask all patients 10–40 years old or in high-risk groups. Count one point for every "yes"; a score of ≥2 indicates a likely case of anorexia nervosa or bulimia.

TABLE 1.4 Diagnostic categories and criteria of eating disorders

Anorexia nervosa

- Substantial self-induced *weight loss*, often losing up to 85% of normal weight, but 85% is only typical case, not a requirement; more important is sufficiently great weight loss that signs of medical starvation are present. In growing children and young adolescents: failure to gain normally so that weight is ≤85% of healthy weight for age and height.
- Duration of >3 months
- Irrational (morbid) fear of fatness, usually with an intense drive for thinness
- Excessive valuation of the importance of thinness for self-esteem
- Frequently, body image distortion, in which the body is perceived to be much larger than actual weight
- Signs of medical starvation for >3 months, especially abnormal gonadotropin hormone functioning. While amenorrhea may be frequently present in females, it is not essential.
- Two subtypes: (a) classic food restriction (ANR) or (b) binge-purge subtypes (ANBP)

Bulimia nervosa

- Binge eating, twice a week (on average) for >3 months. Binges vary in amount from rapidly eaten huge amounts of food to more subjective perception of food intake as bingeing.
- Regret after binges, especially guilt or shame, fear of becoming fat, and/or medical discomfort, primarily gastric fullness
- Compensation for perceived overeating after binges by purging (vomiting, laxatives, diuretics), compulsive exercise, or increased fasting
- Shared psychopathological disturbance with anorexia nervosa of an excessive valuation of thinness for self-esteem and mood regulation
- Two subtypes: purging subtype (80%) or other compensation (20%) such as fasting or exercise
- Weight in broad normal range or overweight, i.e., not anorexia nervosa

Binge eating disorder

- Binge eating (average of >2 binges/week for >3 months), with a spectrum of binges from huge caloric intake to subjectively distressing smaller amounts to almost constant grazing, resulting in psychological distress (regret, guilt, shame) and/or medical discomfort, primarily stomach pain
- No compensatory behaviors to minimize the unwanted consequences of the binges
- Patients often older (30s–50s), frequently medically obese; present in about 25% of medically obese patients

TABLE 1.4 *(continued)*

EDNOS: atypical disorders (eating disorders not otherwise specified)

- Subsyndromal anorexia nervosa: chronic dieting with chronic underweight, showing fewer signs of severe medical starvation (less likely to have amenorrhea), but with typical overvaluation of the benefits and necessity of slimming; mental preoccupation with weight loss and/or shape change. May intermittently purge only. Approximately 8% of female infertility due to being only 10–15 pounds underweight

- Subsyndromal bulimia nervosa (e.g., may binge less than twice a week or for fewer than 3 months)

- Medically unexplained disorders: lack of medical diagnosis to explain weight loss or binge-purge behavior, and denial by patient of typical morbid fear of fatness or relentless drive for thinness, but indirect indications of eating disorder (e.g., parental documentation of signs of vomiting or frequent weighing, mirror gazing, complaints of fatness)

or weakness. The historical requirement of three months of amenorrhea is clearly not essential and should be disregarded anyway if a patient is on birth control. Reduction in weight to below 85 percent of healthy norms is an example listed in DSM-IV of how much weight loss is typical, not a requirement. The three groups of patients most commonly overlooked in making a diagnosis of anorexia nervosa are males, matrons, and minorities (Beck, Casper, and Andersen, 1996). Be cautious of stereotypes of patients' being adolescent Caucasian females.

The diagnosis of bulimia nervosa is made if a patient is binge eating, eating out of control (usually large amounts), and eating faster than normal (most commonly foods of higher fat or sugar content), commonly stopping only after developing medical distress or running out of food or feeling panic about weight gain. People who have bulimia nervosa share the psychopathology of anorexia: an irrational fear of fatness and/or a relentless drive for thinness, and overvaluing weight/shape ideals to excessively determine self-esteem. Patients with bulimia may test a physician with innocuous questions about other symptoms before revealing bulimic symptomatology.

The third, more heterogeneous group consists of atypical eating disorders (technically called "eating disorders not otherwise specified," or EDNOS). They are no less serious. About 50 percent of cases coming to university hospital clinics for eating disorders do not meet the strict criteria for anorexia nervosa or bulimia nervosa because these criteria are narrowly based on research studies. Over the next decade, this group of atypical disorders will be further refined (Strober, Freeman, and Morrell, 1999). (See Table 1.5.)

The most common eating disorder, technically a subgroup of ED-NOS, is binge eating disorder. Binge eating disorder is also often secretive or unapparent, mixed with the frequently comorbid obesity, and passed off as overindulgence, since it lacks the dramatic purging features of bulimia nervosa. Like the other binge subtypes of eating disorders, it produces in those affected a sense of demoralization about the inability to control the binge behaviors. That its presentation is commonly in older patients, in the 30s through the 50s, also makes binge eating disorder a less obvious diagnosis, since it does not conform to the societal stereotypes for anorexia nervosa or bulimia nervosa. The binges may be large—several thousand calories, a source of social embarrassment—or may be subjective and not as obvious externally but cause an internal sense of loss of control and regret, but without compensation. Some patients binge primarily at night, barely remembering their binges in the morning, except for the evidence provided by remnants of food and their containers; this subtype is called the *night eating syndrome.*

TABLE 1.5   Atypical eating disorders (eating disorders not otherwise specified, or EDNOS)

- Approximately 50% of eating disorders are misclassified as atypical (EDNOS) because formal AN/BN criteria (with DSM-IV more out of date than ICD-10) are research-based and overly restrictive. Amenorrhea is not necessary for the diagnosis of anorexia nervosa in females even if all other features are present but is still required by DMS-IV, and therefore anorexia nervosa without menses is often misclassified as EDNOS.
- Atypical eating disorder are no less serious than anorexia nervosa or bulimia nervosa.
- Payment for EDNOS cases is often inappropriately rejected by insurance companies, who sometimes erroneously consider EDNOS a less-serious disorder.
- Binge eating disorder—the most common eating disorder—is classified under EDNOS currently by DSM-IV but more logically belongs with the bulimia nervosa disorder spectrum.
- The EDNOS category is often confusing to clinicians.

Table 1.6 lists a number of clues to secretive eating disorders. In contrast to most medical syndromes, such as flu, diabetes, or a broken ankle, the patient may not see an eating disorder as an illness. It is often a source of pride in anorexia but shame in bulimia. Denial of thinness and denial of the illness are characteristic of anorexia nervosa. Weight loss in an otherwise healthy person beyond the point of medical benefit should be a tip-off to ask about excessive fear of fatness and drive for thinness. Anorexia may present to a gynecologist with signs of amenorrhea or oligomenorrhea, to a gastroenterologist though similarities to malabsorption, to an endocrinologist by the appearance of hyperthyroidism-like symptoms, or to a neurologist by signs compatible with a central nervous system tumor.

A "rule-out" approach to the diagnosis of eating disorders, by focusing on all possible medical causes without appreciating the mental status changes, leads to delay in treatment and iatrogenic morbidity. In not a single case of more than 1,000 anorexia nervosa individuals we have treated did any patient having the core psychological symptoms of eating disorders and typical self-induced weight loss turn out to have a previously undisclosed medical cause for the weight loss or the binge-purge behavior. Occasionally a case may simulate anorexia nervosa in many ways, but without the crucial morbid fear of fatness and drive for thinness and without distortion of body image. For example, consider a case of Crohn's disease in a 25-year-old individual with obsessive personality which manifests itself by avoidance of all solid food and limitation of intake to sports drinks. This case appears at first glance to be anorexia nervosa. The Crohn's disease was correctly diagnosed only after a positive stool evaluation for occult blood and the absence of typical mental symptoms of anorexia nervosa. The value of medical assessment for reasons other than diagnosis should not be underestimated. Medical assessment is vital for understanding the consequences and complications of the disorder, as well as for decision making about the location and intensity of treatment and methods of treatment, but not for diagnosis.

A number of psychiatric syndromes may also imitate anorexia nervosa, primarily by behaviors of food refusal or weight loss. Major depressive illness is frequently accompanied by weight loss of 15–20 pounds. Appetite return and weight restoration with cognitive-behavioral therapy, antidepressants, or electroconvulsive therapy, and the absence of

TABLE 1.6 Clues to secretive eating disorders

Anorexia nervosa

- Unexplained weight loss, especially in adolescents, or failure to gain proportionate to height in preteens and adolescents
- Secondary amenorrhea in adolescents or preadolescents without obvious medical cause
- Membership in avocational or identity groups promoting or requiring weight loss (ballet, wrestling, modeling, female gymnastics, gay orientation)
- Preoccupation with need for additional weight loss or body shape change, despite obvious thinness (females) or muscularity (males)
- Frequent mirror gazing
- Frequent talk of the need for weight loss without a medical basis; negative comparison of self to thinner peers
- Unexplained high TSH, low T3, low LH/FSH from central hypothalamic hypogonadism; feeling cold compared to peers, often with objective hypothermia; unexplained hair loss; development of lanugo hair (fine, downy hair on face and back)
- Hypercarotenemia

Bulimia nervosa or binge-purge form of anorexia nervosa

- Unexplained hypokalemia (low potassium)
- Family report of patient vomiting without medical illness or of finding remains of boxes of laxatives or diuretics
- Swollen or tender parotid glands
- Loss of dental enamel on lingual surface, or large number of new caries
- Gastroesophageal reflux or symptoms of esophageal erosions in young person
- Yo-yo weight pattern

Binge eating disorder

- Obesity
- Continued unexplained steady weight gain or sudden rapid weight gain
- Shame or guilt in discussing eating patterns
- Hopelessness, helplessness about weight

body image distortion or a morbid fear of fatness, usually confirm the correct diagnosis. Patients with obsessive-compulsive disorders or traits may be unable to eat normally because of obsessional ruminations about the nutritional content of food, making decision making about meals difficult. A choking episode may sensitize an individual so that he or she avoids swallowing solid food of any kind and has led to weight loss as severe as in anorexia nervosa in a number of patients. Paranoid states, especially paranoid schizophrenia in adolescents and young adults who have narrowly focused delusions about food being poisoned, may lead to substantial weight loss but be inscrutable because of the patient's suspiciousness prevents him from giving the physician full awareness of the inner delusional process. Treatment with neuroleptics usually leads to improved eating and increased weight as well as the ability of the patient to be more candid in the mental status examination.

Eating disorders seldom occur alone; they almost always have companion disorders (Jordan et al., 2008). Table 1.7 lists the most common associated disorders. Once the diagnosis of anorexia, bulimia, or an atypical eating disorder has been made, brief additional questioning will usually disclose the companion disorders. In virtually all cases of severe eating disorders, the clinician is treating a cluster of disorders, some self-improving, some needing separate treatment.

Classic food-restricting anorexia is accompanied by, on average, two

TABLE 1.7 Psychiatric companion (comorbid) disorders that commonly occur with eating disorders

- Mood disorders (40%–70%): major depression, bipolar II (cycles of depression plus mild highs), dysthymia (low mood >50% of year, but without blocks of ≥2 week periods of depression)
- Anxiety disorders: generalized anxiety disorder with or without panic
- Obsessive-compulsive disorders (especially in anorexia nervosa)
- Alcohol and/or other drug abuse (especially in bulimia nervosa or ANBP)
- Personality disorders
  ◦ Cluster C traits that are common in anorexia nervosa: sensitive, perfectionistic, persevering, self-critical
  ◦ Cluster B traits that are common in bulimia nervosa: impulsivity, unstable moods, dramatic, emotional intensity

additional associated psychiatric diagnoses; the binge-purge subtype of anorexia typically has four associated diagnoses; and bulimia nervosa has three (Margolis et al., 1994). Binge eating disorder is often associated with depression and obesity. Community-based untreated cases of eating disorder may not have as high an incidence of comorbid disorders, but the majority of individuals with eating disorders (50%-70%) who come for treatment will have some form of mood disorder, personality disorder, drug or alcohol abuse, anxiety state, or obsessive-compulsive disorder. It is important to emphasize the assessment of the comorbid syndromes because comprehensive treatment, and certainly management, depend on a combined approach. Anorexia nervosa has an increased chance of suicide (Bulik et al., 2008)

Vulnerabilities of personality, whether traits or disorders, are increased in all eating disorders but are not randomly distributed. Patients with anorexia nervosa are more likely to be sensitive, persevering, self-critical, and perfectionistic, while patients with bulimia nervosa or the binge-purge subtype of anorexia nervosa are more often (but not always) likely to be impulsive and dramatic and to have unstable moods. Monozygotic twins share a 50 percent chance of both having an eating disorder if one is afflicted. There is no conclusion yet as to what is being transmitted for genetic vulnerability—possibly vulnerabilities in personality or mood, such as a predisposition to depressive illness, persevering and sensitive personality traits, and other features that might be related to variations in central nervous system serotonin regulation. It has been estimated that the genetic vulnerability to an eating disorder ranges from 50 to 70 percent (Bulik et al., 2006).

Table 1.8 summarizes features of eating disorders in males. (Eating disorders in males are discussed in Chapter 12.) Males may be slower to be diagnosed because clinicians may not recognize that males can develop eating disorders. Also, males may be sensitive that they will be told they have either a girl's disease or a gay person's disease. (See Fig. 1.2.)

Some "pearls" and tips about diagnosis of eating disorders in general are listed in Table 1.9.

TABLE 1.8   Characteristics of males with eating disorders

- Large community studies indicate that M:F ratio for eating disorders is 1:2–3; thus, 1 out of 10–20 cases in clinics is false ratio. Implication: Many males with eating disorders are undiagnosed or avoidant of diagnosis and/or treatment.
- Dieting usually begins for specific goals rather than general desire for weight loss, as more often found in normal-weight females. Most common specific reasons are
  - to increase athletic performance,
  - to avoid being teased for childhood obesity, in association with sensitive personality,
  - to avoid weight-related medical illness, especially those found in the father,
  - to improve a gay relationship.
- Males usually preoccupied with attaining lean muscularity, and especially concerned with body shape from the waist up; females most commonly concerned with body shape from the waist down.
- Increased probability of gay orientation exists (18%–20%) but homosexuality still constitutes a minority of cases.
- Males usually perceive fatness and a need to start dieting at higher relative weights than females, who feel fat starting at 15%–17% below normal. Males generally perceive fatness at more objective overweight levels.
- Males may fear being told they have a girl's disease or a gay person's disease. They will often delay coming in for diagnostic evaluation. Anorexia nervosa generally ego-alien in males, often ego-syntonic in females. High feeling of shame.
- Males sometimes stigmatized by female eating-disordered patients as typical of problematic males in their past.
- Many health professionals uneducated about eating disorders in males and often do not consider a diagnosis of eating disorders in males, or programs may not accept males, a form of gender discrimination.

Note: See also chapter on males.

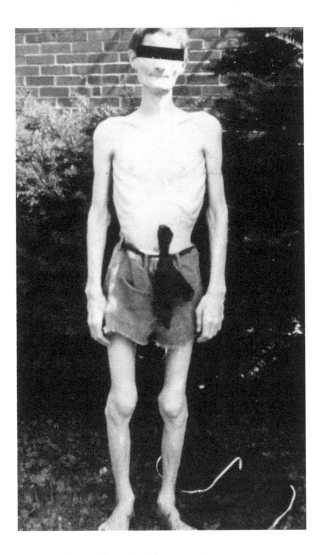

FIGURE 1.2. A typical very ill male with anorexia nervosa.
Source: Reproduced with permission of the patient.

TABLE 1.9   Clinical "pearls" for the diagnosis of eating disorders

- Diagnosis is made by simple history and mental state exam, not by ruling out all possible medical causes.

- Although most common in teens and 20s, eating disorders occur from 7 to 77 years of age. Remember to consider eating disorders in matrons, males, and minorities.

- Females with anorexia are often proud of weight loss, but bulimic behavior is usually shameful or guilt-producing. The patient may test how judgmental you are before disclosing bulimia.

- Purging alone is not diagnostic for bulimia nervosa, but on questioning the clinician discovers that it is usually preceded by subjectively distressing binges and is therefore a form of bulimia nervosa without huge binges. Binges do not have to be large to be distressing.

- Binge eating disorder (binge eating without any compensation) occurs in about 25% of medically obese patients as a contributing factor to total weight burden. Therefore, inquire about symptoms of eating-disordered thinking and behavior in all obese patients.

- Binge eating disorder patients most typically are older patients (30s–50s) This disorder occurs about equally in males and females and may involve compulsive grazing as well as actual binges.

- Eating disorders in older patients are often complicated by concurrent medical or depressive symptoms as well as a failure to consider an eating disorder as a possible diagnosis.

- Once an eating disorder diagnosis is made, assess the patient for the comorbid psychiatric disorders which are usually present, as well as for medical consequences. Decide which are predisposing factors and which are secondary to the eating disorder.

- The most common contributing factor to eating disorders is dieting. "Diet" is a four-letter word.

- Approximately 8% of anorexia nervosa cases have involuntary onset: self-directed additional weight loss is practiced only after initial weight loss from a medical or surgical cause, such as flu, postoperative weight loss, jaw-wiring, etc.

- Younger patients with anorexia nervosa may try to fool the physician about prescribed weight restoration by carrying secret weights in pockets or drinking noncaloric beverages before examination.

- Primary care physicians can be fully competent to treat many cases of eating disorders, especially the earlier and milder cases that are most common.

Case 2

G.M. was an 18-year-old male who had reached a weight of 205 pounds at 6 feet tall. He was teased by his classmates and also advised by his coach to take off weight. He gradually cut down food intake to the point of having only an orange a day plus a health shake, and he lost almost 60 pounds over 3 months. He developed superior mesenteric artery syndrome, becoming nauseated and vomiting after meals. His primary care physician recognized the compressive effect of a full stomach on the superior mesenteric artery, caused by the absence of the abdominal fat pad, which had been lost by starvation. He was promptly treated in the hospital, and though he minimized his drive for thinness, no other cause was found. He fully restored his weight and went on to maintain himself in a healthy range with full relief of abdominal symptoms. He was diagnosed with a probable eating disorder and associated depressive symptomatology.

Therapeutic Interventions

Primary care physicians can, and should, not only diagnose but also treat many early and moderate cases with eating disorders, sometimes in conjunction with colleagues in psychology, nutrition, and social work. After diagnosis, the next step is setting goals for treatment (Table 1.10).

The methods of treatment available to a primary care physician are low in technology, modest in cost, and potentially effective. Patients with anorexia nervosa should be restored to a full healthy weight, which, at a minimum, in women is a weight that leads to normal regular menstrual cycles. Typically, the return of menses occurs at an average of 92 percent of healthy weight. Freedom from feeling colder than peers, improved bradycardia into a normal heart rate, and normalization of T3, LH, and estradiol (testosterone in males) are signs of being close to a healthy weight even if menses are not yet restored. Treatment is not limited to achieving a weight goal. Normal weight is the *beginning*, not the end, of treatment. Normal eating behavior and personal comfort and confident eating in a variety of social situations are essential. The real core of treatment, however, is persuading patients to think differently about the value of thinness and to find ways other than self-starving to deal with stress,

TABLE 1.10   Key goals and methods of treatment for eating disorders

Key goals

1. *Fully normal individualized weight,* not determining weight from an insurance table (useful as an intermediate goal) but prescribing nutritional rehabilitation until the individual has returned to a self-regulating personal "set-point" for weight—indicated by evidence that the patient is not cold and has normal T3, normal hunger and satiety patterns, and normal gonadotropin functioning

2. *Normal eating behavior and normal dietary content* in wide variety of social situations

3. *Healthy thinking about weight, shape, and food* is the overriding goal. When the patient's only concern about weight is "culturally normative distress," treatment is successful. It is unrealistic for most women to have no concerns about weight—or at least not to give lip service to dieting when with friends. Crucially, however, preoccupation with weight loss/shape change no longer dominates mental life.

Methods of treatment

- *Cognitive behavioral treatment* (CBT) is the most effective evidence-based form of psychotherapy for eating disorders and consists in teaching patients to challenge with evidence-gathering their overvalued beliefs about the benefits of slimness/shape change. In its basics, it is simple to learn and practice. Early and mild bulimia nervosa may respond fully to only a few sessions of counseling.

- If no experienced cognitive behavioral therapist is available, *SSRIs* (e.g., fluoxetine, sertraline, escitalopram) often decrease binge-purge symptoms by 50%, but patients may relapse if medications are discontinued or may not respond at all. Primarily for bulimia nervosa and binge eating disorder. Best used if CBT is not by itself fully effective. May be used alone for bulimia nervosa or binge eating disorder if no counseling available.

- *Help patient understand that the core issue is not weight or food,* but emotional distress, for which the eating disorder is a pseudosolution. Therefore, identifying key issues in developmental snags, mood regulation, and distressed relationships, and teaching age-appropriate coping skills is crucial.

- *Provide parents and significant others with psychoeducation* about the nature of the disorder, coping with "burnout" while caring for chronic cases, and maintaining healthy family relationships without being monitors or "food police." They need support and education, not criticism, as well as resolution of family functioning issues they identify as needing therapeutic work.

(continued)

TABLE 1.10 *(continued)*

- *Prevention of relapse* by continued treatment for 2–4 years after initial goals are attained is essential, and particularly in the first year after treatment. Comprehensive integrative treatment can provide full resolution of the eating disorder, especially in younger patients, with the best studies documenting about 75% fully recovered. It is a myth that all cases are difficult or chronic. Realistic optimism is justified.
- *Outpatient treatment can work even in some severe cases.* Evidence-based studies show that some cases of even severe anorexia nervosa (BM of ≥14.5 in teens) can be treated by an experienced outpatient-based family therapist using the LeGrange and Locke method.
- *Comorbid psychiatric diagnoses may remit or diminish with full treatment of the eating disorder* and therefore may not need intensive separate treatment unless they persist after resolution of the eating disorder with the achievement of normal weight and normal thinking about food.

depressed or other dysphoric moods, crises in development or family functioning, and low self-esteem. The most validated psychological treatment is called *cognitive-behavioral therapy* (CBT). CBT is a shorthand term for normalizing patterns of behavior and letting go of the drive for overvalued cognition of the benefits of slimness and fear of healthy weight, to be replaced by a willingness to allow the body to seek its healthy weight and by learning to respond to challenges in development and mood regulation directly instead of using weight loss to deal with these issues (Bowers, 2001). The physician should think of eating disorders not only as an *illness,* but also as a *strategy* promoted by sociocultural norms to deal with issues in mood regulation and challenges in development and relationships. Weight loss and weight control become pseudosolutions to the task of finding a personal identity.

Bulimia nervosa is a heterogeneous spectrum condition, a kind of final common pathway, variable in seriousness and response to treatment. Bulimia nervosa treatment essentially involves "working the binge episodes out of a job." This means assessing the primary purpose that binges serve, beginning with identifying their triggers—a task easily accomplished with a week of daily diaries on 3 × 5 cards, documenting time of eating, food eaten, binge behavior, mood, and events. The three major triggers for binge episodes are (1) hunger from underweight or restricted eating; (2) emotional distress of any kind; and (3) an almost automatic conditioned reflex based on autonomic conditioning for a certain time of day. When any degree of underweight is present, an increase to fully normal weight is essential to decrease the intensity of hunger which helps to drive binge episodes. The psychological core of treatment in bulimia nervosa involves decreasing emotional distress, altering habit patterns, improving distressed relationships, and developing stress management techniques. SSRIs (fluoxetine, sertraline, citalopram) alone *may* (but do not always) decrease binge episodes and purging by about 50 percent within 3 months, but symptoms tend to recur when medications are stopped, or they may break through despite medication use. Recent evidence suggests that use of evidence-based psychological treatment methods like cognitive-behavioral therapy (CBT) or interpersonal therapy (IPT) leads to even better and longer-lasting results than those that can be achieved by use of antidepressants alone. Antidepressants generally are best used in patients who have not responded to CBT or IPT after 10–12 weeks, or where there is a preexisting history of depressive illness before the onset of the eating disorder. Buproprion is generally contraindicated because of possible seizures. The primary care physician or nutritionist colleague will give the patient a nutritional program adequate in energy (calories) and balance (exchanges), teaching the patient healthy nutrition, not endorsing an unbalanced emphasis on fat grams and calories.

The treatment of binge eating disorder usually requires a combination of a lifetime nutritional plan, teaching assertiveness, improved stress management, moderate regular exercise to increase lean muscle mass, and often an antidepressant of the SSRI category at the beginning of treatment. CBT again is the core of treatment of binge eating disorder. An approach to binge eating disorder in obese patients would be to first bring the eating disorder under control, and only then, if body weight is still medically excessive, to consider additional weight-reducing methods for the bedrock of the genetically predisposed remaining obesity. An alternative is to accept BMI up to 30 when further weight loss is fraught with suffering and to emphasize development of lean muscle mass and cardiopulmonary fitness. Normalization of eating behaviors takes priority over weight loss. Fitness within any weight category generally produces more health benefits than weight loss, is more achievable, and is more enduring.

A nonjudgmental view of obesity as a chronic lifetime disorder is timely, but the field awaits long-term pharmacological methods.

Table 1.11 identifies some of the most common reasons for referral to hospital for treatment of an eating disorder. In general, most person with entrenched anorexia nervosa will require some form of hospitalization (either 24-hour or partial hospital, full-day treatment), while most persons with bulimia nervosa can generally be treated as outpatients, with exceptions for severity or medical comorbidity. Lock and LeGrange (2005)

TABLE 1.11   Reasons for 24-hour or partial hospitalization of patients with eating disorders

- Moderate to severe anorexia nervosa: some hospitalization (full or partial hospital or day hospital) usually required
- Patients with bulimia nervosa: outpatient programs usually the best choice except for patients experiencing severe depression or self-harmful behavior.
- Substantial weight loss or rapid weight loss, especially below 75%–80% of normal, or 20%–30% below onset weight, especially if weight loss is rapid in children or teens
- Significant medical symptomatology (low serum potassium, severe malnutrition, unstable vital signs, uncontrolled comorbid diabetes)
- Significant psychiatric comorbidity, especially if impairing outpatient treatment:
  - suicidality
  - borderline personality disorder
  - substance abuse
  - severe comorbid OCD
  - major depression
- Lack of response to outpatient treatment
- Hostile living situation or lack of experienced local therapists
- Diagnostic uncertainty with probable eating disorder present and severe medical symptoms
- Presence of a life-threatening situation (refusal of treatment despite severe weight loss, hypokalemia, suicidality), in which case involuntary treatment may be necessary. Involuntary treatment is as effective as voluntary treatment; generally, insight returns in about 2 weeks.

Note: Treatment on a unit dedicated to eating disorder treatment with an experienced team-oriented, comprehensive approach is more effective than treatment on a general unit with inexperienced staff.

developed an intensive family treatment that allows many adolescents with anorexia nervosa under 18 years of age, and with a BMI over 14, to be treated entirely as outpatients. Full treatment to a healthy normal weight leads to fewer rehospitalizations (Baran, Weltzin, and Kaye, 1995) and is in the long run more cost-effective (Crow and Nyman, 2004). Managed care has made ruthless inroads in the length of stay for psychiatric disorders in general and eating disorders in particular, but hospital care is often essential for good short-term and lasting long-term outcome. Once initial treatment in hospital has been accomplished, the focus of long-term treatment changes to relapse prevention, with planning for aftercare and relapse prevention starting on the day of admission. There is increasingly proven efficacy for CBT (and IPT) as well as for adjunctive antidepressants, especially fluoxetine, for prevention of relapse for inpatient as well as outpatient treatment. In the absence of a clinician skilled in CBT or IPT, continued aftercare treatment with an SSRI is an alternative better than no treatment, but experienced therapy is ideal.

For patients under age 18, treatment of the family unit as a whole after discharge has produced more sustained improvement and relapse prevention than treatment of the young individual alone. Recently, this death rate has come down but is still high in most outcome studies ($\geq 10\%$) and may be the highest death rate of any psychiatric disorder. A few series, such as that by Strober, Freeman, and Morrell (1997), have had no deaths and, in addition, have documented remission in more than 75% of patients. Half of deaths from anorexia nervosa are due to starvation and half to suicide. The positive news is that most patients who do not die become moderately to substantially better, but on the average only after 3–5 years of treatment.

The goals of treatment have to be reasonable and achievable. Being mildly concerned about weight and shape is culturally normative and consistent with otherwise successful treatment: normal weight, normal eating, normal thinking, healthy self-esteem. There is no guarantee that individuals with bulimia will be free from urges to binge or purge. What is *completely possible* is to redirect binge or purge urges in a healthy manner so that the individual never carries out binge or purging behaviors, but chooses healthy alternatives instead. Patients are on the way to wellness when they realize that the crucial issues in their lives are not food, weight, or shape, but individually recognized and treated issues in living, mood regulation, and development.

The Treatment of Comorbid Psychiatric Syndromes

The overall treatment of an eating disorder is often determined as much by the comorbid psychological symptoms as by the eating disorder itself. Once comprehensive diagnosis has been made, a systematic approach to the companion psychological disorders is essential and not overly complex (Woodside and Staab, 2006). As a general guideline, once the patient's medical status has been assessed and stabilized, treatment turns first to the eating disorder with normalization of weight, eating behavior, and resolution of cognitive distortions. Unless comorbid syndromes are severe, it is often prudent to delay treatment of them until the patient's weight is close to normal and binge-purge behaviors are improved, waiting at least 4–8 weeks after the beginning of treatment. The reason is that a fair percentage of depressive symptomatology, anxiety states, and obsessive-compulsive syndromes will improve with weight restoration and cessation of binge-purge behavior. Initially treating both the eating disorder and comorbid syndromes is a failure to appreciate how many of these psychological symptoms are either secondary to or accentuated by the eating disorder.

If comorbid psychiatric syndromes are not improved after treatment of the eating disorder, the following approaches are useful.

1. *Depressive disorders:* Any SSRI (fluoxetine, sertraline, or citalopram) is equally effective, although the most data have been collected with fluoxetine. We recommend starting with one-half the usual minimum maintenance dose for one week and then beginning the standard dosage for 6 weeks; for example, 20–60 mg fluoxetine, 50–150 mg sertraline, 20–40 mg citalopram. Where a seasonal worsening of depression is clear in the lower-light fall and winter months, the addition of bright light therapy (10,000 lux for one-half hour at 18–22 inches each morning) will add incremental benefit. Occasionally a mood stabilizer is helpful for bipolar II disorders.

2. *Anxiety disorders:* Panic disorder responds to the same treatments

as depressive illness—SSRIs and CBT—with additional teaching helpful about the nature of panic symptoms. Generalized anxiety is less responsive to medication but does improve with behavioral relaxation techniques, stress management teaching, and sometimes short-term benzodiazepines in individuals without substance abuse histories. Binge episodes not infrequently are used to treat intolerable anxiety.

3. *Obsessive-compulsive disorder:* Where true OCD exists after improvements in eating disorder, fluvoxamine, or fluoxetine (at higher-than-antidepressive doses, 60–100 mg/d), is often effective. There are contraindications in using Luvox with concomitant administration of some antibiotics, or antifungals, or in the presence of prolonged QT intervals.

4. *Substance abuse:* The first goal is to assess the role of substance abuse in the eating disorder. In perhaps half of cases, the substance abuse is related to the eating disorder, and dependence will be diminished when the eating disorder is treated. For example, some anorexics can allow themselves to eat more than minimal amounts of day food only when they have had several drinks just before bedtime. A substantial percentage of bulimic teenage women using methamphetamines or cocaine are depending on them for suppression of hunger, for interruption of binge urges, and for mood increase. If there is no clear disappearance of the drug craving after treatment of the eating disorder, then referral to drug rehabilitation, inpatient or outpatient, after eating disorder treatment is optimal. The initial treatment of this dual diagnosis is usually best accomplished in an eating disorder program because of the general capability of such programs to treat all psychiatric disorders; substance abuse programs generally do not treat the eating disorder effectively. Nicotine withdrawal can be accomplished skillfully without any feared increase in weight.

5. *Personality disorders:* The guideline is long-term management according to the type of personality disorder. Patients with sensitive, persevering, anxious features generally respond to support, education, and CBT as part of their eating disorder treatment. A common and sometimes challenging combination is the combination of an eating disorder with a borderline personality disorder. These individuals respond best to skilled, experienced group therapists with programs in emotional management, such as dialectic behavioral therapy (DBT).

Three caveats concerning antidepressants should be noted. First, medications should not be used in place of CBT as the core treatment for eating disorders. More antidepressants in total are prescribed by primary care doctors than psychiatrists. Recent studies have documented not only that antidepressants sometimes do not need to be used because the depressive symptomatology may clear with treatment of the eating disorder, but also that even where depressive symptoms are present and nonresponsive to CBT, they do not respond to antidepressants when a patient is starved. There was no difference in the improvement in depressive symptoms in starved anorexic patients given fluoxetine versus placebo. There has been abundant demonstration, however, that antidepressants may play an important role in relapse prevention after in the patient's weight and binge-purge behavior has improved. The second concern is that bupropion (Wellbutrin), often now used either when SSRIs are accompanied by unacceptable side effects or as a primary treatment, is relatively contraindicated in bulimic patients. It is probable that the initial reports of seizures in bulimic patients treated with bupropion were due to electrolyte abnormalities, but the medication should be used cautiously in bulimia nervosa until patients are free of binge-purge symptoms. Finally, the currently less-used but still worthy tricyclics may produce QT prolongation in emaciated anorexics and probably would not be a first choice.

Recent studies have demonstrated that anorexia nervosa is associated with variable, but usually significant, changes in the brain itself (Swayze et al., 1996). Severe cases may appear on magnetic resonance imaging (MRI) to be indistinguishable from the brain of a person with Alzheimer's disease. Ventricles are enlarged and cortical substance is decreased. While anorexic patients often have a surprising degree of accomplishment in school, as weight erodes they become increasingly unable to attend and concentrate on written materials or sustain reasoning. Of concern is the demonstration that weight improvement in the patient is not immediately associated with complete restoration of normality in an MRI brain scan, especially in the gray matter. Work is under way in positron emission tomography (PET) to localize the specific brain regions most affected by starvation so as to determine their response to treatment.

Communicating with Eating Disorder Specialists

Persons with serious, chronic, or complex cases of eating disorder usually do best when referred to established programs. The benefits versus risks of referral need to be weighed. Long-term continuity of treatment with an established primary care physician argues for keeping treatment as local as possible. When an anorexic patient's weight is not restored steadily (at a rate of 1–2 lb per week) or bulimic symptoms are not improved despite the treatment methods described above, then referral to a specialized program, either outpatient or inpatient, is required. The success of treatment is maximized by combining the skills of a primary care physician with concurrent psychotherapy by a psychologically trained colleague, whether a psychiatrist, social worker, psychologist, or nurse clinician. This partnership allows the primary care physician to monitor and treat the medical symptomatology and keep a long-term relationship, while the psychologically trained person works with established methods of treating the core psychological dysfunction, but the motivated primary care doctor may do both the medical management and psychotherapeutic care.

Communicating with the Patient and Family

Both families and clinicians treating persons with eating disorders need to be aware that they may be holding to myths about eating disorders that will interfere with the process of healing or convey undue pessimism if not recognized as untruths and corrected (Table 1.12).

Many patients are not surprised when a diagnosis of an eating disorder is made. Often, patients come to evaluation with ambivalence. Sometimes they actively resist treatment. An anorexia patient may fear she will be forced to become fat. A bulimic patient may not be able to imagine life without the stress-relieving "benefit" of a binge. Unfortunately, a binge episode does produce a substantial temporary autonomic discharge, which serves as a short-term (but ultimately ineffective) way to deal with distressed moods and situations, having some similarities to a "drug fix." We encourage psychological education: eating disorders are a common occurrence in our society; no one is or should be criticizing or blaming a patient or a family for having an eating disorder; treatment

TABLE 1.12 Myths about eating disorders

Myth	Fact
Eating disorders are always chronic.	The large majority of patients improve or show remission; up to 76% remission for younger persons.
Eating disorders are difficult to treat.	Anything is difficult without training and experience. Eating disorders respond well at all levels of severity to a multidisciplinary team approach.
Eating disorders always recur or appear in a different form.	The concept of "symptom substitution" is disproved; recurrence may occur, but with expert treatment, only in a minority of cases.
"Normal" means no concerns about body weight, shape, or food ever.	"Normative cultural distress" is goal, with "lip service" given to peers about dieting; during occasional self-doubt about body, patient learns to respond quickly by identifying feelings and working through cognitive distortions.
Eating disorders are always severe.	Eating disorders occur on a spectrum of severity, with most cases being mild to moderate in severity and responsive to treatment.
It always takes a village to treat an eating disorder.	Sometimes multidisciplinary team treatment is necessary, but a small, coordinated team usually suffices.
Families of person with eating disorders are always abnormal.	Families vary; most are worn out, worried, and have done their best.
Most males with eating disorders are gay.	Most males with eating disorders are heterosexual. Younger males often asexual.
Eating disorders are a form of depression, OCD, or schizophrenia.	Eating disorders "breed true." They are not an indirect expression of other disorders; these disorders may be comorbid.
Eating disorders are a result of past trauma.	Past trauma increases the chance of developing some psychiatric disorder, not specifically eating disorders.
Forcing anorexic patients to eat works.	Persuasion and group role models work.
Finding the right medications works.	No medication has proved effective for anorexia nervosa; medication may be

TABLE 1.12 *(continued)*

Myth	Fact
	adjunctive minority partner for bulimia nervosa and binge eating disorder.
You can scare patients into wellness.	Discovering the benefits of wellness works better; scares for eating disorders or substance abuse seldom last.
Eating disorders are addictions.	While there are some similarities, one can not be addicted to food or learn an abstience model for eating. Eating disorders do not meet WHO definition of addiction.
Eating disorders are purely psychiatric disorders.	Eating disorders begin with dieting, secondary to an overvaluation of the benefits of thinness, but once established are medical disorders also.
Eating disorders are due only to our cultural and voluntary personal choices.	Eating disorders have a 50%–70% contribution from genetic predisposition.
Eating disorders only occur in spoiled white, suburban, upper-class teen girls.	Eating disorders are equal opportunity illnesses occurring at all ages (7–77), in both genders, in all ethnic and racial groups, in all locations.
Anybody can treat eating disorders.	Persons with eating disorders do better with clinicians trained specifically in eating disorders diagnosis and treatment; general competence is not enough.
Eating disorders involve delusions.	Delusions are uncommon. Most patients have strong overvalued beliefs about the benefits of slimness or shape change.
Slow heart rate, low body temperature, and low blood pressure need immediate correction by specialists.	These are generally self-improving with weight restoration and watchful waiting. Other symptoms, such as prolonged QT interval, do need immediate attention.
The reproductive system is ruined.	With recovery, patients who have anorexia nervosa rarely have permanent effects in gonadotropin functioning; "nothing broken, only waiting for normal weight."

involves a partnership, not a "drop off and fix" treatment; eating disorders are not a failure of effort or will; these are illnesses that develop self-sustaining features and serve psychological needs. Our goal is to work with patients to achieve freedom from the symptoms of eating disorders and to prepare them for healthier living with a good and stable mood, appropriate social skills, normal weight, normal eating behavior, and good body image, with adequate self-esteem in a society preoccupied with slimness. Families often receive excess criticism or blame themselves when a family member develops an eating disorder; they need to be reassured that eating disorders are true illnesses.

The biological features of both anorexia and bulimia are fairly predictable for each patient, but the personal developmental and psychological history for each patient is unique. Therefore, the programmatic or protocolized part of treatment will focus on improving the weight and eating pattern and the shared psychopathology, while using more dynamic approaches in psychotherapy to work on the individual personal forces behind the eating disorder. We always tell patients that there are no bad reasons for developing eating disorder; such disorders always spring from understandable human needs: a desire to be free from teasing, to feel accepted by others, to accept one's self, to deal with distressed mood, to help family situations, or to deal with a crisis in development. When eating disorders are treated adequately and promptly, the individual may be, in some ways, better off than if he or she had never had the disorder because effective treatment means coming to terms with powerful forces within the individual, and within society.

Follow-up Care and Prognosis

It is essential for a patient to know that organ functions will not be completely normal for 3–6 months after weight becomes normal. Attaining healthy weight is the *beginning* of comprehensive treatment, not the end. Bulimia nervosa patients may be reassured to know that urges to binge or purge are not, in themselves, indications of ineffective treatment. Continued reflux in formerly bulimic patients may indicate some incompetence of the gastroesophageal junction. When reflux persists despite the usual precautions of avoiding late meals and not lying down after meals, proton pump inhibitors are generally effective in alleviating gastroesophageal reflux disease (GERD) with or without a prokinetic agent such as metaclopramide. During the course of nutritional rehabilitation, if there is persistent bloating from delayed gastric emptying, prokinetic agents such as metoclopramide may give relief. The major drawbacks of using metaclopramide to help gastric emptying are that it frequently causes drowsiness (in that case start giving only 5 mg one hour before supper and 10 mg at bedtime), and occasionally akasthesia.

There is no evidence that these medications are essential in all cases. Our goal regarding medical symptoms is prompt, effective, complete treatment so that we can accomplish changes in thinking and behavior without uncomfortable or serious medical symptomatology interfering with the process of psychological and behavioral change. Severe bloating, painful reflux, or severe hypothermia makes it difficult to concentrate in psychotherapy. Occasionally, a specialist may be needed for assessment and treatment of complex medical aspects of cases.

There is increasing concern that low bone mineral density may be present in patients who have had as little as 6 months of amenorrhea. Therefore, dual-energy X-ray (DEXA) should be requested for patients with a history of 3 months of amenorrhea, 6 months of significant weight loss, and, in males (Mehler et al., 2008), a low weight for 6 or more months. Other chapters in this book deal in more detail with medical evaluation and treatment of endocrine, GI, cardiac, and bone symptomatology.

The goal of treatment is remission, not simply improvement, and certainly not slight improvement in abnormal labs leading to premature discharge from treatment. Numerous studies demonstrate that up to 76 percent complete remission is possible, with no symptomatology of eating disorders at 10- to 15-year follow-ups (Strober, Freeman, and Morrell, 1997), a more optimistic picture than with OCD, childhood-onset diabetes, or schizophrenia.

Summary

Primary care physicians can confidently diagnose eating disorders with a brief set of screening questions and a mental status examination and can treat these disorders with clear, proven treatment goals and methods (Mehler, 2001). Relatively recent cases of mild to moderate severity can be treated comprehensively by the primary care physician alone or in conjunction with psychologically trained colleagues. Medical assessment is important for establishing the severity of illness and treating significant medical complications, but not for diagnosis. The guideline is to "rule in" eating disorders, not to "rule out" all possible cause of weight loss or binge-purge. Families respond well to a combination of education, support, and inclusion in the treatment process, according to the age of the patient and the needs of the family. As noted above, realistic optimism based on comprehensive treatment is entirely warranted. Every aspect of most eating disorders can be improved, especially with up-to-date diagnostic and therapeutic skills of motivated medical and psychological clinicians. For an overview, see Fairburn and Harrison (2003).

REFERENCES

Andersen AE and Jager J. 2005. Eating disorders. In: Sadock BJ and Sadock VA, eds. *Kaplan & Sadock's Comprehensive Textbook of Psychiatry*, 8th ed. Philadelphia: Lippincott Williams & Wilkins, pp. 2002–21.

Baran SA, Weltzin MD, and Kaye WH. 1995. Low discharge weight and outcome in anorexia nervosa. *American Journal of Psychiatry* 152:1070–72.

Beck D, Casper R, and Andersen AE. 1996. Truly late onset of eating disorders: A study of 11 cases averaging 60 years of age at presentation. *International Journal of Eating Disorders* 20:389–95.

Bowers WA. 2001. Basic principles for applying cognitive behavioral therapy to anorexia nervosa. In: Andersen AE, ed. *Psychiatric Clinics of North America*. 24:293–303.

Bulik CM, Sullivan PF, Tozzi F, Furberg H, Lichtenstein P, and Pedersen NL. 2006. Prevalence, heritability, and prospective risk factors for anorexia nervosa. *Archives of General Psychiatry* 63:305–12.

Bulik CM, Thornton L, Poyastro AP, et al. 2008. Suicide attempts in anorexia nervosa. *Psychosomatic Medicine* 70:378–83.

Crow SJ and Nyman JA. 2004. The cost-effectiveness of anorexia nervosa treatment. *International Journal of Eating Disorders* 35:155–60.

Fairburn CG and Harrison PJ. 2003. Eating disorders. *Lancet* 361:407–16.

Jordan J, Joyce PR, Carter FA, et al. 2008. Specific and nonspecific comorbidity in anorexia nervosa. *International Journal of Eating Disorders* 41:47–56.

Keel PK. 2007. Purging disorder: Subthreshold variant or full-threshold eating disorder? *International Journal of Eating Disorders* 40 (Suppl):S89–94.

Latner JD and Clyne C. 2008. The diagnostic validity of the criteria for binge eating disorder. *International Journal of Eating Disorders* 41:1–14.

Lock J and le Grange D. 2005. Family-based treatment of eating disorders. *International Journal of Eating Disorders* 37 (Suppl):S64–7.

Margolis R, Spencer W, DePaulo RJ, Simpson SG, and Andersen AE. 1994. Psychiatric comorbidity in eating disorder patients: A quantitative analysis by diagnostic subtype. *Eating Disorders* 2:231–36.

Mehler PS. 2001. Diagnosis and care of patients with anorexia nervosa in primary care settings. *Annals of Internal Medicine* 134:1048–59.

Mehler PS, Sabel AL, Watson T, and Andersen AE. 2008. High risk of osteoporosis in male eating disordered patients. *International Journal of Eating Disorders* 41:666–72.

Morgan JF, Reid F, and Lacey JH. 1999. The SCOFF questionnaire: Assessment of a new screening tool for eating disorders. *British Medical Journal* 319:-1467–68.

Russell G. 1979. Bulimia nervosa: An ominous variant of anorexia nervosa. *Psychological Medicine* 9:429–48.

Striegel-Moore RH, Dohm FA, Kraemer HC, et al. 2003. Eating disorders in white and black women. *American Journal of Psychiatry* 160:1326–31.

Strober M, Freeman R, and Morrell W. 1997. The long-term course of severe anorexia nervosa in adolescents: Survival analysis of recovery, relapse, and outcome predictors over 10–15 years in a prospective study. *International Journal of Eating Disorders* 22:339–60.

Strober M, Freeman R, and Morrell W. 1999. Atypical anorexia nervosa: Separation from typical cases in course and outcome in a long-term prospective study. *International Journal of Eating Disorders* 25:135–42.

Swayze VS, Andersen A, Arndt S, Rajarethinam R, Fleming F, Sato Y, and Andreasen NC. 1996. Reversibility of brain tissue loss in anorexia nervosa assessed with a computerized Talairach 3–D proportional grid. *Psychological Medicine* 26:381–90.

Woodside BD and Staab R. 2006. Management of psychiatric comorbidity in anorexia nervosa and bulimia nervosa. *CNS Drugs* 20:655–63.

Team Treatment

*A Multidisciplinary
Approach*

COMMON QUESTIONS

Why do patients with eating disorders benefit from team treatment?
Who are the members of the multidisciplinary team?
What role does each discipline play on the team?
How does the primary care physician interface effectively with the
 team?
How does a clinician decide on the appropriate level of care for
 a patient with an eating disorder?
Can one clinician effectively treat all aspects of an eating disorder?
What strategies promote team cohesiveness?
How can interaction with managed care become a win-win situation?
Will machines replace people on teams?
What myths persist concerning eating disorders?
Is group therapy simply less costly than individual care, or is it differ-
 ently effective?
How can staff teach a patient to internalize the multidisciplinary team
 and its functions?

Case

J.M., a 47-year-old female, was admitted to inpatient treatment after a
long history of anorexia nervosa since adolescence, considerably worsened during the 13 years before admission. In addition to food restriction, she abused laxatives to the point where she required a partial colec-
tomy because of rectal prolapse. Her ileostomy has never received

reconstruction due to her persistent anorexia nervosa. By limiting herself to two cans of tuna fish, a few crackers, and occasional carrots over many years, she developed a toxic mercury level of 93 µg/L, as well as lowering her weight to 73 pounds, 53 percent of ideal weight. Her mood and cognition had worsened considerably in the 2 months before admission. J.M. perceived herself to be healthy despite her low weight. Her long course of treatment included Succimer, 10 mg/kg three times a day for 5 days and then 10 mg/kg twice a day for 14 days, to complete a 19-day course of chelation therapy. A second course of chelation therapy was required. She was transitioned to the partial hospital for Monday–Friday care 8:00 a.m.–4:00 p.m. During the treatment phase in partial hospital, the second phase of her treatment, she resisted weight restoration beyond 90 percent of healthy weight, plateauing at 124 pounds (target weight 136–40 lb). Despite considerable weight restoration and decrease in mercury to 13 µg/L (normal 0–10), she complained of persisting difficulty in thinking clearly and had many nonspecific complaints about decreased sensation and tingling in her arms and hands. She obtained some relief from the numbness and tingling in her right hand with a carpal tunnel release performed in orthopedic surgery. She increased her exercise in her residential overnight facility, losing weight to 85 percent of target weight, yet denying she was overexercising. She persisted in asking for a reduced calorie intake.

After 6 weeks of ineffective partial hospital, during which she lost weight and continued overexercising, J.M. was readmitted to the inpatient unit for another intensive period of treatment. She denied suicidal ideation but expressed feelings of depression. Her treatment included sertraline, 150 mg/d. Social workers held conferences with J.M. and her father. After 4 weeks of inpatient treatment, during which she attained 99 percent of her target weight goal, she returned to partial hospital for continued work on relapse prevention, internalization of healthy body image, work on long-term unresolved pubertal issues of femininity, and practice in choosing healthy meals in a supported community setting of restaurants and cafeteria. Her discharge diagnoses from the inpatient phase were as follows:

Axis I: Anorexia nervosa, restricting type; depression, not otherwise specified; anxiety disorder, not otherwise specified; cognitive disorder, due to general medical condition (mercury poisoning), in remission;

Axis II: Cluster C personality traits, especially avoidant and obsessive-compulsive features;

Axis III: History of mercury poisoning from food intake; osteoarthritis; osteopenia, status post-proctocolectomy with ileostomy due to laxative abuse complications; history of left popliteral cyst removal on knee; history of migraines; carpal tunnel syndrome, bilateral;

Axis IV: Severe due to chronic mental and physical illness, poor family support, and being on disability;

Axis V: At admission, 25; upon discharge, 42.

Consider the number of disciplines involved in this patient's care: psychiatry, internal medicine, surgery, nursing, social work, psychology, activities and occupational therapists, registered dietitian, and residential care facility personnel.

Background

Patients with eating disorders benefit from team treatment because of the complexity of the disorders and because evidence demonstrates better results with experienced multidisciplinary team treatment than with single modalities or with efforts by a single clinician. Physicians in cardiology, surgery, and other specialties have long become accustomed to working with coordinated multidisciplinary teams. The cooperative approach of the early years of modern psychiatry, illustrated by Adolf Meyer's advocacy of social work as an integral part of team treatment, yielded in the decades of 1920–60 to a phase of primarily individual therapy based on psychoanalytic theory, with the exception of a custodial team approach to state mental hospitals. This phase was succeeded by an emphasis on monotherapy with psychopharmacological agents beginning in the late 1950s and dominating the next three decades. During and after the 1980s, with the publication of evidence-based studies documenting the effectiveness of cognitive-behavioral therapy (CBT) and interpersonal therapy (IPT) as well as psychopharmacology, and in the context of the growth of systems approaches and quality teams in businesses, the benefits of team treatment became apparent in psychiatry as well. The biopsychosocial model went from theory to implementation and is the current norm for seriously ill patients with most psychiatric disorders, especially when hospital care is needed. The fundamental understanding of eating disorders has progressed from their being regarded as medical disorders only, to being seen as psychiatric disorders only, to the current understanding that they are best understood as the outcome of a combination of genetic, neurochemical, psychosocial, developmental, familial, and comorbid illness factors. Appreciation of the complexity of the origin and treatment of eating disorders plus the cost-effectiveness requirements of third-party payers have validated multidisciplinary team treatment as normative for treatment of serious eating disorders (Garcia de Armusquibar, 2000; Halmi, 2005; Gicquel 2008).

The Members and Function of the Multidisciplinary Treatment Team

Table 2.1 summarizes the needs of the patient, the most closely matched multidisciplinary team member for that need, and the method of care delivery for meeting that need. The multidisciplinary team includes the psychiatrist, internist or pediatrician, psychologist, social worker, nurses, registered dietitian, occupational and activities therapists, educator, clergy, administrators, and others as needed.

The psychiatrist is usually the "captain of the ship," coordinating the team effort and having primary responsibility, often with the psychologist, for diagnosis and treatment planning. The psychiatrist is most often the doctor of record legally and decides on medications that are safe and effective. Depending on the psychiatrist's background, he or she may also carry out primary care medical roles as well. Working closely with the psychiatrist, the psychologist has special training in diagnosis and in treatments emphasizing evidence-based psychotherapy.

The core of the eating disorder psychopathology is the overvaluation of the benefits of slimness or shape change, mandating that the heart of the treatment program be the challenging and changing of these overvalued beliefs that initiate and sustain the illness. The psychiatrist and the psychologist join efforts to remit or diminish these core overvalued beliefs with a combination of psychotherapy and experiential relearning and individualized medications. They also focus on comorbid conditions, observing which are secondary and which are primary. Abundant standardized testing exists to document quantitatively and qualitatively

TABLE 2.1 Patients' needs and the multidisciplinary team

Need	Team member	Function
Weight restoration	Physician, nurse, dietitian	Structured, supported, dietitian supervised refeeding
Medical complications: prevention and treatment	Psychiatrist, nurse, and internist or pediatrician	Assessment and treatment, with specialist consultants as needed
Psychological assessment	Psychologist(s) and psychiatrist	Eating disorders assessment (EDE, EDI, EAT), neuropsychology and general psychology baselines
Changing core cognitive distortions	Psychologist(s), other therapists	Individual and group therapy
Behavioral relearning of everyday activities	Occupational and activities therapists	Shopping for food, meal preparation, shopping for "healthy" clothes (experiential therapy)
Family assessment	Social worker	Family interview for assessment and treatment; education, disposition; community resources
Psychopharmacology	Psychiatrist, nurse	Evidence-based studies and patient education
Recreation and balance in life	Occupational and activities therapists	Structured recreation, daily "balance wheel"
Healthy physical activity	Activities therapist	Establish normative progressive aerobic and strength training; individualized
Education	Educator/teacher	Individual teaching parallel to school assignments and liaison with school
Psychiatric comorbidity	Psychiatrist, nurse, psychologist, social worker	Integrative care, evidence-based studies
Team cohesion and continued growth	Psychiatrist, psychologist	Regular weekly process groups, continued education, ventilation

TABLE 2.1 *(continued)*

Need	Team member	Function
Financial management	MBA and assistants, legal staff, social worker	Maximum advocacy for insurance coverage, state low-income plans, appeals, disability application
Body image normalization	Psychologist, nurse, other therapists	Group and experiential therapy
Patient education	All team members	Group and individual education in meal planning, medications, recreation, relaxation, medical symptoms
Relapse prevention	Psychiatrist, social worker, psychologist	Structured long-term planning for intensive integrative treatment
Milieu management	Psychiatrist, nurse, psychologist, cleaning staff, facilities management	Weekly meetings and liaison
Protocols and discharge or transition criteria	Psychiatrist, nurse, psychologist, social worker, other team members	Advance planning for components of treatment suitable for protocols; specific, ratable criteria

the eating disorder symptoms before treatment. These instruments also are used to follow progress and, at discharge, to score the extent of change compared with the patient's state at admission. Individualized analog scales may be used to rate the severity of binge or purge urges, hunger, satiety, and other measures of improvement.

The only way to validate treatment is to use standardized instruments to rate symptoms, as well as to obtain more subjective team and patient feedback. Instruments validated include the Eating Disorders Examination (EDE), the Eating Attitudes Test-26 (EAT-26), and the Eating Disorders Inventory-2 (EDI-2), as well as standardized general psychological testing such as the SCL-90, the MMPI, and the Beck Depression scale. Neuropsychological assessment is often warranted because of the effect of the primary eating disorder on brain function, because of co-morbid history (drug abuse, head injury), or when there is lack of progress in thinking proportional to weight restoration and diminished binge-purge features. An assessment of intellect, especially in adolescents, may help guide the level of psychotherapeutic intervention and materials used for teaching.

The more medically ill the person with an eating disorder is, however, the less able she or he is to fully use CBT or IPT—hence, the importance of the internist or the pediatrician and subspecialist consultants in preventing and improving medical symptoms (Kreipe and Yussman, 2003; Mehler and Krantz, 2003). The starved person has a starved brain, less capable of learning and subject to shorter attention span and distraction. Restoration of healthy weight needs to be accomplished in a manner that prevents the "refeeding syndrome," a complex of medical symptoms from imprudent resumption of nutrition. A variety of uncomfortable medical symptoms, such as gastric bloating and esophageal reflux, require medical interventions not only for safety, but also so the patient can be freed from discomfort to attend to psychotherapy. Psyche and soma are intimately related. The internist, pediatrician, or other primary care physician, preferably a stable part of the team, is needed to decide which symptoms, such as bradycardia with normal QT interval or hypothermia, need only be passively observed during improvement *pari passu* with weight restoration, and which symptoms, such as tachycardia, hypokalemia, and prolonged QT interval, need immediate intervention. Simple forms of psychotherapy should be started even in the very medically ill patient.

Nurses are the multitaskers in the treatment process. They may function in formal psychotherapeutic roles, especially with advanced registered nurse practitioner training in psychotherapy, as well as in individual support and education. They monitor daily medical and psychiatric conditions with skill, care, and compassion. They function as "eyes and ears" for the rest of the team and form individually meaningful relationships with the patient. Nurses and other team members share a common theoretical orientation to treatment, especially in CBT as a unifying theme. Nurses along with other team members understand the terror many patients with eating disorders face when thinking of or approaching a state of giving up their eating disorder as a strategy for living.

In many states, only the physician and the registered dietitian may legally prescribe nutrition for patients. A decision needs to be made whether the dietitian interacts directly with patients from the beginning or, as in the University of Iowa Program, meets daily only with the small treatment team, and only at the end of transition to the next level of care, with the patient to share information about weight, meal planning, and questions about nutrition. The registered dietician leads group meetings on education about healthy eating, the nutritional complications of eating disorders, and perception of hunger and satiety. The emphasis in teaching meal planning is toward an ADA (American Diabetes Association) approach of choosing food groups, learning exchanges, and estimating portion size, defusing the focus on counting calories or fat grams. In other programs, the registered dietician meets with patients individually from the beginning. The psychiatrist teaches that "food is your medication and is not negotiable as with other medications regarding amount and content." Vegetarianism is allowed only when the family has a faith tradition such as Buddhism or Seventh-Day Adventism. The most knowledgeable cleric of a given faith tradition is consulted when a patient claims the need to fast on religious holidays. These clerics almost always say that health care comes first and overrides use of religion in the service of fasting.

The social worker serves the invaluable role of treating the individual in the context of the family system. Initially, emphasis is placed on support and education, and evaluation of family functioning. Blame is wrested from the family's shoulders, and realistic hope is instilled. Family therapy sessions are planned to meet the needs of the family, without the assumption of any, or a particular type of, psychopathology within the family. Meetings usually include parents or significant others as well as the patient, but at times meetings with the parents only may be needed for the parents' marital issues. The younger the patient, the more important family therapy, although 40-year-olds may still be struggling with boundary issues with parents or other family members. A group meeting of families in treatment allows families to gain support and mutual encouragement from each other. Finally, the social worker makes contact with community resources and joins with the team in planning aftercare.

Occupational and activities therapists direct experiential "hands on" activities. Patients need to learn to shop for and prepare food in a healthy and social manner, without label reading and without the fear of becoming fat dominating the patient's food choices. Shopping for "healthy clothing" may involve rituals of throwing or giving away clothing of inappropriate size. Patients are taught that clothes are our servants, not our masters, and that there is much commercial gamesmanship and economic incentive in sizing clothing. These experiential therapists are instrumental in helping patients diminish body distortion and self-loathing. Compulsive overexercisers and "couch potatoes" are both guided to moderate, regular, individualized exercise. A sound program of aerobic training with strength training will lead to healthier weight restoration, serve as an antidote to anxiety, and free the patient of either the burden of compulsive exercise or the self-view of being incapable of meaningful physical activity. Therapists are guided by their formal training and by the patient's medical status, including bone mineral density.

The younger the patient, the greater the need for a trained educator. Well-established programs allow patients to keep up with school work, as well as remediate deficits in personal education, such as sex education, jointly planned with the school and parents. The educator chooses age-appropriate tools for continued education and liaises with the school system. Individual instruction in computer skills and educational modules is increasingly important.

Deciding on the Level of Care

Table 2.2 describes levels of care ideally available for the treatment of patients who have eating disorders. Eating disorders occur across a spectrum of severity, necessitating a range of choices for care based on the intensity of the illness. The case illustrated at the beginning of this chapter documents a typical pattern of chronic severe illness in which treatment began at the inpatient level with multiple medical services provided. This patient was then transitioned to the partial psychiatric hospital (PPH), but she was not able to maintain self-management of eating or overexercise and was therefore readmitted to inpatient treatment. Finally, the patient returned to PPH, then advanced to an intensive outpatient program (IOP) of three days a week of PPH, and finally, to once-a-week psychotherapy with an experienced advanced registered nurse practitioner, with added medical consultations as needed. Many illnesses include such chronic and less treatment-responsive cases. It is an indication of the nature of the illness, not a lack of treatment effort by clini-

Level of care	General requirements
Inpatient team treatment	Seriously ill patient with eating disorder (see Chap. 1); needs full team multidisciplinary treatment; treatment may be in integrated program for all ages, or in separate adolescent and adult units, with 24/7 treatment by medical staff
Residential care	Full daytime staff treatment and light night-time supervision for safety
Partial psychiatric hospital (5–7 days and/or evenings)	A step down from inpatient treatment for patient too ill for outpatient treatment; patient able to self-regulate eating and exercise, and to avoid substance abuse/self-cutting during nonprogram hours
Intensive outpatient	A step down from partial hospital for patient too ill for weekly therapy alone but not meeting criteria for partial hospital; 1–3 days/week in partial hospital or several weekly outpatient sessions needed; next lower team size
Outpatient treatment	Patient able to benefit from once- or twice-weekly outpatient sessions; continued integrative care with other disciplines
Residential living facility	Supported and supervised living for long-term, graduated approach to full remission while in outpatient treatment
Self-treatment	Newer computerized self-help assessment and/or treatment modules based on evidence-based studies; may supplement formal treatment at outpatient level

cians or good will by the patient, that readmission to some level of intensity other than outpatient is required. Part of discharge planning from any level of care is stipulation of what symptoms will mandate return to the higher level of care. It is better, for example, to readmit a patient to PPH when he or she is steadily going down in weight, or increasing in binge-purge behaviors, than to wait until a medical crisis occurs.

There are several approaches to choosing a level of care. For seriously ill patients with eating disorders, a numbers of programs begin with inpatient treatment; transition to the PPH level occurs only after preestablished criteria are met. For example, in cases of anorexia nervosa, when the patient is at least 85 percent restored in body weight and has the necessary psychotherapeutic skills—especially response inhibition of urges to self-starve or binge-purge, and internal awareness of mood and thoughts—for self-management of eating and behaviors in hours away from programming, she or he will transition to PPH with a high but not certain probability of success. An increasingly common approach is to abbreviate the length of inpatient stay and have all patients, once past medical stabilization, jointly take part in a broader version of PPH, as is done at Johns Hopkins Hospital. Some states require separate programs for adolescents, but several programs with published results integrate adults and adolescents, with appropriate emphasis on the separate educational needs of adolescents.

A gradual therapeutic slope for change in intensity of treatment (inpatient to PPH to IOP to outpatient therapy), rather than a cliff (inpatient directly to outpatient status), is preferred. The model for the PPH level of care was established at the University of Toronto by Piran and Kaplan (1990) for the moderately ill majority of patients who do not need an inpatient level of care. After inpatient and/or PPH care, the optimal next step is intensive outpatient treatment several days a week for a variable period of time before transition to a weekly outpatient program for relapse prevention and continued psychological growth. A relapse prevention and growth enhancement phase should be planned for at least one to two years after acute hospital-based care. Trite but true, failing to plan is planning to fail.

It is important to remember that eating disorders are disorders of behavior as well as disorders of psychopathology and medical disorders. An inpatient level of care may be required because the severity of the behavioral pathology, not, as third-party payers at times demand, only because of abnormal laboratories or suicidality. *Patients can die with normal laboratory values.* The sum total of the complexity of the case, its chronicity, its lack of response to lower levels of treatment, its comorbidity, the intransigence of the behavioral abnormalities, all factor into decision making leading to inpatient care. Figure 2.1 summarizes the possible interactions between different levels of care.

The Use of Protocols and Criteria for Changes in the Level of Treatment

Many phases of the treatment of seriously ill patients with eating disorders can and should be protocolized. The appendix shows one protocol for adults and adolescents during the inpatient phase. Aspects of treatment amenable to protocols include the rate of change of calories and food content, the decrease in amount of time after meals during which patients are supported and supervised, and conditions for therapeutic leaves of absence. The use of protocols frees team members to work individually with patients in those areas that mandate individual attention, such as internalizing CBT and dealing with personal crises, and uncovering dynamics where a psychodynamic approach is appropriate. The protocol can, of course, be overridden when necessary—for example, when a patient has a medical condition requiring a different rate of refeeding. The protocol approach to the routine aspects of treatment leads to better results than multiple individualized approaches not just in eating disorders but also in cardiac surgery, hip replacement, and prevention of infection in the ICU.

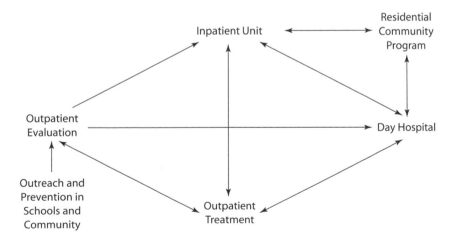

FIGURE 2.1. The spectrum of care for eating disorders.

The Solitary Clinician

Not every clinician treating eating disorders needs, or is close to, a multidisciplinary team. In almost every location, however, a functional equivalent to a designated team can be effectively assembled, and the resulting care will be improved beyond the sum of its parts. For example, if the treating clinician is a psychiatrist, she or he may not have the training or time to do individualized psychotherapy, so will seek out an experienced therapist. In addition, a registered dietician will guide the nutritional rehabilitation with a scheduled nutritional approach. A primary care physician will evaluate the patient medically at the beginning of treatment and intermittently. A decision needs to be made regarding who will weigh the patient. It is crucial for successful treatment and for legal reasons to have regular interactions between team members and to keep adequate records of these interactions.

If the primary diagnosing and treating clinician is a psychologist, then a primary care physician is needed for medical evaluation and care, and that physician, who may be the psychiatrist, may prescribe and monitor psychotropic medications. In both cases, a social worker trained in family assessment and treatment will be an invaluable asset.

Team Cohesiveness versus Burnout

Business and governmental groups have explored and described principles that promote cohesiveness and prevent burnout (Covey, 1989; Bossidy and Charan, 2002). A single integrating theoretical psychotherapeutic approach, CBT being the best demonstrated, but sometimes IPT or DBT (dialectical behavioral therapy), will allow all team members to be reading from the same page and avoid clashing methodologies (Bowers, Evans, and Andersen, 1997). Each team member learns pertinent levels of application of CBT for his or her discipline. Table 2.3 summarizes some of the principles and approaches that foster team cohesiveness. Each team member makes an invaluable contribution. Role functions are drawn up so that the different disciplines intersect in their roles, but do not duplicate or conflict with each other. As the treatment of each patient comes to a conclusion at a given level of care, there is a sense of shared accomplishment when the team has successfully worked together. Often

TABLE 2.3 Principles and approaches for team cohesion and avoidance of team member burnout

- Establish an atmosphere of realistic optimism using evidence-based studies.
- Encourage discipline-specific and integrative continued education within the program and through local and national conferences.
- Hold daily small team meetings for coordinated patient care and weekly large team meetings for assessment of progress and long-term planning.
- Adopt a protocolized approach to specific aspects of treatment that otherwise would be distracting in the number of details, with override for individualized care: dietary progression, level of supervision at meals and other times, level of activity, criteria for therapeutic leaves of absence, criteria for change in level of care. These protocols are designed from large team input in advance of implementation, with agreement from all disciplines.
- Hold progress-in-treatment regular monthly meetings to review changes needed in protocol.
- Apply a single, integrative psychotherapeutic technique at appropriate levels by each discipline, preferably based on principles and practices of cognitive-behavioral therapy. Interpersonal therapy or dialectical behavioral therapy is also suitable.
- Hold ad hoc small team meetings (psychiatrist, nurse, social worker, psychologist) for especially challenging patients.
- Obtain maximum information from previous treatment experiences and from collateral resources.
- Hold off-the-record gripe sessions.
- Recognize special efforts by each discipline in working toward and achieving program excellence.
- Encourage research within and between disciplines.
- Choose new staff members carefully: avoid hiring new personnel with active eating disorders. Make decisions in advance about degree of self-disclosure of past staff illnesses.
- Assess patient ratings of positive and negative aspects of treatment before discharge and at longer-term follow-up (3–12 months).
- Emphasize that the goal is full remission of illness over the long term: "Treatment really begins when you leave the acute intensive treatment program to live in a world preoccupied with an irrational overvaluation of slimness."

the positive feedback from patients does not occur until months or years after treatment has concluded and the patient is on the way toward a life path in which eating disorders offer no pseudosolutions for the journey in a society besotted with overvaluation of the benefits of thinness.

Burnout among individual team members from psychological conflicts sometimes occurs without warning, and usually cannot be prevented, but burnout and demoralization from ineffective team management can be foreseen and prevented. A higher degree of interpersonal involvement is required for successful treatment of patients with eating disorders. Team members must have their own inner resources for self-esteem that do not depend upon receiving immediate thanks from patients. Successful team members will be valued for their unique contributions, be respected for decision making within their disciplines, and be given within-discipline and interdisciplinary continuing education. For example, one activities therapist became interested in the possibility of using aquatherapy for desensitizing patients to wearing a bathing suit, accepting their reflection as they pass mirrors in the locker room without body disgust or mirror gazing, and then learning to relax and be in touch with their bodies below the neck as they recline in gently swirling warm water in a therapeutic pool in the physical therapy section of the hospital. The experience not only has proved successful but also has been approved as a thesis topic. Patients have come to associate aquatherapy with a positive body image and a relaxing experience. In contrast, staff members will more often experience burnout if they are given purely mechanical tasks, when their observations and viewpoints are not solicited, when they receive no continuing education, when the team members are not stable over time, when roles conflict, and when institutional financial considerations come before quality of patient care.

Managed Care: The Good, the Bad, and the Ugly

Table 2.4 sketches out a few approaches that may increase the effectiveness of interactions with managed care. Managed care ranges from reasonableness, with a win-win approach, to the completely unreasonable, with artificial financially driven criteria for admission and continuing care after the case. For example, the patient described in the first case in Chapter 1—who was at 67 percent ideal weight, with a clear diagnosis

TABLE 2.4   Approaches that maximize effective interaction with managed care

- Obtain comprehensive information from current treatment, past treatments, and collateral sources (family, school, friends, as appropriate).
- Take a proactive approach to preapproval and response to reviews during treatment.
- Consider compiling a standardized list of reviewers' most commonly asked questions in advance of reviews.
- Know thoroughly the patient's current status and progress to date, as well as your treatment goals, rationale for continued certification at each level of intensity, discharge plans, or plans for transition to next level of care.
- Advocate for medical insurance coverage for anorexia nervosa until weight is at or greater than 85 percent of target weight, per court decisions. Involve legal staff or personal legal counselor when appropriate to advocate for medical benefits where appropriate.
- Appeal, appeal, appeal. In states where legislative action allows, consider referral to expert outside independent evaluators for non-negotiable definitive decisions when regular appeals are turned down (for example, IMEDECS).
- Be courteous, civil, and fully informed during interactions with reviewers. Advocate assertively, not aggressively, for patients.
- Tape-record telephone conversations with managed care companies. Most managed care companies inform staff that their phone conversations are recorded for "quality assurance"; do likewise, informing reviewers in advance, courteously, "for reference afterward to be sure we have accurate record of information and agreements."
- Follow telephone agreements with e-mail or fax confirmation of positive agreements.

of anorexia nervosa, and had a grave medical status, including a non-united humeral fracture—was denied admission because of the health plan's coverage. This clearly inappropriate denial was later overturned.

We recommend that all interactions be tape-recorded to ensure accuracy of recall and to avoid distracting note taking during the interaction, with notice of the recording given at the beginning of the interview. The tone in conversations with managed care reviewers should be serious, respectful, reasoned, and persuasive. Preparation includes knowing the cases thoroughly, including the patient's history and past treatments, the reason for the current level of care, progress to date, progress in psychotherapy, dynamic conflicts, and plans for continued treatment as well as the criteria for moving to the next lower level of care. At times a collaborative relationship may be formed with specific reviewers in specific large third party organizations. Know whether the reviewer has the ability to decide individually on cases or will slavishly follow the guidelines of the company. The legal rule is, when in doubt, the right belongs to the insured.

Here, the question of the nature of the eating disorder comes into play. Eating disorders are clearly medical disorders, especially when the patient is medically starved or has other medical consequences of the disorder, such as metabolic instability. Court cases have established the following: (1) An eating disorder does not become nonmedical because it is being treated on a psychiatric service or because the person is receiving psychotherapy (*Ronald Simons v. Blue Cross and Blue Shield*, 1989). (2) Body weight below 85 percent of normal for age, height, and gender is a medical diagnosis, metabolic starvation. Until treatment brings the patient's weight up to approximately 85 percent of the target goal, medical insurance benefits, not psychiatric, apply (*Manheim v. Travelers Insurance Company*, 1995).

Consider the following parallel example: A man incurs severe orthopedic injuries, including multiple fractures, in the course of a suicide attempt by jumping from a building onto concrete. He has 30 days of psychiatric coverage and 90 days of medical coverage. At the end of 30 days, he still has severe orthopedic injuries that require inpatient care from multiple services and a long spell of rehabilitation ahead. His health insurance coverage does not expire at the end of 30 days because the origin of the injuries was psychiatric. Likewise, with anorexia nervosa, the medical consequences are diagnostically valid and covered by medical benefits below a certain point of starvation and are not invalidated because there are psychiatric causes for the medical diagnoses. Not all insurance payers accept these facts. In that case, legal backup is needed, and is often persuasive.

Eating disorders have suffered particularly from "carve-outs," an artificial distinction between psychiatric and so-called medical disorders. There is less voluntariness about developing eating disorders than in developing lung cancer from a chosen behavior, smoking. Certainly, insurers understand the nonvoluntary nature of obsessive-compulsive disorder (OCD), schizophrenia, and bipolar disorders. Yet, financial incentives and a lack of clinical training on the part of adjudicating personnel cloud the judgment of companies whose goals, despite lip service otherwise, are financial rather than clinical welfare. Eating disorders have been especially singled out for further limitations of benefits, perhaps because of the lack of advocacy on behalf of the younger and more helpless group of patients. In contrast, inappropriate limitations on hospital services for women after childbirth, narrowing care to 12 hours in hospital, were reversed by organized protests to legislatures beginning at the state level and spreading to the national level. Now, most companies guarantee 48-hour care for normal deliveries and 72–96 hours for Caesarian sections. Legislative mandates for parity in medical coverage for serious psychiatric disorders has led to some improvement in benefits for the treatment of eating disorders, at times substantive, in other cases, fictional.

The Mechanical Approach to Treatment: Does It Work?

Table 2.5 summarizes some of the mechanized approaches to the diagnosis and treatment of patients with eating disorders. We live in an increasingly mechanized world. The question is which aspects of health care can be mechanized and which need individual attention. In the area of diagnosis, computerized versions of diagnostic questions sometimes generate more candidness than in-person interviews. The use of computerized questionnaires appears especially promising for screening large populations, such as colleges, for possible cases. While a firm and clear diagnosis of an eating disorder requires a subsequent in-person, detailed interview, cases that might not otherwise have come to definitive diagnosis may be found with computerized screening.

The core task of treatment is identifying, challenging, and changing the overvalued beliefs about the benefits of weight loss (or muscle gain in "reverse anorexia"). This existentially engaging process involves a clinician with a "dual aspect" approach to the individual. First, the clinician must have a clear, evidence-based view of the person as a diagnostic entity with the eating disorder and its comorbidities and an understanding of evidence-based literature on the best type of treatments suited for this combination of challenges, including statistical probabilities of outcome for 100 such persons. Second, the clinician must also establish an existentially sensitive psychotherapeutic engagement with the individual as if she or he were the only person in the world, entering into that person's phe-

TABLE 2.5   Mechanized approaches to assessment and treatment of eating disorders

Functional goal	Methodology
Psychological assessment	Self-administered versions of EDE, EAT, and EDI tests; computerized versions of general psychological tests; computerized Web-based assessment modules for use in homes, schools
Weight restoration	Liquid meals only, in place of nursing-supervised "normal food eaten normally": not validated, but saves staff time
Behavioral monitoring	Videocameras; automatic recording toilets; automatic door locks
Cognitive-behavioral therapy	Computerized Web-based modules: possibly effective for milder cases
Applying relaxation techniques	Audiotape, CDs, DVDs
Activity monitoring	Wrist or ankle distance monitors for level of activity
Cardiac assessment	24-hour monitors for specialist assessment
Monitoring blood glucose levels	Noninvasive glucose monitors
Pre-post-treatment assessment visually	Pre-post-treatment photographs for chart
Evaluating body image distortion	Computerized assessment of level of distortion; draw-a-person
Psychoeducation	DVDs or computerized modules on healthy nutrition, medication management, diabetes
Answering commonly asked questions	Computerized FAQ modules
Communication with community resources	E-mail availability, monitored for appropriateness
Measuring interval weights and body fat	Self-recording "Tanita"-type scales
Recording patient progress	Speech-to-print computerized programs

Note: The approaches listed here are used in various places. Listing does not imply endorsement.

nomenological experience as a partner in the healing process to form a therapeutic alliance that allows the individual to let go of the eating disorder as a strategy for living and develop healthy coping mechanisms and age-appropriate defenses, as well as internalize CBT, IPT, or DPT skills. Crisp (2006) articulately described the existential fears of maturation that drive many cases of anorexia nervosa among young persons; such fears require one-on-one engagement with the illness. Introducing mechanization must be done with a respect for the core task of treatment and not dissolve into a reductionistic approach of mechanized steps.

Aspects of care that involve mechanization of routine functions—such as toilet doors that lock automatically and toilets that record body eliminations, videotape surveys of distant parts of a unit, and ankle recorders of activity expended—are examples of possible reasonable mechanizations. DVD- and computer-based modules may supplement, but not supplant, small group teaching about nutrition, medical symptoms, healthy exercise, developing media skepticism, and other topics.

Some preliminary studies have supported the practice of computer-based relapse prevention efforts and, at times, core psychotherapeutic work for outpatients with milder forms of eating disorders, especially when the media-based therapy is ancillary to intermittent in-person contact with experienced staff at a treatment center. The possibility of preventive intervention via media-based learning is open to validation, but its efficacy or effectiveness has not yet been confirmed.

Group Approaches to Treatment

Table 2.6 examines group approaches to healing eating disorders. The primary power of groups is their ability to mobilize resources that are less available in one-to-one treatment: the experience of peer support and peer challenge, being able to see parallels in the experience of others, and using peers who are further along in the treatment process as role models. CBT for eating disorders has been markedly effective (Fairburn, Cooper, and Shafran, 2003; Wilson, 2005). Parents, in particular, may wonder whether a patient will "learn bad habits" from groups. With experienced leadership, the benefits of group treatment far outweigh the disadvantages. A predominance of group work over individual work has been validated for day hospital (PPH) and outpatient treatment. Inpa-

TABLE 2.6   Goals of therapeutic groups

Cognitive-Behavioral Group

Goal is group therapy for eating disorders using CBT, with emphasis on periodic review of how to apply CBT personally by connecting behaviors with feelings and thoughts. Teaches how to identify and change most common cognitive distortions. Emphasizes validation of full range of (often split-off) feelings, opening possibility of positive affects and behaviors that increase joy and contentment.

Body-Image Group

Emphasis is on a combination of psychoeducation about body image distortion, validation of treatment-related changes in body weight and shape, CBT-based challenge of body image distortion, development of media skepticism. Establishes a framework for living in a weight-preoccupied society. Provides information about mirror-gazing and identification of automatic thoughts negatively comparing self to others. Validation of normal bell-shaped curve for weight and height.

Nutritional Planning Group

Provides psychoeducation about healthy nutrition vs. weight/fat/calorie-preoccupied approaches; raises awareness of and challenges automatic "cash-register" approach to counting calories and fat grams. Teaches development of flexible meal plans and how to determine healthy serving sizes as an empowerment strategy in new situations. Becoming reacquainted with taste and texture as positive experiences in eating; associating eating with socialization and relaxation.

Relaxation Group

Daily teaching, and practice on mats, of relaxation, stress management, validation of being in touch with entire body ("getting out of your head"); emphasizes lifetime methods using either Jacobson (tense and relax) or Benson (ideational) methods. Considers "body scan" method from Mindfulness groups where qualified personnel available.

Rape Victims Advocacy Group

Where qualified personnel are available, helps women victims come to terms with fearfulness, PTSD, and teaches healthy understanding of body, assertiveness training. Works on detaching emotional reliving from factual memory.

Men's Group

Where two or more males are present at any level of treatment, they benefit from being able to talk about normal "guy" topics not possible in largely female groups, such as sports, cars, dating. Also, more substantive topics emerge as discussions develop, especially father-son relationships, acceptance of feelings. Group leaders are males in any therapeutic discipline.

Sex Education Group

Primarily for adolescents and young adults at any level of treatment, emphasizing acceptance of sexual feelings; responsible sexual behaviors; normative sexual

TABLE 2.6   *(continued)*

behaviors, thoughts, feelings at each stage of development; relationship of starvation to changes in sexual drive and behaviors. Where individuals are comfortable, includes discussion of sexual identity and past experiences. Educators and nurses often most qualified as group leaders.

Expressive Arts Therapy Group

Goal is to learn to express feelings and have a wide, healthy, sense-related experience in music, visual arts, dance, poetry. Practice theme of "anything worth doing is worth doing badly" for perfectionistic individuals who are fearful of trying new experiences; acknowledges variety of learning and expressive styles of individuals; hidden expressiveness found in "Karaoke" evenings. At times, deeper psychological themes of past trauma are best expressed in artwork when it is freely expressed without judgment.

Spirituality Group

Voluntary group with hospital-trained expert clergy who open up discussion of spiritual dimensions of suffering and healing. Nondenominational. Validates a variety of individual faith traditions.

Weekend-Planning Group (for 5 day/week partial hospital programs)

How to structure time, finding a balance between compulsive overplanning and lack of any structure; role-playing interactions with family and friends; validating mild to moderate anxiety of choosing meals out of hospital; developing 3 × 5 index cards for purse or pocket for reminders on dealing with cognitive distortions; practicing techniques for response inhibition of self-starvation, binge, or purge urges; distinguishing urges from behaviors; emergency numbers; self-reliance; renewal of pledge of no-substance use, including alcohol.

Family Support Group

These groups are modeled on the excellent experience in pediatrics with family support groups. The goal is to put families in touch with one another (advance informed consent given) for support, sharing successful problem-solving approaches, psychoeducation about nature of eating disorders, stopping the common "walking on eggshells." These groups give hope to families of newly admitted patients who are encouraged by meeting families of recovered or almost-recovered patients.

Meal Preparation Group

Small groups are taken with support and education on shopping trips to grocery stores, where emphasis is on how to choose healthy food groups without scrutiny of labels. Food is then prepared in a group in hospital, with emphasis on balance and social enjoyment of meals. Desensitization of "dangerous foods" takes place.

(continued)

TABLE 2.6   (continued)

Renewed or new acceptance of taste and texture. Defeats phobias of touching food.

Exercise and Activities Group

Combines a group approach to progressive healthy aerobic exercises and strength training with development of an individual exercise prescription for within-program and after-program completion. Emphasis on lifelong exercise skills and sense of functional efficacy of the body vs. an objectified emphasis on body appearance. Aquatherapy in warm, swirling water leads to adaptation to swimsuits and to learning to feel body relaxation. Validated with before vs. after levels of perceived anxiety.

tients benefit from groups, but because of the acuity of their illness require more individual time from staff in multiple disciplines.

A secondary benefit of group treatment is economy of staff time and some decrease in treatment costs, but these savings are not as much as financial administrators might think. Group sessions are usually longer than individual sessions (often 90 minutes for CBT and body image groups) and require documentation of the individual's behavior in the group setting. The therapist balances topic-based feedback with process comments (in other words, makes the group aware of the processes going on interpersonally, separate from the topic of the group).

Groups differ considerably in their focus. The key core groups are involved in psychotherapeutic orientation—for example, applying CBT. In addition, groups to challenge and change distorted body image are essential, as are psychoeducation groups for teaching healthy nutrition. It is hard to imagine improvement in deeply rooted abnormal behaviors without experiential groups in which patients learn new, healthy patterns of exercise, how to shop for and prepare food, and methods of relaxation. Individual programs may have different names for their groups, but the goals of the groups cluster around the important challenges in the healing process. Life without balance and diversional activities is not life. The ability to discover the self through art, music, and body expression contributes to the normality of life for persons who have often become devoid of humor and recreation. Having fun is not only permitted but is also almost mandated for patients with eating disorders. When a patient improves and no longer spends 50–90 percent of the day thinking about food, weight, and shape, she or he needs to fill that time constructively, not simply develop multitasking work or school activities. For families, groups may be a lifeline and anchor for their sanity, providing them with psychoeducation and the tools to change in needed ways.

As with almost any activity, the effectiveness of a group depends on expert group leaders. It would be unreasonable to expect a surgeon untrained in a specialized operation to achieve results as good as those of an experienced surgeon with hundreds of operations in the area of concern. The treatment of patients with eating disorders requires integrative and sequential skills, sometimes from a formally constituted, continuing team and sometimes from an informally organized, ad hoc team. The potential remission rate of patients with eating disorders can be much higher than remission rates for entrenched OCD, schizophrenia, or bipolar disorder. Strober, Freeman, and Morrell (1997) document a 76 percent remission rate for multidisciplinary team treatment of adolescents with anorexia nervosa. Yet, eating disorders need not be chronic, severe, or difficult to treat, as common but mistaken clinical mythology sometimes suggests. Expert treatment leading to remission is not complex but needs to be well thought out and sustained for several years.

Clinicians treating patients who have eating disorders need to work with a "player-coach" mentality, not a hierarchical, power-oriented approach. Making some predictable functions routine, and being flexible regarding individual variations and needs, is an optimal approach. Few other disorders allow the clinician to participate so much in bringing a patient back from an at times morbid condition to a fully functioning human being, all the while engaging with the patient in the process of change over a long enough time, and with the help of multidisciplinary peers, to see humanity reemerge. An expert in treating eating disorders recognizes personal limitations, engages others in the shared task, and has few egocentric demands. Ethical conflicts in the care of anorexia nervosa patients are described in Chapter 14.

Summary

The biopsychosocial model and the multidisciplinary treatment team are the foundation of state-of-the-art patient care, given the complexity of treating individuals with eating disorders in the context of managed care. Evidence supports the assertion that definitive acute care with a goal of full remission (Crow and Nyman, 2004) is also the most economical care. The "revolving door" for treatment needs to stop (Baran, Weltzin, and Kaye, 1995). Numerous disciplines blend their skills to provide the optimal recovery environment. At times, only months or years after treatment do patients have the perspective to write that the treatment was difficult and intensive, but that they can see no other way to have achieved remission. Optimal treatment involves a combination of shared and fairly uniform components (groups, weight restoration) as well as very individualized components (the individual's life journey, specific medical needs, family environment). The assembly, integration, and ongoing management of the multidisciplinary team provide both challenge and satisfaction for all involved: the patient, the family, and the team.

REFERENCES

Baran SA, Weltzin TE, and Kaye WH. 1995. Low discharge weight and outcome in anorexia nervosa. *American Journal of Psychiatry* 152:1070–72.

Bossidy L and Charan R. 2002. *Execution: The Discipline of Getting Things Done*. New York: Crown Business.

Bowers WA, Evans K, and Andersen AE. 1997. Inpatient treatment of eating disorders: A cognitive therapy milieu. *Cognitive and Behavioral Practice* 4:291–323.

Covey SR. 1989. *The Seven Habits of Highly Effective People: Restoring the Character Ethic*. New York: Simon and Schuster.

Crisp A. 2006. In defense of the concept of phobically driven avoidance of adult body weight/shape/function as the final common pathway to anorexia nervosa. *European Eating Disorders Review* 14:189–202.

Crow SJ and Nyman JA. 2004. The cost-effectiveness of anorexia nervosa treatment. *International Journal of Eating Disorders* 35:155–60.

Fairburn CG, Cooper A, and Shafran R. 2003. Cognitive behavior therapy for eating disorders: A "transdiagnostic" theory and treatment. *Behaviour Research and Therapy* 41:509–28.

Garcia de Amusquibar AM. 2000. Interdisciplinary team for the treatment of eating disorders. *Eating and Weight Disorders* 5:223–27.

Gicquel L. 2008. Management strategies of eating disorders in adults. *Revue du Praticien* 58:167–71.

Halmi KA. 2005. The multimodal treatment of eating disorders. *World Psychiatry* 4:69–73.

Kreipe RE and Yussman SM. 2003. The role of the primary care practitioner in the treatment of eating disorders. *Adolescent Medicine* 14:133–47.

Manheim A v. Travelers Insurance Company. 92–CV-5466 (JG). Sept. 15, 1995.

Mehler PS and Krantz M. 2003. Anorexia nervosa medical issues. *Women's Health* (Larchmt) 12:331–40.

Piran N and Kaplan AS, eds. 1990. *A Day Hospital Group Treatment Program for Anorexia Nervosa and Bulimia Nervosa.* Brunner/Mazel Eating Disorders Monograph Series, No. 3. New York: Brunner-Routledge.

Simons RM v. Blue Cross and Blue Shield of Greater New York. 536 N.Y.S. 2d 431 (A.D. 1 Dept.[A] 1989).

Strober M, Freeman R, and Morrell W. 1997. The long-term course of severe anorexia nervosa in adolescents: Survival analysis of recovery, relapse, and outcome predictors over 10–15 years in a prospective study. *International Journal of Eating Disorders* 22:339–60.

Wilson TG. 2005. Psychological treatment of eating disorders. *Annual Review of Clinical Psychology* 1:439–65.

CHAPTER THREE

Medical Evaluation of Patients with Eating Disorders

An Overview

COMMON QUESTIONS

Are anorexia and bulimia nervosa associated with significant medical issues?

Are there specific physical signs, symptoms, or laboratory results that point to a diagnosis of anorexia or bulimia nervosa?

What questions need to be asked during an initial history and physical examination?

Which examinations are strongly recommended?

Which laboratory tests are strongly recommended?

Which examinations are optional?

How often do the examinations have to be repeated?

This chapter presents a broad general overview of the medical evaluation that is appropriate for the patient with an eating disorder. Many of the medical issues dealt with in this chapter are reviewed in more detail in other chapters. The specific chapters are noted throughout this review and should be consulted for additional in-depth details about these medical issues.

Most of the medical complications of anorexia nervosa and bulimia result either from starvation and weight loss or from the specific purging behavior. *Purging* indicates all forms of self-induced compensation for unwanted calories or methods to lower weight by loss of body fluids. This can be accomplished via self-induced vomiting (which may be induced manually, with an object such as a toothbrush; by simply tightening abdominal muscles; or by ingesting ipecac), laxative abuse, diuretic abuse, or ingestion of thyroid hormone or stimulant-type medications.

The first three methods are the most common, followed by others in descending order of frequency.

These are dangerous illnesses. Anorexia nervosa is a potentially life-threatening disorder and one of the most lethal psychiatric disorders. In a meta-analysis, the aggregate 10-year mortality rate was 5.6 percent (Sullivan, 1995). About 27 percent died from suicide, 54 percent died from a direct effect of the illness, and 19 percent from unknown and other causes. The middle group, which is the largest, died from the medical complications of the illness. The author concluded that the aggregate mortality rate associated with anorexia nervosa is more than twelve times higher than that of 15- to 24-year-old females in the general population and more than two times higher than that of female psychiatric inpatients 10 to 39 years old.

Bulimia nervosa is medically more benign than anorexia nervosa. Death appears to be a relatively rare event; however, the follow-up periods in the literature are short compared to those for anorexia nervosa. When death occurs, it is usually caused by cardiac abnormality from hypokalemia (low potassium) due to some type of purging behavior, or by suicide, which is generally a consequence of the common comorbid personality disorder.

Diagnosis

Most individuals who have an eating disorder will not present with symptoms directly attributable to the eating disorder and may attempt to hide evidence of disordered eating from the physician. This is especially true for individuals of normal weight who have bulimia. However, symptoms, signs, and laboratory results provide appropriate clues for the alert clinician.

SYMPTOMS

Most often, patients with an eating disorder are females in their teens or twenties, and they present for medical care with nonspecific complaints of feeling "bloated" and experiencing constipation, infertility problems, swelling of the hands and feet, or nonspecific cardiopulmonary symptoms such as exertional fatigue, palpitations, or syncope (fainting) (Table

3.1). If the physician misses these subtle clues, he or she can easily overlook the diagnosis.

SIGNS

The most common signs associated with anorexia nervosa and bulimia are listed in Table 3.2. In severe anorexia nervosa, the emaciation of the patient usually alerts the clinician to the diagnosis. However, individuals with anorexia usually try to conceal their low weight. Common strategies include wearing large pants and sweaters to mask their thinness, and carrying hidden objects or ingesting water to artificially inflate their weight. Not infrequently, probably because of society's emphasis on thinness, health care professionals overlook the marked degree of emaciation and thus may fail to recognize the seriousness of the patient's condition.

TABLE 3.1   Symptoms found in individuals with eating disorders

Anorexia nervosa	Bulimia nervosa
Amenorrhea	Irregular menses
Infertility	Heart palpitations
Irritability	Esophageal burning
Depression	Nonfocal abdominal pain
Exertional fatigue	Abdominal bloating
Weakness	Lethargy
Headache	Fatigue
Dizziness	Headache
Chest pain	Constipation/diarrhea
Faintness	Swelling of hands/feet
Constipation	Frequent sore throat
Abdominal pain	Teeth sensitivity
Nonfocal abdominal pain	Depression
Feeling of "fullness" with eating	Swollen cheeks
Polyuria	
Dry skin	
Intolerance of cold	
Low back pain	

TABLE 3.2   Physical signs found in individuals with eating disorders

Anorexia nervosa	Bulimia nervosa
Emaciation	Calluses on the back of the hand
Hypothermia	Salivary gland hypertrophy (swollen cheeks)
Hyperactivity	
Bradycardia (heart rate <60 beats per minute)	Erosion of dental enamel (perimolysis)
	Periodontal disease
Hypotension (low blood pressure, <90 mmHg systolic)	Dental caries
	Facial petechiae (red dots on the face)
Hypoactive bowel sounds	Perioral irritation
Dry skin	Mouth ulcer
Pressure sores	Hematemesis (vomiting blood)
Brittle hair	Edema (ankle, periorbital)
Brittle nails	Abdominal bloating
Hair loss on scalp	Cardiac arrhythmia
"Yellow" skin, especially palms	
Lanugo hair	
Cyanotic (blue) and cold hands and feet	
Edema (ankle, periorbital)	
Heart murmur (mitral valve prolapse)	

People with anorexia nervosa have thinning scalp hair; lanugo hair growth (downy, fine hair), particularly on the face, neck, arms, back, and legs; and a yellowish tinge to the skin. There is bradycardia, hypotension, and hypothermia, which may present as cold intolerance and an inability to compensate for changes in temperature. The hands and feet are frequently purplish-blue due to cyanosis and abnormalities of temperature regulation (acrocyanosis) (Yager and Andersen, 2005).

In contrast to people with anorexia, whose emaciation draws medical attention, people with bulimia nervosa often appear physically healthy. Because binge eating is often done secretively, most patients will not provide this information unless specifically asked. In addition, the associated behaviors of vomiting and of abuse of laxatives, diet pills, diuretics, or ipecac are often concealed from others due to guilt or shame and must be specifically inquired about during the history.

However, certain signs present on physical examination are of some utility in detecting occult bulimia nervosa (Mehler, 2003). A common sign is the erosion of dental enamel in individuals with bulimia who vomit. The erosion is particularly marked on the lingual surface of the upper teeth. This is referred to as perimolysis. Fillings or amalgams, which are relatively resistant to the gastric acid, appear to be raised above the level of the tooth surface. Other types of dental change include increased sensitivity to cold or hot temperatures and a possible increased rate of developing caries (Little, 2002). A second clinical sign is swelling of the salivary glands, particularly the parotid glands on the sides of the face. This swelling is usually bilateral and painless, but can be pronounced (Mandel and Abai, 2004). This is sometimes referred to as "puffy cheeks" by patients and is seen in people with bulimia who engage in excessive amounts of self-induced vomiting. Interestingly, it becomes manifest 2–3 days after a bout of vomiting has ceased (see Chap. 10). A third sign of diagnostic utility is calluses on the dorsum of the hand as a result of irritation by the teeth during repeated induction of self-induced vomiting (Russell's sign). This sign, specific to bulimia, may be more common early in the course of the illness; during later stages of the illness, patients often no longer require mechanical stimulation to induce vomiting and can simply turn their head, bend forward, and initiate vomiting.

In some patients, periorbital petechiae (small red dots around the eyes) may be seen shortly after a forceful vomiting episode, and there may be redness of the skin around the corners of mouth as a result of irritation by acidic stomach contents. This is referred to as angular cheilosis. Fluid retention can be dramatic, particularly in the hands and feet, after withdrawal of laxatives or diuretics or cessation of excessive vomiting. Severe hyponatremia (low sodium level) can result from diuretic abuse in a patient with bulimia who is further volume-depleted from vomiting or in a patient with anorexia who is drinking even as little as 5–10 liters of water per day to obtain a "full" feeling without eating. If therapeutic correction of the serum sodium is too rapid, these patients risk developing the serious neurologic disorder known as central pontine myelinolysis. In both disorders, physical signs of past self-mutilation are not uncommon, especially in bulimia nervosa associated with borderline personality disorder.

LABORATORY RESULTS

Unfortunately, objective measures of the existence and severity of disordered eating behavior do not exist, and clinicians must rely on the self-reports of their patients, who may not accurately describe the frequency of their bulimia-related behaviors. There are no good, consistently reliable screening laboratory tools for occult or denied bulimic behavior. A good patient-doctor relationship, which sets the tone for candid responses to screening questions, is key. There are, however, some helpful clues on blood testing that may speak to the presence of bulimia.

Abnormally low serum potassium levels are specific for purging behaviors but are not highly sensitive for the detection of purging behavior (see Chap. 5) (Greenfield et al., 1995). In general, the body is able to maintain normal serum levels of potassium in the absence of severe gastrointestinal or renal loses of potassium. Pure dietary-induced hypokalemia is relatively rare in the absence of purging behaviors, which deplete the body's potassium stores. The serum bicarbonate level is often abnormal as well in bulimia. High levels (greater than 30 meq/L) are most consistent with either self-induced vomiting or diuretic abuse; low levels are most consistent with diarrhea from laxative abuse. Patients with purely restrictive anorexia nervosa are rarely at risk for hypokalemia, even if their weight is very low. In fact, generally their blood chemistry values are remarkably normal, and they may die from anorexia nervosa starvation with normal blood laboratory values, including a preserved serum albumin level. Therefore, the presence of a substantially low albumin level should prompt the clinician to look for independent medical comorbidities.

Serum amylase levels are frequently raised above the normal range in people who vomit regularly. The hyperamylasemia is mostly salivary-based rather than pancreatic in origin and results from enlarged salivary glands due to overeating and vomiting. As with potassium levels, the role of serum amylase measurements as a diagnostic test is limited. Nevertheless, amylase levels correlate positively with time since the last eating episode and in some patients with frequency of binge-eating and purging. Because an elevated amylase level can also be seen with acute pancreatitis, it is worthwhile to also then check a lipase level. If the lipase is normal, then one can conclude that the elevated amylase level is of salivary origin rather than of pancreatic origin.

In summary, the presence of an abnormally low potassium value and an abnormally high serum amylase level together with an elevated bicarbonate level, in an otherwise healthy young woman, appears to be specific for frequent purging behavior. However, its sensitivity as a screening tool is poor. As with all patients, a careful history, directed toward uncovering problem behaviors that might cause serious medical complications, is the most important source of information, for which no laboratory tests can substitute, especially for patients between the ages of 13 and 30, when eating disorders are most prevalent.

Hypercholesterolemia has been noted in up to 50 percent of patients with anorexia nervosa but is probably clinically insignificant (Table 3.3). It is probably a reflection of an elevated "good" cholesterol subtype (HDL) rather than an elevated "bad" cholesterol subtype (LDL).

Elevations of liver transaminase levels can be seen both before refeeding in severe anorexia nervosa, as well as a result of aggressive refeeding dietary plans containing high dextrose caloric sources (Saito et al., 2008).

Differential Diagnosis

In the food-restricting subtype of anorexia nervosa, the symptoms and signs are usually those that occur secondary to caloric restriction and weight loss. Most of the manifestations are similar to the complications observed in patients with starvation due to other causes. However, there are a few important differences. For example, most starving patients will note lethargy and inability to exercise, whereas patients with anorexia may exercise excessively in attempts to lose weight. Patients with weight loss from other organic causes will express concern about their weight loss, while patients with anorexia will be unconcerned about their marked weight loss. Moreover, other common causes of weight loss due to malabsorption will present with diarrheal symptoms, which are absent in anorexia nervosa, or they will have symptoms of adrenergic excess,

TABLE 3.3 Laboratory results that might point to a diagnosis of eating disorder

Anorexia nervosa (food-restricting subtype)	Bulimia nervosa
Hypercholesterolemia	Hyperamylasemia
Hypoglycemia	Hyponatremia
QT prolongation on EKG	Hypokalemia
Bradycardia (low heart rate, <60)	Hypomagnesemia
Low white blood cell count (leukopenia)	Metabolic alkalosis
Low red blood cell count (anemia)	
Low LH, FSH, estradiol, or testosterone levels	
Hypophosphatemia	
Hyponatremia (low sodium)	
Osteopenia	

such as sweating and rapid heart rates, which are not present in anorexia nervosa. The clinician should also bear in mind that the most common cause of substantial weight loss in young adolescent females in Western societies is anorexia nervosa. Patients with anorexia are often spared the starvation-related complication of the inhabitants of developing countries (kwashiorkor and marasmus) because of their usual ingestion of vitamins, even though their total caloric intake is very low.

Therefore, especially for those patients presenting with atypical features, clinicians should make a careful assessment to exclude other organic pathologies such as occult malignancies, chronic infections, diabetes, or malabsorption syndromes. Selected laboratory tests can facilitate the diagnosis of other illnesses, such as hyperthyroidism (TSH), which may cause weight loss and simulate anorexia nervosa. Inflammatory bowel disease affecting the small intestine can cause abdominal pain associated with eating that may lead to food restriction, incorrectly suggesting the diagnosis of anorexia nervosa; the central psychopathology of anorexia (see Chap. 1) and normal albumin levels are lacking, however. Other common psychiatric disorders are also associated with weight loss, such as depression, schizophrenia, substance abuse, somatoform disorders, and dissociative disorder. When starvation begins with self-induced vomiting and the patient endorses a drive for thinness with a morbid fear of weight gain, a purely medical cause is rarely found. In addition, the patient's menstrual threshold, which is usually at about 85–90 percent of ideal body weight, should be established.

Similarly, a variety of other medical conditions may present with symptoms that are difficult to distinguish from those of bulimia. For example, illnesses such as inflammatory bowel disease and connective tissue syndromes (scleroderma) may cause abnormal gastrointestinal (GI) motility and result in many of the same symptoms as in people who have bulimia and abuse laxatives. Generally speaking, these diagnoses can be made by a thorough medical history and physical examination together with laboratory screening tests. Complex and expensive work-ups are rarely indicated. The guiding principle is that a diagnosis of an eating disorder is made not by a "rule-out" approach of all possible medical disorders but by confident determination of the presence of an eating disorder through screening questions and a brief mental status examination (Table 3.4) (Walsh, Wheat, and Freund, 2000).

Patients frequently complain about constipation. However, a detailed history of the patient's perception of constipation is required because constipation is variably defined by patients and physicians. Experts define constipation as having fewer than three bowel movements per week, with hard and small stools on more than 25 percent of occasions. In bulimia nervosa, constipation is usually caused by dependence on stimulant laxatives, which, in the long run, can result in the death of the colonic wall myenteric nerve plexus and severe constipation. In anorexia nervosa, GI motility is delayed due to lack of oral intake (Mitchell and Crow, 2006) (see Chap. 6).

Given the frequency of comorbid psychiatric conditions, a complete psychiatric evaluation should be performed to diagnose comorbid depression, substance abuse, and personality disorders. The patient should also be evaluated for impulsivity and suicidality.

Physical Examination

There are two distinct reasons for conducting a physical examination of patients with eating disorders. The first is to elicit the signs related to the medical complications of anorexia or bulimia nervosa, and in the pro-

Anorexia nervosa	Bulimia nervosa
Hyperthyroidism	Scleroderma or other connective tissue disorders with GI involvement (and abnormal gut motility)
Addison disease	
Diabetes mellitus	
Malignancy, especially lymphoma, stomach cancer	Inflammatory bowel disease
Chronic infection, especially tuberculosis, AIDS, fungal disease	Esophageal stricture
	Peptic ulcer disease
Hypothalamic lesion or tumor	Gastric outlet syndrome
Cystic fibrosis	Parasitic intestinal infection
Superior mesenteric artery syndrome	Chronic pancreatitis
Malabsorption syndrome	Diabetes
Inflammatory bowel disease (Crohn's disease, ulcerative colitis)	Hypothalamic lesion or tumor
	Zenker diverticulum
Parasitic intestinal infection	Brain tumor
Chronic pancreatitis	
Psychiatric disorders associated with weight loss	

cess to begin to define a treatment plan to stabilize patients medically (Mehler, 2001). The second is to use it in a motivational context and to confront patients with objective evidence that the disordered eating behavior has adversely affected their physical health (see Chap. 13). This information is particularly relevant for physicians in the light of the long-term increased mortality rate, which is especially pronounced for patients with severe anorexia nervosa. The facets of such a physical examination are summarized in Table 3.5.

Obtaining accurate measures of a patient's height and weight and assessing the degree of emaciation are important. For a patient with anorexia nervosa, it is helpful to consider that person's status in the construct of percentage below ideal body weight (IBW). It can be easily calculated, starting with 100 pounds for someone 5 feet tall and then adding 4–5 pounds

TABLE 3.5   Physical examination for patients with eating disorders

Weight and height	Dental examination
Pulse and blood pressure	Cardiac examination
State of hydration	Abdominal examination
Skin examination	Extremity examination (edema)

for each additional inch. Thus, if the patient is 5 feet 5 inches tall and weighs 100 pounds, he or she is 20 percent below the IBW. Severe anorexia nervosa is generally diagnosed for weights that are more than 25 percent below IBW (Chap. 4). The patient's current weight should not be self-reported, because patients with eating disorders are often unreliable in self-estimation of body weight. The clinician should also attempt to establish the patient's premorbid weight, which gives an approximation of the patient's natural weight. For patients with bulimia nervosa, this is often significantly above matched population mean weights for age and height. In contrast, patients with anorexia nervosa without bulimia tend not to have been premorbidly overweight.

Examination of the mucous membranes, skin turgor, and, if indicated, orthostatic blood pressure helps to assess the patient's state of hydration. An examination of the abdomen may be necessary in patients with constipation or other GI complaints (Mehler, 1997). Inspection, auscultation, and light palpation are recommended. In most patients, further evaluation will not be necessary.

For individuals with bulimia, a careful dental examination for evidence of dental caries and enamel erosion should be performed. The erosion has a characteristic pattern, tending to occur on surfaces that have maximum exposure to the vomitus, particularly the palatal surfaces of the maxillary teeth and the occlusal surfaces of posterior teeth, especially on the lingual sides (see Chap. 10).

Pulse and blood pressure should be checked in all patients. Sinus bradycardia of fewer than 60 beats per minute is present in many patients with anorexia nervosa because of an energy-conservation slowing of the metabolic rate and vagal hyperactivity. Hypotension, with a blood pressure of less than 90/60 mmHg, is present in these patients, related to chronic volume depletion, and often results in episodes of dizziness and frank syncope. Sympathetic nervous system hypofunction may also be a contributing factor, including the mechanism of decreased circulating norepinephrine. Orthostatic pubic blood pressure measurements should be taken, including supine, sitting, and standing postures, with subjective as well as objective findings noted (Guarda and Redgrave, 2006).

An electrocardiogram (EKG) with a rhythm strip is desirable for any patient who is abusing ipecac or diuretics, who is severely emaciated or has hypokalemia, or who has signs and symptoms attributable to the cardiovascular system. It is probably worth obtaining a baseline EKG for any patient hospitalized with an eating disorder. The EKG commonly shows sinus bradycardia; low-amplitude P wave and QRS voltages reflecting reduced cardiac size; nonspecific ST segment and T wave abnormalities; and occasionally U waves associated with hypokalemia and hypomagnescmia. QT abnormalities may also be present (see also Chap. 7).

Which Laboratory Tests Are Mandatory?

Several screening procedures and tests are indicated for all people who present with an eating disorder, and several specific procedures and tests are indicated in certain situations. The choice of laboratory tests at the initial evaluation will be guided by the results of the history and the physical examination and the severity of the eating disorder. Most people with eating disorders should have a screening laboratory panel of blood tests performed. A complete blood count with differential, electrolytes, blood urea nitrogen, creatinine, blood glucose, calcium, phosphate, and liver function tests are indicated for most people with eating disorders, especially those being admitted to a hospital or those first engaging in mental health treatment.

Low white and red blood cell counts can occur with anorexia nervosa, reflecting bone marrow suppression due to malnutrition. An increase in leukocyte counts, due to infections, might be overlooked due to low baseline values. Therefore, increased vigilance is necessary with patients who have anorexia and are being evaluated for possible infections. Also, they may not manifest a fever in infectious states because of baseline hypothermia.

Serum electrolytes should be checked routinely for all patients to detect possible electrolyte imbalances. Specifically, elevated serum bicarbonate levels indicating metabolic alkalosis are frequently seen in patients who vomit regularly. Hypokalemia is often present in patients with bulimia. Because hypokalemia is a potentially life-threatening abnormality, it would be suboptimal not to evaluate electrolyte function in patients with bulimia who are actively purging. Furthermore, many patients with electrolyte abnormalities are clinically asymptomatic. As mentioned before, patients who are in a low weight range, and for whom intense purging is acknowledged or suspected, are most at risk. Hypophosphatemia can lead to serious complications and often develops during the early stages of refeeding patients who have anorexia nervosa (see Chaps. 4 and 5).

Liver enzyme abnormalities are relatively uncommon among patients with eating disorders at near-normal weights. However, it is well known that low body weight can cause hepatic damage and that hepatic dysfunction may occur in patients with eating disorders more often than in the general population. Thus, elevated liver enzymes, aspartate aminotransferase (AST) and alanine aminotransferase (ALT), occur in patients with anorexia nervosa and especially if there is concomitant alcohol abuse or medication use. Abnormal liver function tests can also be found during the initial stages of refeeding. In particular, the hepatocellular enzymes ALT and AST, as well as indirect bilirubin, may be increased during refeeding, especially if nutritional intake emphasizes foods with high glucose content (see Chap. 4).

A disproportionate rise in blood urea nitrogen compared with creatinine may be caused by dehydration from diuretics, laxative abuse, or decreased fluid intake in anorexia nervosa. Generally, this ratio is less than 20:1. Blood glucose often decreases with more severe weight loss in anorexia nervosa but is generally asymptomatic in the 40–60 mg/dL level. Hypoglycemia is a bad prognostic sign in anorexia nervosa because it indicates depleted hepatic glycogen and glucose stores.

Because the symptoms and signs of both hyper- and hypothyroidism can mimic eating disorders, thyroid function tests are appropriate. Patients with anorexia nervosa might be misdiagnosed as having hypothyroidism. The pattern of thyroid indices found in patients with anorexia is a normal or low T4, decreased T3, increased reverse T3, and a normal TSH. The most common pattern of low T4, decreased T3, and increased reverse T3, with normal TSH represents a physiologic adaptation to starvation that need not be treated with thyroid supplementation. It is referred to as the euthyroid sick syndrome. Patients may even abuse thyroid

TABLE 3.6   Laboratory tests for patients with eating disorders

CBC with differential	Serum BUN, creatinine levels
Serum electrolytes	Blood glucose level
Calcium, magnesium, phosphorus levels	T_3, T_4, TSH levels
	Urinalysis
Liver function tests	Stool examination if GI bleeding, abdominal complaints, or anemia is present
Serum salivary amylase level	

hormone therapy to further lose weight. Occasionally, TSH is mildly elevated, but it generally returns to normal three weeks after refeeding is under way, and thus should be rechecked before committing a patient to thyroid hormone replacement therapy (Table 3.6).

Young people with insulin-dependent diabetes mellitus sometimes overdose their insulin to compensate for binges or underdose to create ketoacidosis-induced urinary frequency and weight loss.

It is important to remember that conception can occur during recovery from anorexia nervosa and before the return of menstruation. Most females with anorexia nervosa have amenorrhea, which generally remits once weight restoration has raised their weight within 90 percent of IBW.

Which Examinations and Laboratory Tests Are Optional?

The specific items of the history, the complaints of the patients, and the findings on physical examination should direct the physician to the necessity for further evaluation, such as chest or abdominal X-rays, electromyography (EMG), examination of muscle enzymes (CPK), computed tomography (CT) or magnetic resonance imaging (MRI) scans of the head, or GI endoscopy if there is evidence of GI blood loss or significant esophageal, gastric, or abdominal pain.

If abuse of diuretics or laxatives is suspected but is denied by the patient, urine samples to detect the surreptitious use of these agents may be considered, as well as stool samples for phenolphthalein as evidence of laxative use. The presence of possible neurologic dysfunction would necessitate an electroencephalogram (EEG) and computerized tomography

(CT) to rule out seizure disorder or structural brain illness, especially in atypical eating disorders.

Screening for osteoporosis should be a standard part of the management of those with anorexia nervosa of more than one year's duration, and the results can often be used as a motivational tool. Recently, it has been recommended to perform a dual-energy X-ray absorptiometry (DEXA) scan for bone density of hip and spine for all women with a history of six months or more of anorexia nervosa. These findings may be used to guide the physician in giving advice about the level of physical activity suitable for the patient and to support recommendations for adequate calcium intake and full restoration of body weight to restore normal menstrual activity. Unfortunately, most studies to date have not found estrogen administration to starved patients with anorexia and deficient bone mineral density to be effective in mitigating the risk of osteoporosis (see Chap. 8).

On the basis of the initial evaluation, judicious use of medical subspecialists to evaluate any identified major medical complications may be indicated. Certainly, at a minimum, a primary care physician who is well versed in the medical issues of these patients should be closely involved in their care.

Ongoing Medical Management

The majority of the above-mentioned abnormalities and complications are fully reversible with weight restoration and cessation of purging behavior. Osteoporosis may be the glaring exception. However, careful, ongoing medical management on a regular basis is an essential component of the treatment plan for patients with eating disorders. The frequency and content of medical follow-up visits must be individualized for each patient, depending on the severity and chronicity of the eating disorder and the associated medical complications. For medically stable patients, return visits approximately every two to three months may be appropriate. These visits should include routine evaluation with a history, a physical, and relevant laboratory tests. However, it is occasionally necessary to see patients who have severe anorexia or bulimia a few times per week during the early phases of their treatment plan or weight-restoration program or when a nonmedical therapist expresses concern for the patient's appearance or new complaints.

Regular monitoring of weight and blood pressure with judicious usage of EKG is strongly advised in all markedly underweight patients who have anorexia or are purging. For many patients with eating disorders, especially those who have bulimia, electrolyte abnormalities are the most prominent medical complication. The clinician should closely follow these patients to ensure adequate correction of electrolyte values. Asymptomatic hypokalemia should be treated with oral potassium supplementation, and intravenously if severe (see Chap. 5).

Follow-up evaluations should be performed more frequently if medical complications have been identified, if the anorexic patient is being aggressively refed or is more than 25–30 percent below IBW, if the patient's condition has deteriorated, or if medical interventions are planned that might affect these parameters. All health care workers caring for these patients must be aware that eating disorders pose serious medical risks and predispose the patient to the development of serious medical complications.

Summary

Eating disorders can have a deleterious effect on many different body systems. It is imperative that patients with eating disorders have a health care provider who is well versed in the medical complications of eating disorders, especially as the prevalence of eating disorders increases.

REFERENCES

Greenfeld D, Mickley D, Quinlan DM, et al. 1995. Hypokalemia in outpatients with eating disorders. *American Journal of Psychiatry* 152:60–63.
Guarda AS and Redgrave GW. 2004. Eating disorders: Detection, assessment, and treatment in primary care. *Advanced Studies in Medicine* 4:468–75.
Little JW. 2002. Eating disorders: Dental implications. *Oral Surgery, Oral Pathology, Oral Radiology and Endodontics* 93:138–43.
Mandel L and Abai S. 2004. Diagnosing bulimia nervosa with parotid gland swelling. *Journal of the American Dental Association* 135:613–16.

Mehler PS. 1997. Constipation: Evaluation and treatment. *Eating Disorders: The Journal of Treatment and Prevention* 5:41–46.

———. 2001. Diagnosis and care of patients with anorexia nervosa in primary care settings. *Annals of Internal Medicine* 134:1048–59.

———. 2003. Clinical practice: Bulimia nervosa. *New England Journal of Medicine* 349:875–81.

Mehler PS, Gray MC, and Schulte M. 1997. Medical complications of anorexia nervosa. *Journal of Women's Heath* 6:533–41.

Miller KK, Grinspoon SK, Ciampa J, et al. 2005. Medical findings in outpatients with anorexia nervosa. *Archives of Internal Medicine* 165:561–66.

Mitchell JE and Crow S. 2006. Medical complications of anorexia nervosa and bulimia nervosa. *Current Opinion in Psychiatry* 19:438–43.

Saito T, Tojo K, Miyashita Y, et al. 2008. Acute liver damage and subsequent hypophosphatemia in malnourished patients: Case reports and review of literature. *International Journal of Eating Disorders* 41:188–92.

Sullivan PF. 1995. Mortality in anorexia nervosa. *American Journal of Psychiatry* 152:1073–74.

Walsh JM, Wheat ME, and Freund K. 2000. Detection, evaluation, and treatment of eating disorders: The role of the primary care physician. *Journal of General Internal Medicine* 15:577–90.

Yager J and Andersen AE. 2005. Clinical practice: Anorexia nervosa. *New England Journal of Medicine* 353:1481–88.

CHAPTER FOUR

Nutritional Rehabilitation

Practical Guidelines for Refeeding Anorexia Nervosa Patients

COMMON QUESTIONS

How is ideal body weight calculated?

What classification is used to define the severity of anorexia and the need for inpatient versus outpatient treatment?

Are there risks inherent in the refeeding process?

What is the "refeeding syndrome," and which patients are at risk?

Are there general guidelines to follow in formulating a dietary plan when refeeding a patient who has anorexia?

What laboratory tests should be checked, and how often should they be checked, when refeeding a patient who has anorexia?

How are calorie needs ascertained and calculated?

What physical findings should the clinician follow during the refeeding process?

What alternative nutritional approaches help reverse the course of refractory, severe anorexia?

What do enteral nutrition and total parenteral nutrition mean?

How does one know if one is providing adequate calories for the nutritional repletion of the patient with anorexia nervosa?

How does one approach a patient's lack of expected weight gain on a specified dietary regimen?

Refeeding the patient who has anorexia nervosa is essential to achieving a successful treatment result. Judging by outcome studies from around the world, most experts agree that one cannot effectively treat anorexia nervosa without first restoring body weight. It is also clear that without a concerted refeeding effort, no meaningful psychotherapy can take place because anorexic patients have starvation-induced cognitive deficits. However, weight restoration may be one of the most challenging and frustrating parts of the recovery process for many patients with anorexia nervosa.

Traditionally, centers that treat patients with moderate and severe degrees of anorexia nervosa have used a combination of behavioral techniques, cognitive restructuring, and a progressive structured program of oral caloric intake to achieve the goal of weight restoration. Different types of gastric feeding and total parenteral nutrition (TPN) may be indicated on a rare basis for more refractory cases. TPN is a specialized procedure and should be undertaken only when medically necessary and by an experienced clinician, with the support of an experienced nursing and nutritional staff. Clinicians caring for these patients must be cognizant of the art of the refeeding process, given the multitude of potential clinical and biochemical caveats that can develop. Two cases illustrate some of these points.

Case 1

S.C., a 41-year-old female, had a 20-year history of anorexia nervosa. She had had multiple unsuccessful inpatient admissions for treatment of this condition. Over the preceding 18 months, she had lost 29 pounds and was infected with a fungal pneumonia. In addition, she complained of cold intolerance, fatigue, and an inability to concentrate. She was therefore readmitted to an inpatient eating disorders unit for the treatment of her anorexia nervosa.

Despite intensive psychotherapy and a defined nutritional plan in the hospital's regimented eating disorder program, S.C., who was 5 feet 10 inches tall, remained at her initial admission weight of 89 pounds. She also developed purulent bronchitis caused by the virulent bacteria *enterobacter* and *klebsiella*. Because of her persistent refractory anorexia nervosa, with a body weight more than 40 percent below ideal, and refusal of a gastric tube, the decision was made to judiciously initiate therapy with an alternative mode of nutritional rehabilitation using TPN.

S.C. received a total of 9 weeks of TPN. When the TPN was discontinued, she had gained 28 pounds, which she has maintained for the 2 years since the TPN was completed. The TPN, consisting of a solution containing 50 percent dextrose and an amino acids solution of 8.5 percent, was started at a rate of 25 cc/hour, and the infusion rate was cautiously advanced over the course of 5 weeks to achieve a maximum intake of 3,600 kcal per day. Calories were also partly derived from a 10 percent intralipid solution for the first week of TPN, which was then advanced to an every-other-day 20 percent infusion of 500 mL. Laboratory values were checked every other day for the first 2 weeks, biweekly for the next 3, and ultimately weekly for the last 2 weeks of therapy. Aside from some minor elevations in serum liver transaminase levels, there were no other significant biochemical changes. During the course of the TPN, S.C. also worked intensely with a dietician to choose oral foods at each meal. By the time the TPN was discontinued, the number of calories she derived from oral feeding had increased from 300 per day to 1,700 per day. During the last 2 weeks of TPN therapy, the rate of the infusion was progressively reduced, and weight gain was successfully maintained after 6 months of follow-up.

Case 2

J.W., a 40-year-old female, had a 15-year history of anorexia. She was transferred to an inpatient eating disorders program after an apparent suicide attempt through self-inflicted stab wounds. On admission, she was found to be almost 40 percent below her IBW (height 5 feet 6 inches, weight 83 pounds). Significant laboratory data included a low hematocrit of 21 percent (normal 38–45) secondary to recent blood loss, sodium of 127 mg/dL (138–43), and serum albumin of 3.4 g/dL (3.5–5.0). Her diet history indicated an average intake of 400–600 kcal per day. She reported weekly use of laxatives and daily exercise of 1 to 2 hours' duration. Her predicted resting energy expenditure (REE) was 1,050 kcal per day based on the Harris-Benedict formula.

J.W. was started on 1,000 kcal per day divided into three meals and progressed to 1,400 kcal per day during the ensuing 7 days. After the first week, she developed slight edema in her legs, which was felt to be secondary to her lacerations and not a manifestation of the refeeding syndrome. Her liver function tests became slightly elevated (AST and ALT), and she had intermittent problems with asymptomatic hypoglycemia, with a fasting venous blood sugar of 38 mg/dL (normal 60–100 mg/dL).

An evening snack was added, but her calories were held at 1,400 kcal per day.

By the end of the second week, her liver function tests began to improve and her edema resolved. Her blood sugar level remained low. Calories were progressively increased to 2,000 per day, but her weight remained unchanged. An indirect calorimetry study was obtained at a local community hospital. It calculated an REE of 911 kcal per day, which indicated that she should have been gaining weight on her current diet plan. J.W. subsequently admitted to covert excessive exercise during evening hours. Once this was addressed in her treatment plan, her hypoglycemia resolved, and she gained a total of 11 pounds over the next 4 weeks. She subsequently gained an additional 18 pounds after discharge on a dietary plan that provided 2,100 calories per day, and she has maintained a weight of 105 pounds over the past 3 years. She did not, however, have resumption of her menses.

Background

In general, the nutritional needs and goals of individuals with anorexia are based on attaining a healthy IBW. For a female, IBW may be calculated at 100 pounds for 5 feet of height, and 4–5 pounds for each inch greater than 5 feet. For a male, the only difference in the calculation is to use 5 pounds per inch. Thus, patients can be classified as mild, moderate, severe, or critical based on whether they are 10 percent, 20 percent, 30 percent, or more below IBW. An alternative way of classifying patients is based on body mass index (BMI), which is calculated on the basis of height and weight and is readily available in tables for an array of heights and weights. Specifically, the BMI value is obtained by dividing an individual's weight in kilograms by height in meters squared. It is limited, however, in that it does not provide any measure of body composition or of nutritional status (Yates, Edman, and Aruguete, 2004). In addition, standardized tables of "ideal body weight" may not be appropriate for use with adolescents. Normative data from the National Center for Health Statistics height and weight tables may be better suited for adolescents 12 to 18 years of age.

When a patient is set to begin the refeeding process, there must be, from the onset, an earnest attempt to achieve agreement among the caregiver, the dietitian, and the patient as to what the target weight is going to be. Also, spending time educating a patient with anorexia nervosa about metabolism and how it may change during the process of weight restoration may prevent future difficulties and reduce stress for the patient. Generally, weight gain to within 10 percent of IBW is an acceptable goal, regardless of the mode of refeeding. Some view a healthy weight as being the weight at which normal menstruation occurred in the past. However, if amenorrhea persists, it may be necessary for the patient to achieve IBW or even a little above it. Discharging patients before they reach a minimum normal weight is associated with an increased rate of readmission (Castro et al., 2004; Weisman et al., 2001). Many practitioners will admit a patient to the hospital for inpatient treatment and nutritional restoration when the patient's weight is more than 30 percent below IBW. This is both to minimize morbidity during the early stages of refeeding and because the rate of severe complications seems to markedly increase at these low weights.

Refeeding Syndrome

Before describing the specifics of refeeding, we should describe a potentially catastrophic complication that can occur during this process. It is referred to as the refeeding syndrome. This syndrome occurs in significantly malnourished patients during the early phase of nutritional replenishment, whether it is by the oral, enteral, or parenteral route. The risk of the refeeding syndrome is directly correlated with the degree of weight loss that has occurred as a result of the anorexia nervosa. Thus, those patients who are more than 30 percent below the IBW should be initially refed during an inpatient hospitalization (Solomon and Kirby, 1990; Bermudez and Beightol, 2004). Earlier in the twentieth century, the heart was believed to be immune to the effects of chronic malnutrition. However, during World War II, experiments were performed using conscientious objectors who voluntarily agreed to lose a certain percentage of their body weight. As a result of this weight loss, they developed low blood pressure, and cardiac size, as seen on a simple chest radiograph, diminished. This led to the progressive realization that the heart can be adversely affected by weight loss as well as by subsequent refeeding.

The mechanism of the potential cardiovascular collapse that occurs with the refeeding syndrome is multifactorial. First, the reduced heart mass that accompanies weight loss makes it difficult for the heart to handle the increase in total circulatory blood volume seen with refeeding. The end result of this can be heart failure. Even though the heart mass does revert toward normal with weight gain, the first few weeks of refeeding require close attention to an anorectic patient's cardiovascular status until this normalization process has occurred. Studies in anorexia nervosa have shown diminished cardiac output as a result of the atrophy of the heart muscle which accompanies unhealthy weight loss (Goldberg, Comerci, and Feldman, 1988).

Second, changes in serum levels of phosphorous as well as potassium and magnesium are key variables in the refeeding syndrome. The mechanism by which hypophosphatemia (low phosphorous levels) develops during refeeding is mainly due to the glucose content of the food substrate. The glucose load increases insulin release, which in turn produces

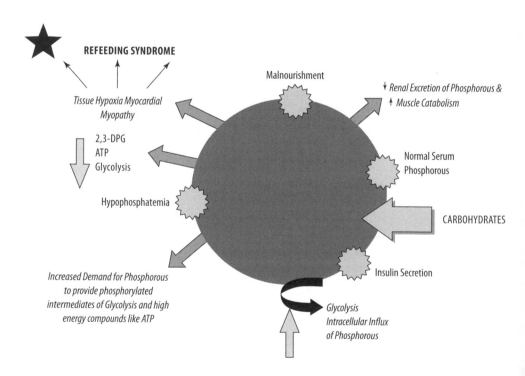

FIGURE 4.1. Refeeding hypophosphatemia.

TABLE 4.1   Strategies to avoid refeeding syndrome

- Identify patients at risk (e.g., any patient who is chronically malnourished, is severely underweight, or has not eaten for 7 to 10 days).
- Measure serum electrolyte levels and correct abnormalities *before refeeding.*
- Obtain serum phosphorus and electrolyte values every other day for the first 7 to 10 days, then biweekly during the remainder of refeeding.
- Attempt to slowly increase daily caloric intake by 300–400 kcal every 3 to 4 days until the level of caloric intake is adequate to produce 2–3 pounds of weight restoration per week.
- Monitor the patient carefully for the development of tachycardia or edema.

shifts of phosphate and potassium into the intracellular space. There is also an incorporation of phosphate into newly synthesized tissues during refeeding. The resultant low phosphate levels are accompanied by depletion of the high-energy chemical adenosine triphosphate (ATP), which impairs the contractile properties of the heart and can evolve into congestive heart failure (Fig. 4.1). Refeeding-induced hypophosphatemia can also result in diaphragmatic muscle fatigue and respiratory failure. Other sequelae of refeeding-induced hypophosphatemia include red and white blood cell dysfunction, skeletal muscle injury (rhabdomyolysis), and seizures. Rhabdomyolysis is diagnosed by finding an abnormally high level of the muscle enzyme creatinine phosphokinase (CPK) on a simple blood test. Low levels of serum potassium and magnesium can also cause cardiac irritability and arrhythmias along with skeletal muscle weakness.

Practical Tips for Refeeding

The medically worrisome refeeding syndrome is usually preventable (Table 4.1). The general dictum to follow with regard to dietary calorie repletion is "Start low, advance slow." The caloric requirements for the female patient with anorexia can be accurately calculated with the Harris-Benedict equation for basal energy expenditure (BEE):

BEE = 6.55 + (9.6 × body weight in kg) + (1.8 × height in cm)
– (4.7 × age in years).

Dieticians are most familiar with this calculation. The basal energy expenditure can be measured by indirect calorimetry, a relatively simple procedure involving a breathing test. It is available in many hospitals through the nutrition department. Calorimetry is based on measurement of carbon dioxide production and oxygen consumption. The BEE value basically reflects the energy used when the body is at rest; in clinical practice the terms BEE and REE are used interchangeably (Cuerda et al., 2007). The BEE must be multiplied by an activity factor (1.2–2.0) to determine total energy expenditure (TEE). In general, the TEE exceeds the BEE/REE by 10–60 percent, depending on how active the patient is. The TEE should not be the starting point of caloric repletion, due to the risk of the refeeding syndrome. Rather, it is a target to achieve days to weeks after the initiation of refeeding. BEE/REE measured by indirect calorimetry gives a slightly lower value for caloric needs than the values estimated by the Harris-Benedict formula. Therefore, if indirect calorimetry is not obtained to define caloric needs early in the refeeding of these malnourished patients with anorexia nervosa, it may be prudent to err on the low side of estimates derived from the Harris-Benedict formula to avoid the refeeding syndrome. Approximately 3 weeks following the beginning of the refeeding period, this discrepancy is no longer an issue in predicting BEE/REE.

Although it is clearly important for patients, especially hospitalized patients, to experience a significant degree of weight gain to maximize recovery, the optimal dietary intervention for effectuating weight gain is unknown. There has been a distinct and surprising paucity of research on nutritional interventions in anorexia nervosa. After the first week or two of an inpatient hospitalization, the usual goal is a weight gain of 2–3 pounds per week. Several different approaches have been promoted. The main tenet is to avoid overly aggressive refeeding protocols early in the refeeding process. Intake levels usually begin at approximately 600–1,000 kcal per day and are increased by 300–400 kcal every 3–4 days. The treatment corollary of this is to individualize intake based on the rate of weight gain. Supplementing the diet with a liquid supplement in the early stages of refeeding to achieve the prescribed calorie goal is an effective strategy to achieve weight gain. Liquid supplements can also be of value when added to achieve large caloric intake. Some programs recommend ultimately attaining an intake of 4,000–5,000 kcal per day, while others peak at 3,000–3,600 kcal per day. Even for normal-weight

TABLE 4.2   Rules for refeeding patients with anorexia nervosa

- The TEE should never be more than twice the BEE.
- Start refeeding at 20–25 kcal/kg/day.
- Intake should rarely exceed 70–80 kcal/kg/day.
- Limit protein intake to 1.0–1.5 g/kg/day.
- Aim for 2–3 pounds per week of weight restoration for inpatients and 1–2 pounds per week for outpatients.

adults, weight gain does not correlate exactly with the total excess calories ingested over basal requirements. Therefore, it may be difficult to define precisely the factors that consistently correlate with the number of calories needed to gain one pound. In general, starved patients who have anorexia are metabolically inefficient and may require a little more than the expected 3,500 kcal beyond maintenance caloric needs to restore a pound of body weight.

Some simple general rules to follow (summarized in Table 4.2) are

1. The TEE should never exceed twice the BEE.

2. Caloric intake should rarely exceed 70–80 kcal/kg of body weight.

3. With the patient who has severe anorexia, begin a diet at 20–25 kcal/kg.

4. Protein intake should not exceed 1.5–1.7 g/kg of body weight and is generally in the 1– to 1.5-g range.

5. If TPN or enteral feedings are being used, carbohydrate intake should not exceed 7 mg/kg/min.

6. Weight gain should be in the range of 2–3 pounds per week.

Males generally peak at 4,000 kcal per day and females at 3,500 kcal per day. All approaches require vigilant clinical and laboratory monitoring and individualization of the dietary plan depending on the rate of weight gain and the laboratory and clinical course of the patient (Table 4.3).

Currently, on most eating disorder units, caloric intake is slowly increased. These increases should always be guided by the patient's actual pattern of weight gain versus the standard goal of 2–3 pounds per week.

TABLE 4.3   Practical guidelines for refeeding

- Start at 800–1,000 kcal/day.
- Advance by 300–400 kcal every 3–4 days.
- Maximum is usually 3,500 kcal/day for females and 4,000 kcal/day for males.
- Follow clinical examination and phosphorus/electrolyte levels closely.
- Begin with low-lactose, low-fat, no-added-salt diet.
- Gradually introduce more dairy products and fats.

It is not uncommon, however, to see no weight gain, or even only 1–2 pounds of weight loss during the first week of nutritional repletion. Drastic increases in dietary calories should not be instituted in response to this. Similarly, caloric intake must be occasionally modified because of changes in the REE during the course of refeeding, and such modifications will affect the rate of weight gain. Change in REE seems to be a real phenomenon: REE is often lower in anorexia nervosa patients early on in the refeeding process than at later stages (Van Wymelbeke et al., 2004; Forman-Hoffman, Ruffin, and Schultz, 2006). It is possible that these changes contribute to the difficulty of ongoing, sustained weight gain during the latter stages of refeeding (Salisbury et al., 1995). Caloric requirements for weight restoration are best determined by monitoring an individual's rate of weight gain. Given this dynamic process, caloric requirements may have to be recalculated if weight gain is not being achieved as expected during the refeeding process, or consideration given to potential confounding sources of weight loss, such as covert exercise or other modes of purging. Recalculation of the REE with indirect calorimetry may be reasonable whenever this clinical scenario is manifested.

It has recently been shown that refeeding a patient with anorexia nervosa may be associated with an increase in REE during the weight gain process. This change in the REE value may be responsible for observed plateaus in the desired rate of achievement of a patient's target weight. Although the mechanism of this phenomenon is currently unknown, its clinical implications are clear: unusually high-calorie diets (70–80 kcal/kg) may be necessary to provide continued weight gain toward the end of the weight-restoration process. As noted above, the optimal treatment strategy should be predicated on regularly monitoring an individual's pattern of weight gain and adjusting the dietary plan because of these inherent individual variations. All of these principles apply regardless of whether refeeding is by customary oral feedings or an alternative such as TPN or enteral feeding.

Potential Complications

From a clinical standpoint, rates of weight gain greater than 2–3 pounds per week are usually not nutritionally sound and may represent edematous fluid retention or retained bowel contents from constipation. Aside from this numeric guide to weight gain, there are clinical parameters that are worthy of being closely followed. Specifically, vital signs contribute useful daily information. Individuals with anorexia generally have bradycardia (heart rate of <60 beats/minute). Although there are other potential reasons for tachycardia (heart rate of >100 beats/minute), the presence during refeeding of an elevated heart rate, even if just in the 80–90 heart rate range, can be a harbinger of the refeeding syndrome and cardiac compromise. Thus, even if patients technically do not have tachycardia, a sudden sustained increase in the pulse to greater than 80–90 deserves evaluation, given anorectic individuals' typical baseline heart rates of 50–60 beats per minute. Thus, daily monitoring of vital signs a few times per day is crucial during the first few weeks of the refeeding process.

In addition, checking for the presence of edema in the ankle and shin areas is also a worthwhile practice during the early refeeding stages; its presence can be an ominous sign of the refeeding syndrome. However, edema may also occur as a minor complication because during the early stages of refeeding, insulin secretion normally increases. Insulin induces sodium retention by increasing kidney tubular sodium reabsorption (Yucel et al., 2005). Low-sodium diets should therefore be used as part of the nutritional plan. The presence of rales on pulmonary examination or evidence of elevated jugular venous pressures are uncommon, but if present may imply true cardiac failure. Any of these clinical findings deserves a thorough medical evaluation with consideration given to possibly decreasing the rate of refeeding. In addition, because of the delayed stomach emptying and prolonged colonic transit time found in the severe stages of anorexia nervosa, these patients often complain of abdominal bloating and constipation. A bowel regimen, with a judicious amount of fiber and adequate hydration, may help alleviate these symptoms during the early refeeding process (see Chap. 6).

A multitude of possible fluid and electrolyte aberrations can occur during the refeeding process, especially in cases of more severe anorexia. As the body shifts from a catabolic to an anabolic state, potassium, phosphorous, and magnesium are incorporated into the newly synthesized muscle tissue and are used for intermediary metabolism; this phenomenon can cause low serum levels, namely, hypokalemia, hypophosphatemia, and hypomagnesaemia. Phosphorous is the key electrolyte in the refeeding syndrome (Ornstein et al., 2003). Frequent monitoring of the patient's blood chemistry values (potassium, phosphorous, magnesium, sodium, and glucose) can avert these problems. Early in the refeeding process, checking serum chemistry values every day or every other day is a reasonable plan. These checks can be advanced to biweekly once the patient has consistently gained weight and has a relatively stable blood profile. Ultimately, with continued weight gain and stable laboratory results, monitoring can be even less frequent. However, the major emphasis should be on serum phosphorous levels, because refeeding hypophosphatemia is the main chemical cause of the refeeding syndrome.

Other metabolic complications might be encountered during the refeeding process. Mild elevations of the liver enzymes aspartate aminotransferase (AST) and alanine aminotransferase (ALT) can be seen during refeeding. Elevated AST and ALT are more common in those patients being refed enterally or with TPN. Generally, the abnormalities are noted after the first few weeks of refeeding. AST and ALT rise first, followed by alkaline phosphatase, and then bilirubin. Usually, these abnormalities have little clinical significance and resolve with a slowing of the rate of the refeeding process. Many hypotheses have been suggested as to the etiology of these abnormalities; much evidence points to excessive dextrose calories causing fat accumulation in the liver cells, a condition known as hepatic steatosis. On occasion the elevations can be more pronounced (more than three times normal) and necessitate consultation with a dietician to reduce carbohydrate-dextrose calories.

Another condition that has been associated with anorexia is hypoglycemia, which is related to depleted hepatic glycogen reserves and gluconeogenesis substrates. Large glucose loads contained in aggressive re-feeding protocols stimulate substantial amounts of insulin release from the pancreas, which cannot be offset by the depleted hepatic reserves of glycogen. Clinicians must always be cognizant that inadvertent or intentional abrupt cessation of TPN or enteral feeds in any patient can result in dangerous hypoglycemia.

Alternative Modes of Refeeding

Although progressive oral refeeding programs are the basic modes of refeeding a patient with anorexia nervosa, it is worthwhile to briefly discuss alternatives to the traditional oral refeeding mode. The oral refeeding plan, with a strict behavioral protocol, is the first choice of treatment because it provides a less invasive, safer, and more therapeutic method of treatment. The dietary goal must be to move from the reduced calorie approach to a truly balanced nutritional program with adequate calories to balance energy expenditures and the patient's developmental stage. There are definite, albeit *infrequent*, indications for TPN and enteral feedings in anorexia nervosa (Mehler, 2008). However, these alternative modes of refeeding are not a panacea for the treatment of anorexia nervosa, and they cannot be recommended as routine therapy for all individuals who have anorexia. Some potential criteria for their use are (1) persistent failure to gain weight with other standard dietary therapies, (2) life-threatening weight loss, and (3) worsening psychological state despite standard treatments (Table 4.4). A patient's odds of recovery decline as the time spent continuously ill with anorexia nervosa lengthens, and thus, on rare occasions these alternative modes of weight restoration might be reasonable.

Controlled studies of nutritional treatments for anorexia nervosa are essentially nonexistent. Enteral nasogastric feedings (NG) or percutaneous endoscopic gastrostomy-based feeding (PEG) have both been used in refractory cases of anorexia. Both of these enteral modes of nutritional delivery use liquid supplements that contain 1–1.5 kcal/cm^3. The only difference is whether the tube that delivers the enteral feed is inserted through the nose and down the esophagus into the stomach or through the skin above the stomach and bored into the stomach and secured. These two modes of enteral feeding can be used either with a 24–hour continuous

TABLE 4.4 Potential indications for TPN or enteral feeding

- Multiple previous unsuccessful attempts at dietary treatment
- Life-threatening weight loss of more than 40 percent below ideal body weight
- Worsening and severe psychological or physical state or complete noncompliance despite standard therapy
- Patient is unwilling or unable to cooperate with oral feedings

flow of supplement or as a bolus feed, which takes only ten minutes to push in, with the daily caloric amount divided into two or three rapid feeds. Dieticians are invaluable in calculating the rates and amounts of enteral feeds necessary to achieve weight gain. The advantage of bolus enteral feeds is that the patient is not tied to the pump all day long. The disadvantage is that the bolus mode may cause gastric discomfort and diarrhea and thus be less well tolerated. Anecdotally, although some physicians promote these modes of refeeding, patients often find them unpleasant, and some clinicians view them as psychologically harmful. Also, patients may complain of gastric fullness with enteral feeds; this sensation is further exacerbated by the delayed gastric emptying that is found in more severe cases of anorexia nervosa. These problems are not associated with TPN, which is nutritionally comparable. However, TPN is more expensive and fraught with catheter-related infection complications. There are no randomized trials to guide the use of TPN versus enteral nutrition in anorexia nervosa. These different modes of nutritional support have been compared in other medical patients, however, and absent unique mitigating circumstances, enteral nutrition is the preferred route, given its reduced rate of infectious complications (Marik and Zaloga, 2004).

Although standard protocols exist, TPN must be viewed as a treatment modality that is prescribed only for severe and refractory cases with utmost discretion on an individual basis. It is beyond the scope of this chapter to discuss all of the specifics. Briefly, with TPN, dextrose and lipid preparations are the main source of energy substrate. This solution is administered on a continuous 24-hour-per-day basis via a catheter, which is surgically placed either in the forearm or in the upper chest and can remain in place for many months. Patients can receive more than 3,000–4,000 kcal per day, in addition to some oral feeds, via TPN. Although TPN is a powerful tool and has been used successfully in the care of patients with refractory, severe anorexia or patients with anorexia who have comorbid gastrointestinal issues that preclude oral caloric intake (Mehler and Weiner, 1993, 2007), its administration may be associated with a plethora of mechanical, infectious, and metabolic difficulties. It is therefore best reserved for use in medical centers where expertise in dealing with these potential difficulties exists and for patients who are truly refractory to more traditional refeeding programs. Also, both enteral and parenteral nutrition should rarely supplant the expectation that the patient will resume normal and adequate eating.

Similarly, enteral nutrition may infrequently play a role in the treatment of a select group of patients who have anorexia. It may also play a role as a supplemental nocturnal refeeding assist for patients whose rate of weight gain is slow or plateaued (Silber et al., 2004). It can be given either via a mercury-tipped nasogastric tube or via a percutaneously placed endoscopic gastrostomy tube. Notwithstanding possible patient aversion to this mode of refeeding, a small series of successful outcomes using enteral programs have been reported in the literature. Generally, a polymeric formula is started at a slow rate, with gradual increases in the rate and tonicity of the solution. Potential problems include diarrhea, blockage of the tube, and electrolyte imbalances. Some centers administer enteral nutrition by continuous-drop infusion for 14 hours per day, while others recommend a 24-hour-per-day continuous infusion and some use the bolus mode mentioned above. If the 14-hour infusion or bolus protocol is used, hypoglycemia may be a problem during the time when the infusion is stopped, especially early in the weight restoration process. Again, given the added potential complications, some level of special expertise is necessary when enteral feeds are considered. There has been debate about the ethics of the "involuntary" feeding of patients with anorexia nervosa (Beaumont and Carney, 2004). Grave medical danger may suffice to trump this concern in severe anorexia nervosa.

Summary

Although nutritional support of the malnourished patient is a most important component of the patient's care plan, nutrition regimens can worsen the patient's condition if used injudiciously. Because rapid refeeding of these patients can result in a catastrophic sequence of events, caution and restraint must be used when initiating therapy, together with careful monitoring of blood chemistry values and of the patient's pattern and rate of weight gain. A well-balanced and nutritional oral diet plan is generally the optimal approach for refeeding malnourished patients, but alternative modes also have a limited role.

REFERENCES

Bermudez O and Beightol S. 2004. What is refeeding syndrome? *Eating Disorders* 12:251–56.

Beaumont P and Carney T. 2004. Can psychiatric terminology be translated into legal regulation? The anorexia nervosa example. *Australia and New Zealand Journal of Psychiatry* 38:819–29.

Castro J, Gila A, Puig J, Rodriguez S, and Toro J. 2004. Predictors of rehospitalization after total weight recovery in adolescents with anorexia nervosa. *International Journal of Eating Disorders* 36:22–30.

Cuerda C, Ruiz A, Velasco C, Breton I, Camblor M, and Garcia-Peris P. 2007. How accurate are predictive formulas calculating energy expenditure in adolescent patients with anorexia nervosa? *Clinical Nutrition* 26:100–106.

Forman-Hoffman VL, Ruffin T, and Schultz SK. 2006. Basal metabolic rate in anorexia nervosa patients: Using appropriate predictive equations during the refeeding process. *Annals of Clinical Psychiatry* 18:123–27.

Goldberg SJ, Comerci GD, and Feldman L. 1988. Cardiac output and regional myocardial contraction in anorexia nervosa. *Journal of Adolescent Health Care* 9:15–21.

Marik PE and Zaloga GP. 2004. Meta-analysis of parenteral nutrition versus enteral nutrition in patients with acute pancreatitis. *British Medical Journal* 328:1407.

Mehler PS. 2008. Use of total parenteral nutrition in severe anorexia nervosa complicated by gastrointestinal illness. *Current Nutrition and Food Science* 4:41–43.

Mehler PS and Weiner KL. 1993. Anorexia nervosa and total parenteral nutrition. *International Journal of Eating Disorders* 14:297–304.

Mehler PS and Weiner KL. 2007. Use of total parenteral nutrition in the refeeding of selected patients with severe anorexia nervosa. *International Journal of Eating Disorders* 40:285–87.

Ornstein RM, Golden NH, Jacobson MS, and Shenker IR. 2003. Hypophosphatemia during nutritional rehabilitation in anorexia nervosa: Implications for refeeding and monitoring. *Journal of Adolescent Health* 32:83–88.

Salisbury JJ, Levine AS, Crow SJ, et al. 1995. Refeeding, metabolic rate, and weight gain in anorexia nervosa: A review. *International Journal of Eating Disorders* 17:337–45.

Silber TJ, Robb AS, Orrell-Balente JK, Ellis N, Valadez-Meltzer A, and Dadson MJ. 2004. Nocturnal nasogastric refeeding for hospitalized adolescent boys with anorexia nervosa. *Journal of Developmental Behavior and Pediatrics* 25:415–18.

Solomon SM and Kirby DF. 1990. The refeeding syndrome: A review. *Journal of Parenteral and Enteral Nutrition* 14:90–97.

Van Wymelbeke V, Brondel L, Marcel Brun J, and Rigaud D. 2004. Factors associated with the increase in resting energy expenditure during refeeding in malnourished anorexia nervosa patients. *American Journal of Clinical Nutrition* 80:1469–77.

Wiseman CV, Sunday SR, Klapper F, Harris WA, and Halmi KA. 2001. Changing patterns of hospitalization in eating disorder patients. *International Journal of Eating Disorders* 30:69–74.

Yates A, Edman J, and Aruguete M. 2004. Ethnic differences in BMI and body/self-dissatisfaction among whites, Asian subgroups, Pacific Islanders and African-Americans. *Journal of Adolescent Health* 34:300–307.

Yucel B, Ozbey N, Polat A, and Yager J. 2005. Weight fluctuations during early refeeding period in anorexia nervosa: Case reports. *International Journal of Eating Disorders* 37:175–77.

CHAPTER FIVE

Evaluation and Treatment
of Electrolyte Abnormalities

COMMON QUESTIONS

Which electrolyte abnormalities are most commonly seen in patients
with eating disorders?
Does the particular pattern of electrolyte abnormalities predict
a specific mode of purging?
How common are these abnormalities?
What is pseudo-Bartter's syndrome, and how is it managed?
How does the clinician differentiate between the various causes
of metabolic alkalosis?
How does the clinician differentiate between the various causes
of metabolic acidosis?
How does the clinician treat the metabolic abnormalities encountered
in these patients?
How does the clinician treat severe hypokalemia?
What are critical levels for potassium, sodium, and bicarbonate
that require urgent care?
How is edema avoided and/or treated during the correction
of electrolyte abnormalities in patients with bulimia?

Case

T.C. was a 24-year-old female tennis player who presented to her primary care provider complaining of progressive weakness of four months'
duration. She denied having fever, chills, weight loss, or gastrointestinal

complaints. Her only medication was birth control pills. Over the preceding week, her weakness had progressed to the point where she found it necessary to curtail her tennis matches soon after starting them.

Her examination revealed a regular pulse of 84 and blood pressure of 90/60 mmHg. She was 5 feet 6 inches tall and weighed 122 pounds. The remainder of her examination, including a detailed cardiac and neurologic examination, was completely normal.

Laboratory tests revealed a normal complete blood count and chemistry panel aside from a low potassium level of 2.9 mEq/L (normal 3.5–5.0) and an elevated bicarbonate level of 34 mEq/L (22–28). Her physician prescribed oral potassium with the instructions to take one 20–mEq tablet twice daily for one week and to return for a repeat blood test at that time.

One week later, she continued to complain of fatigue. Repeat blood tests revealed her potassium to be lower, at 2.7 mEq/L. Her bicarbonate level was now 37 mEq/L. Her physician recommended that she go to the local emergency room for intravenous fluids. In the emergency room she was given 3 L of saline with 40 mEq/L of potassium chloride over 8 hours. Labs drawn at the end of the infusion revealed that her potassium was almost normal at 3.4 and her bicarbonate level had dropped to 29 mEq/L. She was discharged to home.

Three days later, she called her physician complaining of severe leg swelling. In the office she was found to have marked pitting edema of both legs to the level of her knees. Additional questioning revealed that she had been abusing diuretics in an effort to control her weight for the previous 6 months. She was prescribed a low-salt diet, instructed about the need to elevate her legs as much as possible for the next 7–10 days, and counseled to seek professional mental health care. Three days later she returned to her physician complaining of worsening of her leg swelling and a weight gain of 14 pounds. She denied ongoing abuse of diuretics.

The examination again revealed more marked peripheral edema with clear lungs and a normal cardiac examination. A chemistry panel was now completely normal, including tests of renal function. She was prescribed 50 mg/d of spironolactone for 2 weeks. Over the ensuing 2 weeks, she had a gradual resolution of her edema, and her weight declined to her baseline.

Frequency

Metabolic abnormalities are essentially limited to people with bulimic eating disorders, including self-induced emesis, diuretic misuse, and laxative abuse. Restricting anorectic patients almost always have normal blood electrolytes even when they are at a markedly reduced body weight. A study by Crow and others (1997) documented the frequency of fluid, electrolyte, and acid-base disturbances encountered in purging bulimic patients. Out of 168 patients, almost 50 percent had electrolyte abnormalities. The most common abnormality was an elevated serum bicarbonate (metabolic alkalosis), present in 46 (27.4%) of the patients. Other abnormalities observed were hypochloremia (23.8%), hypokalemia (low potassium; 13.7%), decreased serum bicarbonate (8.3%), and hyponatremia (decreased sodium; 5.4%). The electrolyte abnormalities either were isolated findings or were found in combination with other abnormalities. Other studies have reported that hypokalemia and hyponatremia were the most frequently abnormal electrolytes (Miller et al., 2005). Table 5.1 shows the normal laboratory ranges for the electrolytes that are most frequently altered by bulimic behaviors. Another observed abnormality is hypomagnesemia (low magnesium), which is most commonly seen in individuals who have bulimia and abuse diuretics. It is generally accompanied by hypokalemia because both of these cations are handled in a similar fashion by the kidney.

Electrolyte abnormalities are far less common in patients who have anorexia nervosa without associated purging behavior. Warren and Vande Wiele (1973) studied 42 patients with anorexia nervosa and found that electrolytes were normal in all but one of the patients. The single patient with abnormal electrolytes was determined to have also engaged in vomiting. Forty percent of the patients did have azotemia (elevated blood urea

TABLE 5.1   Normal laboratory electrolyte ranges

	Range (mmol/L)
Bicarbonate (HCO_3^-)	22–28
Chloride (Cl^-)	101–12
Potassium (K^+)	3.6–5.2
Sodium (NA^+)	138–47

nitrogen [BUN] and creatinine), which was felt to be due simply to dehydration. In general, a BUN/creatinine ratio of greater than 20 to 1 is indicative of marked dehydration. Unlike patients with bulimia, patients with anorexia do not have a metabolic alkalosis along with the elevated BUN levels. If hypokalemia, hypochloremia, or a metabolic alkalosis is present in a patient who has anorexia, it is more than likely due to the presence of a coexistent covert purging behavior disorder (Wolfe et al., 2001). In contrast, the electrolyte values for anorectic patients who are only restricting intake are remarkably and consistently found to be normal, as are their serum albumin and protein levels. This is an important clinical fact. Thus, the presence of a low albumin level in a patient who is thought to have anorexia or the finding of electrolyte abnormalities as defined should prompt a thorough search for additional causes aside from the diagnosis of anorexia nervosa (Krantz et al., 2005).

Clinical Manifestations

The clinical manifestations of electrolyte abnormalities are nonspecific and vague. Patients may complain of weakness, lassitude, constipation, dizziness, and/or depression. Hypokalemia ([less thann]3.6 mmol/L) causes generalized muscle weakness and fatigue, as well as constipation and occasionally heart palpitations. If severe (<2.5 mmol/L), it can also cause significant cardiac arrhythmias and sudden death. Typical electrocardiographic (EKG) changes may include flat or inverted T waves, ST segment depression, and prominent U waves, which can exceed the amplitude of the T waves. Cardiac complications and EKG abnormalities due to hypokalemia are rare if the potassium level is greater than 3 mmol/L unless there is concomitant heart disease, in which case complications increase in patients with a serum potassium level less than 3.9 mmol/L. Hypomagnesemia may also complicate these symptoms and contribute to arrhythmias and sudden death. Although hypomagnesemia and hypocalcemia are less commonly seen in bulimia, they can, when severe, also result in tetany.

Pathogenesis

As discussed above, metabolic alkalosis is one of the most common metabolic abnormalities seen in patients with bulimia. In patients who have a metabolic alkalosis due to active purging through diuretic abuse or self-induced vomiting, the serum bicarbonate level, which is normally 22 to 28 mmol/L, ranges between 30 and 40 mmol/L. The pathogenesis of this metabolic alkalosis varies according to the particular mode of purging behavior used. With self-induced vomiting, the metabolic alkalosis develops in part because of the acid lost in the vomitus. More important, however, sodium chloride (NaCl) is lost in the presence of vomiting, resulting in a state of decreased intravascular volume from dehydration. This, in turn, stimulates the kidney's renin-angiotensin system, which results in high levels of aldosterone being secreted to prevent low blood pressure and fainting. Aldosterone, a hormone produced in the adrenal glands, increases salt absorption and bicarbonate reabsorption by the kidney, which contributes to the maintenance of the metabolic alkalosis. Thus, this type of metabolic alkalosis is occasionally referred to as a "contraction alkalosis." This whole cascade is a normal protective response by the body to prevent dehydration in the presence of ongoing and frequent purging behaviors.

The metabolic alkalosis seen with surreptitious use of diuretics is also the result of intravascular volume depletion. Diuretics, through their actions on the kidney, cause increased sodium and chloride excretion, which again, through the resultant decreased intravascular volume in the body and dehydration, stimulate increased aldosterone secretion. In general, the metabolic alkalosis seen with diuretics is milder than that found with vomiting, which is associated with the most severe cases of metabolic alkalosis. A good rule to remember is that serum bicarbonate concentrations greater than 38 mEq/L are almost always due to self-induced vomiting. Elevated bicarbonate levels can also be a useful covert laboratory finding when a patient is denying purging behaviors and is almost always indicative of excessive vomiting or abuse of diuretics.

Although laxatives are an ineffective means of weight control, their abuse is also common in people with bulimia (Steffen et al., 2007). Laxative abuse can give the picture of a metabolic alkalosis or a mild metabolic acidosis, in contrast to vomiting or diuretic abuse, which cause only a metabolic alkalosis. Significant acute diarrhea typically causes a hyperchloremic metabolic acidosis (also called a nongap acidosis) as a result of the large amount of bicarbonate lost in the stool. The acid-base abnormality seen with chronic, or even intermittent, laxative abuse is more commonly a metabolic alkalosis, with low serum chloride and potassium levels. The alkalosis tends to be mild, with bicarbonate levels in the range of 30 to 34 mEq/L, whereas the hypokalemia is usually more marked. The primary reason for the hypokalemia is also the marked loss of potassium in the diarrheal stools.

The typical serum and urinary electrolyte findings in the three types of purging disorders just discussed are summarized in Tables 5.2 and 5.3. Engaging in purging behaviors one or two times per week may not cause any significant electrolyte disorders, and thus normal electrolytes do not completely rule out the presence of symptoms of bulimia. The corollary of this fact is that finding an abnormally low potassium level or an elevated bicarbonate level is not consistent with a patient's history that he or she rarely purges or that the purging behaviors have receded. Therefore, appropriate medical assessment of a patient with bulimia should always include obtaining a serum electrolyte panel.

Fortunately, the diagnosis of electrolyte abnormalities is usually straightforward. A set of electrolytes with serum magnesium and amylase can be drawn as part of the clinical evaluation, and this analysis is readily available in all laboratories. It is always wise to check an EKG to look for changes secondary to significant hypokalemia, hypomagnesemia, and hypocalcemia. The common EKG changes seen with a decreased serum potassium are T-wave flattening, U waves, and ST-segment

TABLE 5.2   Serum electrolyte levels in purging disorders

Purge type	Electrolyte				
	Sodium	Potassium	Chloride	Bicarbonate	pH
Vomiting	Increased, decreased, or normal	Decreased	Decreased	Increased	Increased
Laxatives	Increased, decreased, or normal	Decreased	Increased or decreased	Decreased or increased	Decreased or increased
Diuretics	Decreased or normal	Decreased	Decreased	Increased	Increased

TABLE 5.3   Urinary electrolyte levels in purging disorders

Purge type	Electrolyte		
	Sodium	Potassium	Chloride
Vomiting	Decreased	Increased or decreased	Decreased
Laxatives	Decreased	Decreased	Normal or decreased
Diuretics	Increased	Increased	Increased

depression, as mentioned above. Both hypomagnesemia and hypocalcemia can cause a prolonged QT interval and nonspecific T-wave changes. If there is a need to differentiate between the different types of purging behaviors, serum and urine electrolytes can be helpful. In general, once again, metabolic alkalosis (elevated bicarbonate level) indicates vomiting or diuretic abuse, and a metabolic acidosis (low bicarbonate level) indicates laxative abuse. It may be necessary in some cases, when there is a suspicion of laxative abuse despite patient denial, to check the feces or urine for phenolphthalein, an ingredient in some laxatives. Similarly, when there is suspicion of diuretic abuse, a laboratory can test the urine for the presence of common diuretics.

Treatment

Treatment of the metabolic abnormalities observed in eating disorders requires a basic understanding of the pathophysiology of these problems. There are basically two important concepts to always keep in mind. First, because potassium is primarily an intracellular cation, the serum measurement can be misleading in estimating the degree of *total* body potassium depletion. Rough estimates of total body potassium deficits are displayed in Table 5.4. A common mistake is to underestimate the amounts of potassium necessary to correct hypokalemia.

Second, efforts to replete potassium are often unsuccessful if a coexisting metabolic alkalosis induced by dehydration is not treated first. As discussed above, the dehydration stimulates aldosterone production, which not only causes the metabolic alkalosis but also leads to ongoing renal potassium excretion. Treatment of dehydration with intravenous or oral sodium-containing solutions will stop aldosterone production and allow potassium repletion to be successful. The metabolic alkalosis seen in patients who abuse diuretics or engage in self-induced vomiting, with resultant volume contraction and elevated bicarbonate levels, is also termed *chloride-responsive*. This means that saline is the appropriate corrective treatment. Intravenous infusions of sodium chloride restore intravascular volume and lead to the cessation of excessive aldosterone production. This is an important point to remember when attempting to correct hypokalemia in bulimic patients. The efficacy of potassium repletion will be abrogated unless the dehydration state is corrected due to the central role of volume depletion in the hypokalemia associated with severe purging. Treatment of severe metabolic alkalosis (>33–35 mEq/L) with salt water usually needs to be done intravenously at a *slow* rate of 50–75 cc/hr for 1–2 L. Milder cases can be successfully treated with aggressive oral hydration using fluids other than plain water. Restoring plasma volume and providing sufficient sodium are required to shut off renal loss of potassium, which will continue as long as the patient is volume-depleted.

A word of caution is in order: Excessive amounts of intravenous saline (>2–3 L per day) given at a rapid rate of infusion can lead to marked edema and volume overload. This is, in part, due to these patients' poor nutritional status and possible cardiac muscle weakness. In addition, the return of elevated aldosterone levels back to normal may take one to two weeks after the cessation of purging. Therefore, with high ambient serum aldosterone levels, the intravenous saline is avidly reabsorbed in the kidney, a process that can also contribute to the body's retention of salt and water, with resultant edema. In fact, the edema can be severe during the early period after these purging behaviors are discontinued, even

TABLE 5.4 Total body potassium deficits (mEq/L)

Serum potassium	Potassium deficit
3–3.5	100–150
2– 3	200–300
<1.5	400–600

TABLE 5.5 Pseudo-Bartter's syndrome

- Characterized by hypokalemia and metabolic alkalosis
- Volume depletion plays a central role
- Efficacy of potassium repletion is abrogated unless volume is restored
- Restore volume with IV normal saline slowly (50–70 cc/h)
- Edema may be alarming to the patient
- Risk dissipates by 2–3 weeks after cessation of purging

without the use of intravenous fluids, because of increased serum aldosterone levels. This condition, termed *pseudo-Bartter's syndrome* (Table 5.5), is an important clinical entity to be aware of (Mitchell et al., 1998). Some individuals with bulimia who need to frequent emergency rooms for electrolyte replacement therapy may be reticent to seek additional help if their previous visits have been punctuated by the development of significant edema. Emergency department staff, who are used to rapid infusion of intravenous saline for states of dehydration, must be warned about the dangers of this practice in the case of bulimic patients. Generally, the edema can be overcome or prevented during this period with dietary salt restriction, leg elevation for 10–15 minutes a few times a day, a slowed infusion of saline, and a detailed explanation to the patient of the nature of this potential problem (Mehler and Linas, 2002). Occasionally, an aldosterone antagonist, such as spironolactone, has been prescribed in a dose of 25 mg daily, for one to two weeks, to both treat and prevent the severe edema, as described in the case at the beginning of the chapter.

One further word of caution when repleting a dehydrated patient. If the patient also has significant hyponatremia (serum sodium <120 mmol/L), the saline infusion should be slow so that during the initial 24 hours, the serum sodium is corrected to only approximately 125–30 mmol/L. More aggressive correction of the serum sodium level may result in a devastating neurologic complication termed *central pontine myelinolysis* (CPM). A targeted rate of correction that does not exceed 8–10 mmol/L on any day of treatment is recommended (Adrogue and Madias, 2000). In addition, although a healthy person with normal kidney function would need to drink a large amount of plain water (25–30 L) to dilute the serum sodium and experience marked hyponatremia as a result, patients with anorexia nervosa are different. Their ability to tolerate water is severely limited by their extremely limited solute intake, similar to older men and women who live on tea and toast. Therefore, amounts as little as 5–7 L per day can cause hyponatremia (Caregaro et al., 2005).

In most cases, potassium repletion can be accomplished orally. When the serum potassium level is below 3.5 mmol/L, supplementation is warranted. If the potassium level is less than 2.7 mEq/L, it should generally be replaced cautiously by the intravenous route at a rate of 10 mEq/L per hour. If the patient has severe or life-threatening hypokalemia, the rate can be increased in an acute care hospital setting. Oral repletion is generally acceptable for milder forms of hypokalemia and for cases where the metabolic alkalosis is not severe (bicarbonate level <33 mEq/L). Based on the estimated deficits listed in Table 5.4, a reasonable range for oral potassium repletion is 20 to 40 mEq of a potassium chloride preparation twice a day with daily monitoring of blood levels until the potassium level returns to normal (Cohn et al., 2000). Table 5.6 lists various oral potassium preparations available for repletion.

In addition to the central role of volume depletion in the treatment of hypokalemia associated with severe purging, undetected magnesium deficiency can also cause refractory potassium repletion. Magnesium deficiency should especially be considered in those individuals with bulimia who purge through the use of potent diuretics. All diuretics cause some loss of magnesium in the urine (Whang, Whang, and Ryan, 1992). Ongoing magnesium deficiency, if not treated, can impair efforts at potassium repletion.

TABLE 5.6   Oral potassium preparations

Preparation	mEq/tablet (or preparation)
K-Dur (KCl)	10 or 20
K-Tab (KCl)	10
Micro-K Extencaps (KCl	8 or 10
Slow-K (KCl)	8
K-Lor Powder Packets (KCl)	20
Polycitra-K Oral Solution (Kcitrate)	10/tsp (5 cc)
Rum-K syrup (KCl	20/2 tsp (10 cc)

Summary

Metabolic abnormalities are common in patients with eating disorders, especially those who engage in bulimia through various purging behaviors. Metabolic alkalosis and hypokalemia are the most common abnormalities encountered clinically. The treatment of these metabolic derangements requires repletion of potassium and treatment of the volume contraction that causes hyperaldosteronism. A clinician who has skills and familiarity with the treatment of these potentially dangerous electrolyte disorders in this population is necessary for all but the mildest abnormalities.

REFERENCES

Adrogue HJ and Madias NE. 2000. Hyponatremia. *New England Journal of Medicine* 342:1581–89.

Caregaro L, Di Pascoli L, Favaro A, Nardi M, and Santonastaso P. 2005. Sodium depletion and hemoconcentration: Overlooked complications in patients with anorexia nervosa. *Nutrition* 21:438–45.

Cohn JN, Kowey PR, Whelton PK, and Prisant LM. 2000. New guidelines for potassium replacement in clinical practice: A contemporary review by the National Council on Potassium in Clinical Practice. *Archives of Internal Medicine* 160:2429–36.

Crow SJ, Salisbury JJ, Crosby RD, and Mitchell JE. 1997. Serum electrolytes as markers of vomiting in bulimia nervosa. *International Journal of Eating Disorders* 21:95–98.

Krantz MJ, Lee D, Donahoo WT, and Mehler PS. 2005. The paradox of normal serum albumin in anorexia nervosa: A case report. *International Journal of Eating Disorders* 37:278–80.

Mehler PS and Linas S. 2002. Use of a proton-pump inhibitor for metabolic disturbances associated with anorexia nervosa. *New England Journal of Medicine* 347:373–74.

Miller KK, Grinspoon SK, Ciampa J, Hier J, Herzog D, and Klibanski A. 2005. Medical findings in outpatients with anorexia nervosa. *Archives of Internal Medicine* 165:561–66.

Mitchell JE, Pomeroy C, Seppala M, et al. 1988. Pseudo-Bartter's syndrome, diuretic abuse and eating disorders. *International Journal of Eating Disorders* 7:225–37.

Steffen KJ, Mitchell JE, Roerig JL, and Lancaster KL. 2007. The eating disorders medicine cabinet revisited: A clinician's guide to ipecac and laxatives. *International Journal of Eating Disorders* 40:360–68.

Warren MP and Vande Wiele RL. 1973. Clinical and metabolic features of anorexia nervosa. *American Journal of Obstetrics and Gynecology* 117:435–49.

Whang R, Whang DD, and Ryan MP. 1992. Refractory potassium repletion. A consequence of magnesium deficiency. *Archives of Internal Medicine* 152:40–45.

Wolfe BE, Metzger ED, Levine JM, and Jimerson DC. 2001. Laboratory screening for electrolyte abnormalities and anemia in bulimia nervosa: A controlled study. *International Journal of Eating Disorders* 30:288–93.

CHAPTER SIX

Gastrointestinal Complaints

COMMON QUESTIONS

What clues from the gastrointestinal history and physical examination
are helpful during both early (occult) and later stages of eating
disorders?

What gastrointestinal symptoms occur with early weight loss?

What common laboratory abnormalities may signal the presence
of an eating disorder?

What symptoms develop as weight loss becomes more severe?

What treatment strategies can be used for common gastrointestinal
symptoms (i.e., bloating, fullness) that may interfere with nutritional
rehabilitation?

How do symptoms improve with time, and how can this be used
to reassure patients?

What can you tell patients about any long-term consequences for
the gastrointestinal tract?

When are gastrointestinal studies, such as upper or lower gastrointestinal endoscopy or barium studies, indicated?

What role is there for acid suppression through H2 antagonists
(cimetidene or ranitidine) or proton pump inhibitors (omeprazsole
or lansoprazole)?

Case 1

W.H., a 19-year-old female, presented with pure restricting anorexia nervosa, having had a 20-pound weight loss (height 5 feet 6 inches; weight
originally 115 pounds). She had no prior history of intestinal disease. At

the nadir of her weight loss, she complained of epigastric bloating and constipation. Physical examination revealed a normal abdomen, no evidence of distention and hemoccult-negative stool.

Outpatient psychiatric treatment enabled W.H. to gain 15 pounds over a 10-week period. She was reassured that the bloating and constipation would improve with time. Bulking agents, which can often increase bloating, were avoided so as not to worsen her complaint of bloating. Her bloating and constipation spontaneously improved without the use of laxatives or need for any GI studies.

Case 2

A.D., a 25-year-old female with bulimia who was undergoing outpatient psychotherapy continued intermittent, self-induced emesis twice a week. She had no weight loss and did not engage in laxative use.

A.D. complained of sore throat, hoarseness, dyspepsia, and intermittent odynophagia. She was empirically placed on omeprazole 20 mg once a day. The hoarseness, dyspeptic symptoms, and sore throat resolved after four days, and the odynophagia after 2 weeks. One month later she denied any swallowing problems. With intensive psychotherapy, her purging ceased, as did all of the aforementioned symptoms. She was concerned about the previous difficulty with swallowing and wondered if additional testing was necessary. Her omeprazole was discontinued, and her symptoms did not recur. No further testing was recommended.

Background

People who have eating disorders commonly complain of gastrointestinal (GI) symptoms (Waldholtz and Andersen, 1990). Such symptoms are often a consequence of, rather than an etiologic factor for, the eating disorder. However, early in the course of the illness, GI complaints may so preoccupy the patient and the physician that they may interfere with and deflect attempts at psychological treatment. There may even be some question as to whether a primary GI disease exists in addition to the eating disorder. Moreover, an eating disorder may exacerbate a preexisting intestinal disease, especially irritable bowel syndrome, which is seen in approximately one-third of women between the ages of 15 and 35 and is one of the most commonly encountered GI disorders in the general public (Drossman et al., 1993); this is also the age range in which eating disorders commonly present.

The primary care physician and the primary therapist may be confronted with a wide spectrum of GI complaints in patients with eating disorders. To care for these patients, clinicians should be somewhat familiar with the following:

1. the prevalence of these GI symptoms;
2. the time course of the evolution for these GI symptoms during illness and recovery;
3. the effect of GI symptoms on treatment;
4. common laboratory abnormalities associated with eating disorders;
5. possible long-term GI sequelae in individuals who recover from eating disorders;
6. therapeutic modalities available to treat these different GI issues.

Both anorexia nervosa and bulimia are associated with specific GI symptoms that are uniquely attributable to the food restriction, bingeing, and/or purging behaviors that characterize these eating disorders. An initial complete medical history and physical examination is part of the evaluation for patients with eating disorders. It is important to elicit any history of GI disease and current symptoms and to look for clues of an ongoing eating disorder. A history of gastroesophageal reflux (acid reflux), for example, may be exacerbated by weight gain or by the self-induced vomiting of bulimia and may require aggressive treatment. Similarly, patients with preexisting irritable bowel syndrome may develop worsening symptoms of pain or altered bowel patterns at some time during the eating disorder. Patients with irritable bowel syndrome who are already inherently predisposed to focus on intestinal complaints may have the development of altered motility from weight loss, which often causes them to develop more severe bloating or constipation.

Physical signs of bulimia and vomiting include excoriation over the back of the hands (Russell's sign) as well as loss of dental enamel. The abdominal examination itself is often normal except for epigastric tenderness (pain in the upper abdomen) if there is severe reflux disease. A rectal examination should be done if the patient is complaining of severe constipation or diarrhea to rule out fecal impaction or occult blood. Hemoccult-positive stools may be due to GI reflux, peptic ulcer disease, hemorrhoids, or, far less likely, Crohn's disease (inflammatory bowel disease), which may need to be evaluated with barium studies or endoscopy.

Anorexia Nervosa

Table 6.1 lists common GI symptoms associated with the weight loss seen in anorexia nervosa that improve with weight gain (Wiseman, Harris, and Halmi, 1998). Patients with anorexia nervosa who present to gastroenterologists are often heavy consumers of health information because they are hoping to rule out organic causes for their litany of somatic complaints (Emmanuel et al., 2004).

GASTROPARESIS

With pure food restriction, once a weight loss of approximately 10–20 pounds occurs, there is almost universal development of gastroparesis (Kamel et al., 1991). *Gastroparesis* refers to delayed emptying of the stomach. Bloating is the main symptom, and it may be severe. Figure 6.1 demonstrates gastric dilation, which should be screened for with an abdominal X-ray if the patient complains of severe left upper quadrant pain or has significant vomiting or early satiety. The bloating can be worsened by a high-fiber diet, such as the vegetarian diet that these patients often resort to, to treat their slow gastrointestinal transit, or by fiber-based

TABLE 6.1   Common gastrointestinal symptoms with weight loss

- Bloating
- Fullness
- Nausea
- Constipation
- Abdominal pain and distension
- Distension

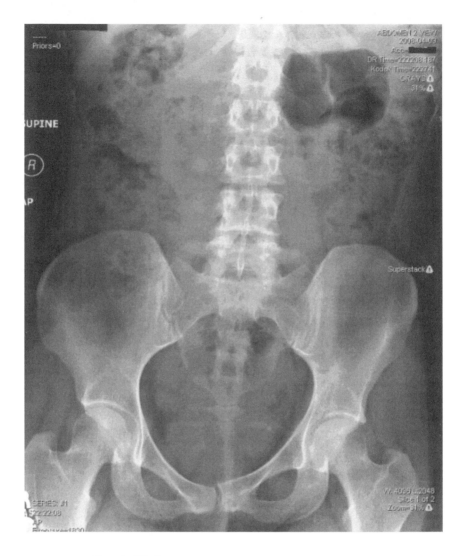

Priors=0

UPINE

R

P

ABDOMEN 2 VIEW
2008-04-09
Acc=
DR Time=222208.187
Kodak Time=2227.11
C-RAYS
31%

Superstack

W: 4095 L:2048
Slice 1 of 2
Zoom=31%

SERIES #1
522:22:08
AP

FIGURE 6.1. Gastric dilation.

laxatives. Once gastroparesis develops, early satiety, nausea, bloating, and even reflux and vomiting that is no longer self-induced may occur. This may hamper attempts at weight restoration. Heartburn may occur as a result of acidic vomitus-induced esophagitis from food remaining in the stomach for prolonged periods of time. In some cases it may be difficult to tell whether spontaneous and/or self-induced vomiting is occurring. Although the bloating improves with weight restoration, improvement often takes 4–6 weeks. Therefore, it is crucial to offer reassurance to these patients and instruct them to avoid legume-type foods, which promote gas and distention, as well as excessive fiber or bran products, which induce similar symptoms. This will enable them to understand that their symptoms will pass with time and that they are not "causing" the pain by eating. Likewise, patients should be informed that refusal to eat and regain weight will only delay improvement in their symptoms.

Useful approaches to the problem of gastroparesis-induced bloating in patients with anorexia include the following: (1) the use of liquid food supplements as half of the daily calories (one can three times per day for a total of 750 calories) for the first week or two of refeeding, since gastric emptying of liquids is generally normal even in severe anorexia nervosa; (2) taking liquid components as opposed to solids earlier in the meal, which generally results in less bloating, so the patient is able to continue eating; and (3) dividing the daily caloric intake into two to three snacks and three smaller meals per day, so that meal-induced bloating will not result in the termination of a meal and loss of a major portion of the daily caloric intake.

Gastroparesis induced by weight loss will generally improve with partial weight restoration. Thus, the severe bloating initially complained of, which will often prevent the patient from eating an adequate meal, progressively improves for most patients. A significant improvement often occurs with a 10-pound weight gain and, in general, largely resolves with weight gain back to 80–90 percent of ideal body weight. However, if there is residual psychopathological distress, symptoms of bloating may remain despite short-term refeeding (Benini et al., 2004). Thus, in rare cases it may be necessary to obtain a nuclear medicine gastric emptying study to investigate prolonged symptomatology after refeeding and weight restoration.

Metoclopramide is an oral medication that stimulates stomach contraction and hastens emptying of the stomach. In a dose of 5–10 mg, 30 minutes before meals and at bedtime, it is clinically useful in bloating and early satiety, secondary to weight loss in anorexia nervosa. It is also a well-established antiemetic medication. Caution must be exercised when using metoclopramide for anorexia nervosa, however, because it can exacerbate neck cervical muscle spasm (torticolis), especially at higher doses.

GASTROESOPHAGEAL REFLUX

Gastroesophageal reflux (heartburn, or acid reflux) may often begin secondary to the gastroparesis. It also improves with time as weight is restored. In contrast to the gastric emptying abnormalities noted above, esophageal emptying has been shown to be normal in anorexia nervosa. Therefore, swallowing complaints by these patients are often of a functional nature. Gastroesophageal reflux may be treated with an antacid (e.g., Tums), two pills a few times a day, or with liquid antacids in mild cases; but it usually also requires histamine-2 antagonists (such as cimetidine 400–800 mg or ranitidine 150–300 mg) twice a day, or a proton-pump inhibitor (such as omeprazole 20–40 mg per day), which is often most effective. The maintenance dosage usually used for peptic ulcer disease (only a nighttime dose) will often be inadequate to control symptoms secondary to reflux. Treatment should be continued for 2 weeks after symptoms resolve because improvement in esophageal inflammation lags behind that of symptomatic improvement. Any patient with persistent vomiting, reflux symptoms, or dysphasia that does not respond after 3 weeks of these treatments should undergo an upper endoscopy (EGD) procedure to evaluate for peptic ulcer disease or for ongoing severe esophageal inflammation, which can progress over years to esophageal carcinoma, especially if there is ongoing esophageal reflux disease. Patients with significant esophageal inflammation may require long-term maintenance therapy with either a histamine-2 antagonist twice a day or a proton pump inhibitor once to twice per day.

Gallstones should also be rarely considered in the differential diagnosis of anorectic patients with vomiting and/or right upper quadrant pain because of an increased incidence of gallstones in patients with weight loss. However, if no right upper quadrant symptoms accompany the vomiting, gallstones are less likely because reflux and/or gastroparesis is usually responsible for these symptoms. A painless right upper quadrant abdominal ultrasound is a simple way to exclude the presence of gallstones.

CONSTIPATION

Constipation will also invariably accompany the weight loss of anorexia nervosa. Patients may complain of bowel movements that are too infrequent or too small. It is helpful to reassure patients that bowel patterns in healthy ambulatory patients may normally vary anywhere from two or three times per day to three times per week and that persons with weight loss issues are expected to have even fewer bowel movements. Patients may incorrectly respond to their perceived problem with constipation by starting treatment with bulking, fiber-containing laxatives or dangerous stimulant laxatives. This may worsen the constipation by inducing bloating and distention or through diarrheal losses of potassium or by making the bowel dependent on these stimulant laxatives. Because individuals often take laxatives in the mistaken belief that they will cause substantial weight loss, it is also useful to educate patients that laxatives act in the colon, after caloric absorption has already occurred, and are thus ineffective as a means of weight loss. Others may take laxatives because they mistakenly believe that the abdominal pain is due to decreased bowel movements. Patients may need frequent reassurance that there is nothing fundamentally wrong with their bowels other than a need for weight restoration. They must be encouraged to focus on the expected slow return, over weeks, to their prior bowel pattern with weight restoration. Daily preoccupation with the lack of bowel movements is not unusual, but reassurance is essential in preventing a return to patients' prior laxative regimen. Generally, with weight restoration and refeeding, there will be resumption of normal bowel transit time within 3 weeks.

In most patients with anorexia, constipation is due either to drastically reduced caloric intake, which results in *reflex hypofunctioning* of the colon, or to slow colonic transit. It is useful to educate patients that (1) constipation is normal and (2) bowel motility will improve with time due to improved GI transit associated with increased caloric intake. Medications, such as the older tricyclic antidepressants, with their anticholinergic side effects, are another common cause of constipation is medications. Likewise, electrolyte abnormalities seen in purging, such as hypokalemia and hypomagnesemia, may also slow colonic transit by interfering with nerve function in the bowel wall.

Treatment options for constipation, in addition to education and progressive weight restoration, include (1) adequate water intake (6–8 glasses of water per day); (2) fiber in low doses (10 g per day), avoiding high doses, which can cause bloating; (3) polyethylene glycol powder, at a dose of 1–3 tablespoons daily; and (4) lactulose, a nonabsorbable synthetic disaccharide that is similar to polyethylene glycol products in its efficacy and mode of action, 30–60 mL one to two times per day. If lactulose is used, it is useful to tell patients that, although this medication tastes sweet, it is devoid of calories because it is not absorbed. Rather, it reaches the colon in an unaltered form and, because of its highly osmotic nature, draws water into the bowel, resulting in a bowel movement. Polyethylene glycol products work in a similar manner and have a long record of efficacy for gut cleansing in preparation for colonoscopy and surgery (Rankumar and Rao, 2005). (See Table 6.2 for a classification of laxative therapies.)

In general, it is best to avoid the use of any stimulant laxatives that contain senna, cascara, or bisocodyl because of the potential for long-term abuse and dependence after weight restoration. Long-term use of stimulant-type laxatives may cause direct damage to colonic nerve cells and result in more difficult cases of constipation when the patient becomes older. This syndrome is termed the *cathartic colon syndrome*. Occasionally, however, early in the refeeding process a glycerin suppository or a laxative derived from senna may be necessary to "jump-start" normal peristaltic motion in the bowel, but always in a limited manner (Mehler, 1997). Colonic transit returns to normal once these patients are consuming a balanced diet and gaining weight.

ABDOMINAL PAIN

Abdominal pain is a frequent complaint in anorexia nervosa but is generally diffuse, unaccompanied by tenderness, and more consistent with gastroparesis or an irritable bowel syndrome. Persistent pain not accompanied by bloating may need further evaluation. Epigastric pain or lower chest discomfort, if unresponsive to 3 weeks of acid-suppression therapy, should be evaluated by upper endoscopy. Abdominal pain accompanied by diarrhea should be evaluated to rule out fecal impaction, infectious causes, and other pathology, especially if accompanied by fever, extreme pain, or an elevated white blood cell count.

Routine laboratory studies are occasionally important in patients with eating disorders who are experiencing abdominal pain. Iron deficiency anemia or concurrent hemoccult-positive stools may indicate significant GI disease. Elevated amylase levels are almost always due to a

TABLE 6.2 Classification of laxative therapies

Class	Mechanism of action	Site of action	Example	Cost (relative to bisacodyl)
Osmotic	Attracts/retains water in intestinal lumen, increasing intraluminal pressure	Small and large intestines	Magnesium hydroxide (saline osmotic)	4.5
		Large intestine—colon	Lactulose	25.0
			Sorbitol	16.0
			Polyethylene glycol	30.0
Irritant or peristaltic (use with extreme caution)	Direct action on mucosa; stimulates myenteric plexus, and alters water and electrolyte secretion	Colon	Senna	5.5
			Bisocodyl (Dulcolax)	1.0
			Danthron	1.0
			Cascara	1.0
				1.0
Bulk or hydrophilic	Holds water in stool and causes mechanical distention	Small and large intestines	Plantain derivatives	3.0
			Methylcellulose	3.0
			Psyllium	14.0
			Ispaghula	3.0
			Dietary bran	0.5
			Celandin	3.0
			Aloe vera	3.0
Stool softener	Softens stool by facilitating a mixture of fat and water (largely ineffective)	Small and large intestines	Docusate	1.2

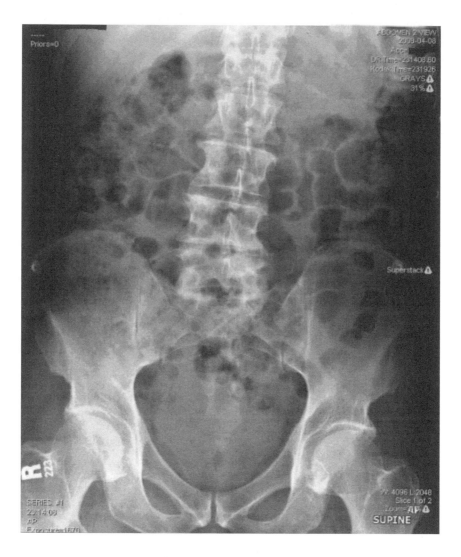

FIGURE 6.2. Excessive stool in colon.

salivary source from excessive vomiting and are not indicative of pancreatitis. This can be confirmed by a lipase measurement, which is elevated in pancreatitis but normal in patients in whom the amylase elevation is due to a salivary source, as seen with purging. In some rare cases, however, the refeeding process, if too aggressive, can induce refeeding pancreatitis early in the course of the refeeding process. In addition, gallstone pancreatitis can develop because gallstones develop with weight loss; these patients have extremely high amylase measurements (>1,000 mg/dL), along with elevated lipases. They require a cholecystectomy because of their risk of recurrent gallstone pancreatitis. However, asymptomatic gallstones, likely due to weight loss, do not generally warrant surgery.

A supine and upright simple abdominal X ray may be useful to exclude bowel distention when symptoms of constipation persist after an adequate trial of medications aimed at alleviating constipation (Fig. 6.2). The absence of excessive stool on these radiographic studies provides the clinicians caring for these patients with proof that bowel function is normal and no longer deserves ongoing concern. This is especially helpful because the interplay of functional gastrointestinal disorders is significantly prevalent in patients with anorexia nervosa (Porcelli, Leandro, and De Carne,1998). These disorders include syndromes such as irritable bowel syndrome.

ABNORMAL LIVER FUNCTION TESTS

Routine liver studies (AST, ALT, alkaline phosphatase, and total bilirubin) are important for patients with eating disorders. Weight loss and fasting can produce mild elevation of transaminase (AST/ALT) and bilirubin. One of the best indications of periods of food restriction is an elevated fasting indirect bilirubin level. Mild transaminase and alkaline phosphatase elevations can also occur early in the course of refeeding if dextrose calories are excessive. These elevations usually resolve and normalize if the daily caloric intake is decreased by 300–500 kcal; a higher level of calorie intake can then be reintroduced at a later date once the liver tests have normalized. Rarely, the transaminase may be markedly elevated with severe anorexia nervosa even before refeeding has started and may be a sign of serious multiorgan failure (De Caprio et al., 2006). Nutritional support may result in improvement.

SUPERIOR MESENTERIC ARTERY SYNDROME

One other rare syndrome to be aware of in people with anorexia nervosa is the superior mesenteric artery (SMA) syndrome. It results from compression of the third portion of the duodenum between the aorta and the vertebral column posteriorly and the SMA anteriorly. Anything that narrows the angle can cause entrapment of the duodenum as it passes between these vessels. The SMA is normally covered with fatty tissue; reduction in the fat pad narrows the angle. Weight loss can thus cause the syndrome. Patients with the SMA syndrome typically present with intermittent vomiting and abdominal pain soon after starting to eat. Weight gain of as little as 5–10 pounds can lead to tolerance of normal feeding (Mehler and Weiner, 2007). The diagnosis is made by upper GI series tests.

Bulimia Nervosa

Bulimia nervosa leads to a different set of GI symptoms (Table 6.3). Severe GI reflux symptoms— namely, heartburn, spontaneous vomiting, acid regurgitation, chest pain, dysphagia and nocturnal chocking when laying supine—and their complications often occur in bulimia owing to self-induced vomiting. These reflux symptoms may be among the few clues to the ongoing illness. Spontaneous vomiting is the effortless return of stomach contents into the mouth without retching. Food-restricting patients who do not have bulimia may also develop reflux due to weight loss-induced gastroparesis, but reflux in these cases generally involves only reflux into the distal esophagus and thus is milder. By contrast, patients who induce vomiting have the acid contents going back through the entire esophagus and mouth, and they are more likely to complain of more severe dyspeptic symptoms and the symptoms of reflux. Specifically, acid-induced inflammation of the vocal cords may produce hoarseness, which will persist for several days even after only a brief exposure of the vocal cords to acid; laryngitis; sore throat; or cough. These patients may also have symptoms of *odynophagia* (painful swallowing) or *dysphagia* (difficulty in swallowing), also caused by the acid-induced esophageal inflammation.

A cessation of self-induced vomiting without concomitant acid-suppressing medication generally will not alleviate these symptoms. In addition, these patients will also often not respond to antacids. Rather, they need either higher-dose histamine-2 blockers (ranitidine 150–300 mg twice a day) or proton pump inhibitors (omeprazole 20–40 mg one or two times a day). Prokinetic agents such as metoclopramide are also

TABLE 6.3   Common gastrointestinal symptoms associated with bulimia

Vomiting-related

    Heartburn

    Odynophagia

    Dysphagia

    Hoarseness

    Sore throat

    Hematemesis (vomiting bright red blood)

Laxative-related

    Diarrhea

    Abdominal cramping

    Hematochezia (passing bright red blood per rectum)

---

effective for controlling the reflux symptoms found in patient with bulimia. In general, evidence from well-controlled trials have established the superiority of the proton pump inhibitors over the histamine-2 receptor antagonists (Sontag, 1993).

Because of the incessant exposure of their esophageal mucosa to the acidic vomitus, patients with bulimia are at risk for Barrett's esophagus, a precancerous transformation of the esophagus. Therefore, refractory heartburn-type symptoms, unresponsive to 4–6 weeks of a proton pump inhibitor, in these patients mandate an upper endoscopy. Barrett's esophagus is found in 10 percent of patients with gastroesophageal reflux disease who undergo upper endoscopy (Ronkainen et al., 2005). However, many patients with Barrett's esophagus may not have typical symptoms of reflux, and there is no current test other than an upper endoscopy to establish the diagnosis. Therefore, endoscopy may be reasonable in patients who have bulimia with a long-standing history of self-induced vomiting.

Bulimic individuals who purge through laxative abuse often have a distinct set of GI problems. The diarrhea that commonly occurs during periods of excessive usage results in blood chemistry abnormalities (see Chap. 5) along with dehydration and dizziness. The bigger problem, however, involves trying to help the patient cease the abuse of laxatives. This is difficult because if stimulant laxatives have been abused, the bowel may have become dependent on them, and cessation of their use can result in rebound constipation and fluid retention (cathartic colon syndrome). The result is a dilated, atonic colon, which is manifested by slowed or absent transit through some or all segments of the colon. Basically, the colon becomes an inert tube, incapable of propagating fecal material. This leads to hard, infrequently passed stools and occasionally a state of refractory constipation. In addition, it is always difficult to convince patients to stop using laxatives because of their psychological dependence on laxatives and anxiety about losing the feeling of weight control that laxatives gives to them (Kovacs and Palmer, 2004). It is important for these patients to understand that the range of normal bowel function, as defined by the Rome II criteria, includes three bowel movements per week or more (Thompson et al., 1999). Also, it is important to point out that laxatives are an ineffective means of achieving weight loss because most of the caloric absorption occurs before the site in the colon which laxatives affect.

Restoration of normal bowel function may take a few weeks. Patients should be encouraged to completely cease their use of stimulant laxatives. There is no scientific basis to support a gradual tapering off because any ongoing exposure to stimulant laxatives can harm the neurons that oversee bowel peristalsis. They must be made to understand that patience is a key virtue when attempting to become independent from stimulant laxatives. If constipation lasts more than three to four days, a short course of a mild *nonstimulating* laxative (see Table 6.2), together with ample oral fluids are important. Daily polyethylene glycol should be started as soon as the decision is entertained to cease stimulant laxatives. An occasional glycerin suppository may be needed early in the "detox"

TABLE 6.4   Ancillary treatments for constipation

- Ample hydration and judicious exercise
- Distraction-free 10–15 minutes on the toilet rather than sitting and straining
- Elevating the legs onto a footstool during defecation
- Substitution of less-offending laxatives
- Measured amount of fiber rather than undefined high-fiber diet
- *Tailoring medications to the complaint!*

process. Patients should be discouraged from using diuretics for the temporary fluid retention that may occur with cessation of laxative abuse. Although diuretics will lessen edema formation, when they are stopped, the edema will recur to a greater degree than initially present. In fact, increased fluid intake is a useful adjunct for reestablishing normal bowel function along with osmotic laxatives such as polyethylene glycol, which are safe and effective with regard to the integrity of bowel function (DiPalma et al., 2007). A judicious amount of exercise is also beneficial for normal bowel function (Table 6.4).

Tegaserod, a new selective agonist that works at 5-hydroxytryptanine receptors to increase small bowel transit, may be another mode of therapy for those trying to cease using stimulant laxatives (Kamm et al., 2005). The effect of Tegaserod on bowel function is seen rapidly after treatment initiation (6 mg twice a day). Lubiprostone is another new medication which may be efficacious for chronic constipation.

In general, most GI symptoms due to vomiting and purging associated with bulimia, in the absence of significant weight loss, resolve fairly quickly after the cessation of bulimic episodes, compared with patients with severe weight loss, who have ongoing symptoms.

Summary

The gastrointestinal system is adversely affected by both anorexia nervosa and bulimia. With anorexia nervosa, the complications are manifest in the state of food restriction but are more prominent as the patient begins the process of refeeding. Similarly, the effects of bulimia on the gastrointestinal system are present during purging behaviors as well as during the treatment phase when the purging tendencies are being controlled. Thus, it is important for clinicians to become familiar with the gastrointestinal complications of anorexia nervosa and bulimia because effective treatment will increase the chances of successful treatment. The guidelines presented in Table 6.5 are useful in the treatment of these patients.

REFERENCES

Benini L, Todesco T, Dalle Grave R, et al. 2004. Gastric emptying in patients with restricting and binge/purging subtypes of anorexia nervosa. *American Journal of Gastroenterology* 99:1448–54.

TABLE 6.5   Guidelines for care of patients with GI complaints

- It is important to reassure the patient that the intestinal symptoms will generally improve with weight gain.
- Educating patients about the physiologic basis for their constipation will help to decrease laxative abuse.
- Lack of improvement in GI symptoms should lead to consideration of an ongoing occult illness and/or underlying primary GI disease.
- Prokinetic agents may be useful in some patients with bloating associated with weight loss. Metoclopramide (5–10 mg before meals and at bedtime) is often effective.
- Constipation is best treated with polyethylene glycol (1–3 tablespoons per day).
- Symptomatic reflux may be treated with H2 blockers (such as oral cimetidine, 400–800 mg, or ranitidine, 150–300 mg) twice a day. Proton pump inhibitors (such as omeprazole, 20 mg one or two times a day) are probably more effective.
- Gallstones may develop due to weight loss but are often not the cause of the patient's pain. Surgery should not be undertaken on a routine basis.
- Mild abnormalities shown in liver studies should resolve with weight gain and adjustments in caloric intake. If they do not, further evaluation is needed to exclude hepatitis B or C, autoimmune hepatitis, hemochromatosis, or Wilson's disease.
- Avoid gastrointestinal barium and endoscopic studies with most patients unless their symptoms fail to improve with psychiatric recovery or if iron deficiency anemia is present.

DeCaprio C, Alfano A, Senatore I, et al. 2006. Severe acute liver damage in anorexia nervosa: Two case reports. *Nutrition* 22:572–75.

DiPalma JA, Cleveland MV, McGowan J, et al. 2007. A randomized, multicenter, placebo-controlled trial of polyethylene glycol laxative for chronic treatment of chronic constipation. *American Journal of Gastroenterology* 102:1436–41.

Drossman DA, Li Z, Andruzzi E, et al. 1993. U.S. householder survey of functional gastrointestinal disorders: Prevalence, sociodemography, and health impact. *Digestive Diseases and Sciences* 38:1569–80.

Emmanuel AV, Stern J, Treasure J, et al. 2004. Anorexia nervosa in gastrointestinal practice. *European Journal of Gastroenterology Hepatology* 16:1135–42.

Kamel N, Chami T, Andersen A, et al. 1991. Delayed gastrointestinal transit times in anorexia nervosa and bulimia nervosa. *Gastroenterology* 1011:1320–11324.

Kamm MA, Muller-Lissner S, Talley NJ, et al. 2005. Tegaserod for the treatment of chronic constipation: A randomized, double-blind, placebo-controlled multi-national study. *American Journal of Gastroenterology* 100:362–72.

Kovacs D and Palmer RL. 2004. The associations between laxative abuse and other symptoms among adults with anorexia nervosa. *International Journal of Eating Disorders* 36:224–28.

Mehler PS. 1997. Constipation: Diagnosis and treatment in eating disorders. *Eating Disorders: The Journal of Treatment and Prevention* 5:41–46.

Mehler PS and Weiner K. 2007. Use of total parenteral nutrition in the refeeding of selected patients with severe anorexia nervosa. *International Journal of Eating Disorders* 40(3):285–87.

Porcelli P, Leandro G, and De Carne M. 1998. Functional gastrointestinal disorders and eating disorders: Relevance of the association in clinical management. *Scandinavian Journal of Gastroenterology* 33:577–82.

Ramkumar D and Rao SS. 2005. Efficacy and safety of traditional medical therapies for chronic constipation: Systematic review. *American Journal of Gastroenterology* 100:936–71.

Ronkainen J, Aro P, Storskrubb T, et al. 2005. Prevalence of Barrett's esophagus in the general population: An endoscopic study. *Gastroenterology* 129:-1825–31.

Sontag SJ. 1993. Rolling review: Gastro-oesophageal reflux disease. *Aliment Pharmacology Therapy* 7:293–312.

Thompson WG, Longstreth GF, Drossman DA, et al. 1999. Functional bowel disorders and functional abdominal pain. *Gut* 45:1143–47.

Waldholtz BD and Andersen AE. 1990. Gastrointestinal symptoms in anorexia nervosa: A prospective study. *Gastroenterology* 98:1415–19.

Wiseman CV, Harris WA, and Halmi KA. 1998. Eating disorders. *Medical Clinics of North America* 82:145–59

CHAPTER SEVEN

Cardiac Abnormalities
and Their Management

COMMON QUESTIONS

Why do patients with anorexia nervosa suffer sudden cardiac death?

What cardiac complications are associated with anorexia nervosa?

What are "normal" vital signs in patients with anorexia nervosa?

Why do patients with anorexia nervosa have bradycardia?

Do patients with bradycardia require cardiac monitoring?

What degree of bradycardia is concerning?

What EKG abnormalities are seen with anorexia nervosa?

Why do patients with anorexia nervosa have chest pain?

What is the significance of heart palpitations in patients who have bulimia?

What cardiac toxicities are associated with abuse of ipecac?

Case

K.L. was a 21-year-old female with a 6-year history of anorexia nervosa. She denied purging behaviors. Her chief complaint was chest pain of 6 months' duration, which was sharp and substernal and lasted 5–10 minutes. The pain occurred at rest and was not exacerbated by exertion. She denied fainting, shortness of breath, palpitations, or use of ipecac. There was no family history of premature coronary artery disease. Her exercise tolerance had diminished over the preceding 2 years, but she remained active and jogged 2 miles per day. She had been in an eating disorder program for 2 weeks. A refeeding program had been initiated, and she had gained 3 pounds. Her physical examination was notable for a blood pressure of 80/50 mmHg, a pulse of 48, and a respiratory rate of 10. She was 5 feet 4 inches tall and weighed 93 pounds. Physical examination revealed a cardiac midsystolic click, clear lungs, no edema, and a benign abdominal examination.

Blood electrolytes revealed normal potassium, magnesium, and bicarbonate levels. Electrocardiogram (EKG) showed sinus bradycardia with a heart rate of 50, normal intervals, and no ST-T wave changes. In view of the cardiac click heard on auscultation of her heart, an echocardiogram is ordered. It revealed mitral valve prolapse with billowing of the mitral valve, a normal left ventricular ejection fraction, and no dyskinetic wall abnormalities. K.L. was educated about mitral valve prolapse and continued to refeed successfully. She had no recurrence of chest pain once she gained a total of 12 pounds. The cardiac click was also no longer audible.

Sudden Death

Anorexia nervosa has the highest mortality rate of any psychiatric disorder (Roche et al., 2005). Initially, there was a concern that anorexic patients were dying as a result of heart attack due to elevated cholesterol levels and atherosclerosis. However, autopsy studies published almost 20 years ago did not reveal evidence of obstructive coronary disease (Isner et al., 1985). Studies then focused on QT interval prolongation, which predisposes patients to torsade de pointes, a serious, life-threatening ventricular arrhythmia that can degenerate into fatal ventricular tachycardia and fibrillation. Some studies have documented QT interval prolongation in severe anorexia nervosa (Cooke et al., 1994). This has not, however, been a consistent finding (Facchini et al., 2006). Current thinking is that the QT interval may not be inherently prolonged in anorexia nervosa nor is it independently the cause of sudden death in these patients. Thus, current teachings are that if the QT interval is found to be prolonged in a patient with anorexia who is strictly restricting, this finding should prompt a search for potential independent causes, including electrolyte (potassium or magnesium) disturbance and congenital long-QT syndrome.

Another marker of increased arrhythmic risk is a measure known as QT dispersion. This is defined by interlead variation in the QT segment length on a routine 12-lead EKG. Normally the length of the QT interval is similar between each of these leads. QT dispersion refers to the difference between the maximum QT interval and the minimum QT interval occurring in any of the 12 leads. QT dispersion reflects heterogeneous ventricular depolarization and, when abnormally increased, may indicate a heightened propensity to develop serious ventricular arrhythmias (Krantz et al., 2005).

Over the last several years, increased QT dispersion has been found in young women with anorexia nervosa before refeeding (Mont et al., 2003). The etiology of increased QT dispersion in anorexia nervosa is unknown but might relate to impairment of myocardial function, which may be due to direct injury of the cardiac muscle cell during the acute metabolic insult of starvation. These patients may have a twofold or greater increase in QT dispersion, which correlates with the severity of their weight loss and reduced metabolic rate. QT dispersion is a widely available and inexpensive measure that may reflect both metabolic status and the potential for arrhythmia. Resting metabolic rate and QT dispersion normalize with refeeding.

Therefore, a definite cause for the increased risk of sudden death in anorexia nervosa is unknown. It is known that it is not due to atherosclerotic heart disease and heart attack, or solely to the QT interval. Increasing attention is currently focused on abnormalities in QT dispersion; these studies may develop a useful measure to help make clinical decisions regarding hospitalization and cardiac monitoring in the patients with more severe degrees of anorexia nervosa.

Cardiac Complications

Overall, with substantial weight loss there is concomitant shrinkage of skeletal and cardiac muscle, a reduction in cardiac chamber volumes, and a decrease in cardiac mass and cardiac output. As a result, there ensues a state of reduced exercise capacity, an attenuated blood pressure response to exercise, and subjective fatigue. These abnormalities improve with weight gain and generally normalize with clinical recovery. Most of these changes become significant only once the patient is below 20 percent of ideal body weight (Olivares et al., 2005) (Table 7.1). Two of the most prominent and consistent findings seen in patients with anorexia

TABLE 7.1   Spectrum of cardiac consequences of starvation and anorexia nervosa

Microscopic changes
      Mitochondrial swelling
      Decreased glycogen content
      Interstitial edema
      Myofibrillar atrophy and destruction
Physiologic changes
      Decreased myocardial contractile force
      Decreased cardiac output
      Reduced cardiac chamber size
Clinical signs
      Bradycardia
      Hypotension
      Nonspecific EKG changes
      Ectopic rhythms
      Mitral valve prolapse
      Diminished exercise capacity
      Heart failure worsened or precipitated by refeeding

nervosa are bradycardia (heart rates <60 beats per minute) and hypotension, defined as a systolic blood pressure less than 90 mmHg and/or a diastolic blood pressure less than 50 mmHg. In reality, both of these changes are predictable results of the weight loss found in this population and are teleologically felt to be due to an attempt by the body to conserve calories. Certainly from a blood pressure standpoint, it is expected that with loss of cardiac muscle mass, the force of cardiac contraction will be diminished and the blood pressure will therefore be reduced. Also, the normal circadian rhythm of blood pressure, in which there is a sharp rise in blood in the morning and a nadir during the night, is absent in people who have anorexia nervosa. This state of a weakened heart muscle is generally normalized after weight recovery (Awazu et al., 2000). Moreover, in overweight individuals with hypertension, weight loss is associated with a reduction in both systolic and diastolic blood pressure values. The hypotension in anorexia nervosa is therefore an expected finding.

The progressive bradycardia seen with increasing severity of anorexia nervosa has recently been an area of scientific inquiry with regard to the influence of the parasympathetic and sympathetic nervous systems on cardiac function. These two systems are components of the autonomic nervous system, which influences many different body systems. Increased sympathetic tone causes increased heart rate and blood pressure. Conversely, conditions in which there are high levels of parasympathetic tone are characterized by low blood pressure and bradycardia. Some studies have shown a marked reduction in both parasympathetic and sympathetic tone in anorexic patients (Rechlin et al., 1998). Others have demonstrated an increase in parasympathetic activity with unchanged sympathetic tone (Galetta et al., 2003). This increased parasympathetic tone, also referred to as increased vagul tone, is the accepted prevailing explanation for the bradycardia so commonly seen with anorexia nervosa and may be deemed an adaptive response to caloric deprivation as the body compensates to avoid having to use energy for cardiac function.

The bradycardia of anorexia nervosa will generally increase into the normal range of 60–90 beats per minute as weight is restored to a level greater than 80 percent of ideal body weight or even earlier once a stable pattern of nutritional replenishment and progressive weight gain ensues (Shamim et al., 2003). However, although clinicians might find comfort in a "normal" heart rate, it is worth noting that a "relative tachycardia" (pulse of 70–100) in a patient with moderate to severe anorexia nervosa may have more sinister implications (Derman and Szabo, 2006). Indeed, because bradycardia is such a constant finding in nutritionally depleted patients with severe anorexia, these "normal" heart rates, even if not strictly in the elevated range (pulse >100), are likely either a side effect of medication or an impending medical complication and should be viewed as a warning sign in need of expert medical evaluation (Krantz and Mehler, 2004). This is especially germane during the early stages of refeeding, as the relative tachycardia for a patient with anorexia nervosa (pulse of 80–90) may be a harbinger of incident heart failure.

An additional sequela of the abnormal autonomic nervous system function found in patients with anorexia nervosa is diminished heart rate variability. The moment-to-moment fluctuations in heart rate reflect the underlying stability of autonomic nervous system function through the integration of sympathetic and parasympathetic modulation. Emerging data demonstrate lower heart rate variability in anorexia nervosa (Melanson et al., 2004). Reduced heart rate variability is a known predictor of sudden death in patients with heart failure from coronary artery disease. Women with depression, independent of anorexia nervosa, have also been shown to have significant reductions in heart rate variability, although the exact pathophysiologic mechanism linking depression and cardiovascular disease has not been fully elucidated (Kim et al., 2005). Reduced heart rate variability may also be correlated with an increased incidence of sudden death in anorexia nervosa. There may thus be clinical utility to obtaining a measurement of heart rate variability through a cardiologist. An abnormal rate may be indicative that the patient needs more comprehensive cardiac evaluation and ongoing cardiac monitoring during the early stages of refeeding. However, issues related to heart rate variability and QT dispersion are not relevant in patients with anorexia nervosa whose weight is less than 20 percent below ideal body weight.

An important clinical dilemma that is commonly discussed is what absolute degree of bradycardia is of concern, and when do patients with bradycardia need intensive-care-unit or telemetry-based cardiac monitoring? There has never been a study performed that definitely speaks to this question. Nevertheless, essentially everyone agrees that a heart rate of less than 30 beats per minute mandates hospital admission, at least telemetry monitoring, and perhaps a stay in an intensive care unit. Some treatment facilities extend this practice to any anorexic patient with a heart rate of less than 40 beats per minute. Certainly, the presence of any cardiac rhythm other than sinus bradycardia, or a heart rate between 30 and 40 beats per minute and hypotension or symptoms of lightheadedness, mandates formal cardiac monitoring. Marked orthostatic hypotension, with an increase in pulse of 20 beats per minute or a drop in blood pressure of 20 mmHg upon standing, may also be indicative of the need for acute care hospitalization (Yager et al., 2006). The only area in which there is a difference of opinion is at what lower level of heart rate hospitalization becomes mandatory. Because bradycardia is expected with anorexia nervosa, it should not, in and of itself, result in therapy directed to increase the heart rate. Rather, the only intervention that may be needed is additional cardiac monitoring to screen for degeneration into more ominous abnormalities and cardiac arrhythmias. Typically, the patient does not complain of specific symptoms related to the bradycardia aside from overall fatigue and perhaps lightheadedness with standing. Similarly, the nonspecific symptoms of weakness, dizziness, and cognitive impairment may be related to hypotension. All of these symptoms become more prevalent when the patient changes position from sitting to standing or from being supine to sitting.

EKG Findings

There are no EKG findings that are specific to anorexia nervosa. Aside from the indications of bradycardia, the EKG is often normal. There have been sporadic reports of cases with atrioventricular block and even dangerous ventricular arrhythmia, especially in connection with purging behaviors that result in low potassium or magnesium blood levels. Cases of nonspecific ST and T-wave changes, along with a prolonged QT-interval, have also been reported, but these are not consistently a result of anorexia nervosa (Figure 7.1). A baseline EKG should be obtained on all patients with moderate or severe anorexia nervosa to screen for these potential abnormalities. Finding any of these would suggest a need for serial EKGs over the ensuing days, depending on their clinical significance, until they dissipate with weight restoration. However, there is no requirement to obtain a cardiac-echocardiogram on all anorexic patients

Patient X		12 Dec 2007	8:11:31 PM
65 yrs	Male		
PR	162		
QRSD	78		
QT	417		
QTc	510		
	*Compared to 12/12/07 8:11 pm ANTERIOR T WAVE ABNORMALITIES HAS IMPROVED		
	—ABNORMAL ECG—		
--AXES--			
P	66		
QRS	45		
T	69		
	PREVIOUS ECG: 12 MAR 2005 8:46:53 AM, CONFIRMED		

FIGURE 7.1. EKG finding.

except in cases where a patient has overt signs of congestive heart failure (pulmonary edema, severe peripheral edema, or hypoxia) or complains of worrisome chest pain.

Chest Pain

On occasion, an individual with anorexia nervosa will complain of chest pain. Typical atherosclerotic-induced cardiac chest pain (angina) is not seen in this young population. Rather, the organic cardiac cause for chest pain in these patients is due to the presence of mitral valve prolapse, which may be seen in 30–50 percent of patients who have severe anorexia nervosa. This syndrome is defined by prolapse of the mitral valve because the heart muscle decreases in size with weight loss while the structural supporting tissues that comprise the mitral valve not decrease in size. The valve is therefore becomes relatively redundant compared to the cardiac chamber and prolapses (Johnson et al., 1986). The physician often hears a systolic murmur and click when a cardiac examination is performed on a patient with mitral valve prolapse, but no EKG findings are associated with it. As a consequence of mitral valve prolapse, these patients can complain of chest pain and palpitations. Mitral valve prolapse is not indicative of any imminent danger to the patient, but if bothersome symptoms persist, beta blocker, given cautiously to patients with baseline bradycardia and hypotension, can mitigate the chest pain and palpitations. A good history and a physical examination on initial presentation should therefore focus on the vital signs, heart and lung auscultation, and checking for the presence of signs of congestive heart failure such as edema, jugular venous distention and rales in the lungs, and low oxygen saturation (<90%).

Bulimia and the Heart

In general, fewer cardiac complications are found in normal-weight individuals with bulimia nervosa than in individuals with anorexia nervosa. However, someone who has bulimia and a prior history of anorexia nervosa may be more prone to ventricular arrhythmia, even after the anorexia has resolved (Takimoto et al., 2006). In contrast with anorexia nervosa, there are no consistent findings from the cardiac examination, vital signs, EKG, or echocardiogram in bulimia nervosa. Rather, the cardiac concerns are due to the metabolic sequelae from the different modes of purging. Hypokalemia is the main culprit that can result in serious and even fatal cardiac arrhythmias. Once the potassium level is lower than 3.0 meq/L, the risk of serious arrhythmias begins to rise. At levels below 2.5 meq/L, continuous cardiac monitoring may be indicated to preemptively screen for arrhythmias and should continue at least until the potassium level is in the low threes. All types of arrhythmia are possible when the potassium level is significantly reduced, but ventricular tachycardia and ventricular fibrillate are the most worrisome. Atrial tachycardia and atrial fibrillation are also precipitated by a low potassium level. The risk of a cardiac arrhythmia secondary to hypokalemia is much higher in a patient who purges six or eight times per day versus the patient with bulimia who abuses laxatives once or twice a week. It is also logical to surmise that if a patient has some features of anorexia nervosa and has lost a significant amount of weight, even milder degrees of hypokalemia might precipitate the onset of serious cardiac arrhythmias.

Essentially, any abnormal cardiac rhythm that is detected on EKG necessitates urgent review by a competent primary care provider, especially if there are symptoms such as palpitations, fainting, and lightheadedness. In addition, severe alkalosis, which often accompanies the hypokalemia seen with self-induced vomiting or diuretic abuse, or acidosis from excessive laxative abuse and its attendant diarrhea, lowers the threshold for the development of cardiac arrhythmias. Any patient with bulimia who purges more than two times per day should have a baseline EKG and a repeat if the purging behaviors accelerate in duration or frequency (Table 7.2).

TABLE 7.2   Electrolyte abnormalities that can cause arrhythmia in people with bulimia

Hypokalemia
Hypomagnesemia
Metabolic alkalosis
Metabolic acidosis

Ipecac

Ipecac is a potent cardiac toxicant. Those individuals with bulimia who induce vomiting by ingesting ipecac are at risk for an irreversible cardiomyopathy (cardiac muscle disease). One of main ingredients in ipecac is the alkaloid emetine, which is a direct cardiac toxicant. Each bottle of ipecac contains 32 mg of emetine. Once the heart is exposed to a cumulative dosage of 1,250 mg of emetine over the period of a few months, the heart muscle-weakening process may ensue. The damage to the heart muscle may be irreversible, even after the bulimia subsides. Individuals with bulimia have died from ipecac cardiotoxity and the ensuing congestive heart failure.

Summary

Cardiac complications contribute significantly to the morbidity and mortality seen in patients with anorexia nervosa, and less so in bulimia. Most of these complications occur with the severe stages of these eating disorders. A thorough cardiac history and meticulous physical examination should be performed and basic chemistry panels (CHEM 7) and a baseline EKG obtained for all these patients after the first visit to screen for abnormalities that need ongoing evaluation and treatment.

Anorexia nervosa is associated with a number of serious cardiac complications. In general, the more severe the anorexia nervosa, the more serious the cardiac issues. The vast majority of these issues resolve with timely weight restoration and do not leave permanent sequelae. With anorexia nervosa, not only are cardiac issues present in the untreated state, but there are also issues that arise as a result of the refeeding process. With bulimia, most of the cardiac issues are due to electrolyte abnormalities related to purging behaviors.

REFERENCES

Awazu M, Matsuoka S, Kamimaki T, Watanabe H, and Matsuo N. 2000. Absent circadian variation of blood pressure in patients with anorexia nervosa. *Journal of Pediatrics* 136:524–27.
Cooke RA, Chambers JB, Singh R, Todd GJ, Smeeton NC, Treasure J, and

Treasure T. 1994. QT interval in anorexia nervosa. *British Heart Journal* 72:69–73.

Derman T and Szabo CP. 2006. Why do individuals with anorexia die? A case of sudden death. *International Journal of Eating Disorders* 39:260–62.

Facchini M, Sala L, Malfatt G, Bragato R, Redelli G, and Invitti C. 2006. Low-K+ dependent QT prolongation and risk for ventricular arrhythmias in anorexia nervosa. *International Journal of Cardiology* 106:170–76.

Galetta F, Franzoni F, Prattichizzo F, Rolla M, Santoro G, and Pentimone F. 2003. Heart rate variability and left ventricular diastolic function in anorexia nervosa. *Journal of Adolescent Health* 32:416–21.

Isner JM, Roberts WC, Heymsfield SB, and Yager J. 1985. Anorexia nervosa and sudden death. *Annals of Internal Medicine* 102:49–52.

Johnson GL, Humphries LL, Shirley PB, Mazzoleni A, and Noonan JA. 1986. Mitral valve prolapse in patients with anorexia nervosa and bulimia. *Archives of Internal Medicine* 146:1525–29.

Kim CK, McGorray SP, Bartholomew BA, et al. 2005. Depressive symptoms and heart rate variability in postmenopausal women. *Archives of Internal Medicine* 165:1239–44.

Krantz MJ, Donahoo WT, Melanson EL, and Mehler PS. 2005. QT interval dispersion and resting metabolic rate in chronic anorexia nervosa. *International Journal of Eating Disorders* 37:166–70.

Krantz MJ and Mehler PS. 2004. Resting tachycardia, a warning sign in anorexia nervosa: Case report. *BMC Cardiovascular Disorders* 4:10.

Melanson EL, Donahoo WT, Krantz MJ, Poirier P, and Mehler PS. 2004. Resting and ambulatory heart rate variability in chronic anorexia nervosa. *American Journal of Cardiology* 94:1217–20.

Mont L, Castro J, Herreros B, Pare C, et al. 2003. Reversibility of cardiac abnormalities in adolescents with anorexia nervosa after weight recovery. *Journal of the American Academy of Child and Adolescent Psychiatry* 42:808–13.

Olivares JL, Vazquez M, Fleta J, Morena LA, Perez-Gonzalez JM, and Bueno M. 2005. Cardiac findings in adolescents with anorexia nervosa at diagnosis and after weight restoration. *European Journal of Pediatrics* 164:383–86.

Rechlin T, Weis M, Ott C, Bleichner F, and Joraschky P. 1998. Alterations of autonomic cardiac control in anorexia nervosa. *Biological Psychiatry* 43:-358–63.

Roche F, Barthelemy JC, Mayaud N, Pichot V, Duverney D, German N, Long F, and Estour B. 2005. Refeeding normalizes the QT rate dependence of female anorexic patients. *American Journal of Cardiology* 95:277–80.

Shamim T, Golden NH, Arden M, Filiberto L, and Shenker IR. 2003. Resolution of vital sign instability: An objective measure of medical stability in anorexia nervosa. *Journal of Adolescent Health* 32:73–77.

Takimoto Y, Yoshiuchi K, Kumano H, and Kuboki T. 2006. Bulimia nervosa and abnormal cardiac repolarization. *Journal of Psychosomatic Research* 60:105–7.

Yager J, Devlin MJ, Halmi K, et al. 2006. American Psychiatric Association Practice Guidelines for the treatment of patient with eating disorders. *American Journal of Psychiatry* 160 (suppl):1–128.

CHAPTER EIGHT

Osteoporosis and Gynecological Endocrinology

COMMON QUESTIONS

What characteristic hypothalamic-gonadal hormonal alterations occur in patients with anorexia nervosa who have amenorrhea?

When does amenorrhea occur during the course of anorexia nervosa?

What is the relationship between weight loss and the onset of the functional amenorrhea in anorexia nervosa?

What other hypothalamic hormonal responses occur in patients with anorexia nervosa? How are they similar to the hormonal responses of acute stress?

What therapeutic interventions may help treat the amenorrhea? Is this important?

What body weight predicts the resumption of menses?

Do patients with a history of an eating disorder have additional problems with pregnancy?

How common is osteoporosis in patients with eating disorders?

What are the clinical consequences of low bone mass in patients with eating disorders?

What features of eating disorders contribute to bone loss?

How is the diagnosis of osteoporosis made?

What therapeutic interventions are indicated to prevent bone loss and attenuate the risk of fracture?

How is osteoporosis treated and monitored?

Case 1

A.H. was a 20-year-old female presenting with secondary amenorrhea. She underwent normal puberty at age 12, initially having regular menstrual cycles. Secondary amenorrhea began at 18 years of age. Family members had typically undergone normal growth and sexual development. A.H. was "overweight" in grade school and in the first two years of high school. She expressed a dislike for obesity, as her mother and sister were "fat." Subsequently she began dieting and exercising to achieve weight loss. In addition to the amenorrhea, she complained of cold intolerance, brittle hair, dry skin, and fatigue. A.H. weighed 102 pounds and was 5 feet 6 inches tall. Pubic hair and breast development were scant, but normal. On careful questioning, she indicated that she was adhering to a strict 500-calorie-per-day diet with use of laxatives to promote weight loss. She exercised daily for 1–2 hours but denied self-induced vomiting. She initiated this dieting at the age of 16; within the next three years, when her weight reached 108 pounds, her menstrual periods stopped. The diagnosis of anorexia nervosa, purging subtype, was made, and she was referred to an internal medicine specialist for further evaluation.

Case 2

C.R. was a 28-year-old female 5 feet 6 inches tall weighing 98 pounds. She had a 12-year history of anorexia nervosa. She initially weighed 164 pounds; after a 35 percent loss in body weight, she developed secondary amenorrhea. Over the course of her illness, she had lost 2 inches in height. She had recently been seen by her primary care provider for evaluation of low back pain. X-rays showed an L2 compression fracture, which a radiologist interpreted to be acute.

Background

People with bulimia and anorexia nervosa may present with an extremely complex medical disorder, resulting from the sociocultural pressures for thinness and attractiveness. This results in numerous psychoneuroendocrine-nutritional medical stresses while the patient relentlessly pursues thinness. Specifically, people with anorexia nervosa experience marked weight loss with resultant amenorrhea, defined as having missed at least three consecutive menstrual cycles.

Manifestation of Stress Reactions

Hypothalamic hormonal activation in response to acute stress reflects an internal adaptive mechanism, which characterizes the well-known "flight-or-fight" state. This stress response may occur in relationship to a major life crisis or acute situational reactions. Severe anorexia nervosa qualifies for either. The hormonal consequence is reasonably well characterized as a hypothalamic-pituitary-mediated secretion of ACTH, cortisol, growth hormone, prolactin, epinephrine, and norepinephrine. Similar hormonal alterations have been noted to accompany marked psychological stress, exercise, and severe chronic illness. The inflammatory cytokines interleukin-1, interleukin-2, and tumor necrosis factor, and other inflammatory mediators such as eicosanoids and platelet-activating factor, are also released. These inflammatory mediators may also act as osteoclastic-activating factors in bone, promoting bone resorption. The currently identified osteoclast-stimulating cytokines are interleukin-1, interleukin-6, interleukin-11, and tumor necrosis factor.

Gynecological Effects of Eating Disorders
THE MENSTRUAL CYCLE IN ANOREXIA NERVOSA

The neuroendocrine regulation of normal female reproductive functions depends on a rhythm of nerve impulses generated within the medial basal hypothalamus, which governs the pulsatile release of gonadotropin-releasing hormone (GnRH) from nerve terminals. Pulsatile GnRH release is the central controller of pituitary luteinizing hormone (LH) and follicle-stimulating hormone (FSH) secretions, which determine the timely onset of normal menstrual function (Doufas and Mastorakos, 2000). At puberty, normally an increase in both the frequency and the amplitude of GnRH induces LH-FSH secretion. Patients with anorexia nervosa have a characteristic "hypothalamic amenorrhea syndrome" with a variable reduction in pulsatile hypothalamic GnRH gonadostat signaling to the pituitary gland, resulting in a failure of ovulation. The degree of impairment varies among patients with anorexia nervosa, but in general, the frequency and amplitude of the LH-FSH pulses are diminished, with a reversion to a prepubertal pattern and the development of the commonly found amenorrheic state. Thus, this functional amenorrhea seen in anorexia nervosa reflects a temporary, reversible disturbance of hypothalamic-pituitary function. Moreover, most amenorrhea seen with anorexia nervosa is of the secondary type, meaning the patient previously had normal menstrual periods, in contrast with primary amenorrhea, in which there was never onset of menses.

Of patients with anorexia nervosa, 20–25 percent may experience amenorrhea before the onset of significant weight loss, and 50–75 percent will experience amenorrhea during the course of dieting and its weight loss (Katz and Volenhowen, 2000). In some anorexic patients amenorrhea occurs only after more marked weight loss. Menstrual irregularities are also common in bulimia nervosa, albeit much less severe and less prevalent than in anorexia nervosa (Gendall et al., 2000). Conversely, on restoring weight toward normal, many patients will have resumption of the normal menstrual cycle. More than 30 years ago, Frisch and McArthur (1974) noted a critical relationship between body mass index, body fat, percentage of body weight loss, and the occurrence of amenorrhea. This relationship was more recently confirmed in a study demonstrating that menses can be expected to resume in anorexic patients at a weight approximately 90 percent of ideal body weight (Golden et al., 1997). Other studies have found the weight requirement for resumption of menses to be more variable and better predicted by the weight at which menstruation ceases (Swenne, 2004). A recent cohort study of 56 adolescent females determined that there was return of menses at a mean BMI percentile of 27 (Golden et al., 2008).

Although these relationships exist, features other than weight loss may also be causing the amenorrhea. Because the onset of amenorrhea precedes significant weight loss in about one-quarter of anorexic women, amenorrhea can persist even after weight restoration in some women, and menstruation even resumes in some women despite a low body weight (Miller et al., 2004b). Other adaptive hormonal responses to sociocultural-psychic stress, excessive exercise, and chronic nutritional energy deficiency may also promote this process (Warren et al., 2002), along with reduced thyroid hormone and leptin levels. Stress, anxiety, exercise, smoking, and abnormal eating habits may contribute. However, as a result of the gonadotropin failure, individuals with anorexia nervosa will have decreased blood levels of the sex hormones (estradiol, estrone, progesterone, and testosterone) (Miller et al., 2007). Therefore, women with anorexia nervosa may not always have withdrawal bleeding to a diagnostic progesterone challenge, indicating a more profound hypothalamic-pituitary gonadotropin deficiency state.

Thus, a critical weight may be necessary, but not sufficient, for menstrual function, and other factors may also be of importance (Gendall et al., 2006). The variegated patterns of menstrual disturbance with anorexia nervosa are in part the basis of the recent impetus to reevaluate the prudency of amenorrhea remaining a criterion for the diagnosis of anorexia nervosa (Pinheiro et al., 2007). Rather, a broader definition of menstrual irregularity, as an associated feature of all eating disorders without a specified duration, is being evaluated.

GENERAL HYPOTHALAMIC DYSFUNCTION

An additional disorder of hypothalamic hormonal function seen in patients with anorexia nervosa is an enhanced activation of the hypothalamic-pituitary-adrenal axis with increased hydrocortisone secretion from the adrenal gland. In these patients, there is both an increased production rate of hydrocortisone and a decrease in its metabolic clearance rate. Subsequently, and importantly, blood cortisol levels are elevated, as will be discussed with regard to osteoporosis. In contrast, adrenal production of male sex hormones is diminished with decreased blood levels of DHEA sulfate. These reduced androgen levels result in a diminished anabolic state and may adversely affect bone remodeling, causing osteoporosis as well as diminished sexual drive.

Further, hypothalamic abnormalities are apparent in thermoregulation and in vasopressin and growth hormone secretion. As a result, 50 percent of patients with anorexia nervosa have an elevation in basal growth hormone levels with a decrease in the production of insulin-like growth factor 1 (IGF-1), a profile characteristic of a starvation state. Reduced IGF-1 levels also impede bone formation. The low vasopressin levels found in some patients may on rare occasions give rise to a diabetes insipidus presentation with failure to concentrate the urine and resultant excessive urination and elevated serum sodium levels.

IMPLICATIONS FOR THE TREATMENT OF AMENORRHEA

Treating a patient with functional (hypothalamic) amenorrhea is not easy. The underlying cause of the amenorrhea, as it relates to sociocultural and environmental psychic stress, needs to be evaluated and primarily addressed. Assessment for clinical or subclinical depressive illness is warranted. A detailed history concerning parental relationships, self-image, social and environmental issues, stressors, sexuality, interpersonal relationships, and support systems is important. Spontaneous recovery of menstrual periods may occur following psychological guidance and correction of the eating disorders and psychopathology. The corollary of this, however, is that even with weight gain, menstruation may not recur if there is persistence of the abnormal eating behaviors or psychogenic factors.

The progestin challenge test is sometimes used in the evaluation of amenorrhea to determine if there is adequate estrogen. The patient is given 10 mg of medroxyprogesterone (Provera) daily for five days. Withdrawal bleeding within 10 days of progesterone administration indicates adequate estrogen levels and is consistent with functional amenorrhea; conversely, a lack of withdrawal bleeding connotes a state of profound estrogen deficiency. Estrogen-progesterone therapy might be considered, but only for those patients not manifesting withdrawal bleeding. A serum leutenizing hormone (LH) level below 5 mIU/mL is indicative also of hypothalamic dysfunction in patients who do not have withdrawal bleeding.

However, in the clinical setting of anorexia nervosa with substantial weight loss, the progestin challenge test is not a crucial diagnostic exercise for evaluating the commonly found amenorrhea. Rather, efforts should be directed toward overall treatment of the eating disorder because there may be little inherent value in the administration of female sex hormones to patients with anorexia nervosa. Although, withdrawal bleeding can be calming because it reassures the patient that her uterus can still function, it may also promote a false sense of well-being and minimize the urgency of engaging in therapy for the eating disorder.

REPRODUCTION

People with anorexia nervosa have self-imposed starvation, concerns about gaining weight, and often a phobia of pregnancy and difficulty conceiving. Approximately 5–10 percent of the women seen in infertility clinics are found to have covert anorexia nervosa or bulimia. The presence of an active eating disorder is commonly felt to be a contraindication for pregnancy and infertility treatments. When pregnancy occurs, it is more often in patients with bulimia nervosa of near-normal body weight, although there are rare patients with anorexia nervosa who ovulate and become pregnant despite their amenorrhea. During the course of the pregnancy, many patients will subdue their binge eating and purging behaviors (Crow et al., 2008). However, there is return to these behaviors in the puerperium in one-half to three-quarters of the patients (Norre, Vanereycken, and Gordts, 2001). Others have worsening of symptoms of bulimia during pregnancy, although this is less common and probably due to a fear of weight gain.

If pregnancy does occur, both the pregnancy and lactation impose a tremendous stress on the maternal skeleton for mineralization of the fetal and newborn skeleton. Hence, it is important to provide vitamin D and calcium supplementation and to emphasize a diet enriched in protein and phosphate. Moreover, pregnancy in eating disorder patients is associated with a greater incidence of premature birth, smaller head circumference, miscarriages, and low-birth-weight infants, especially if the disease is active (Kouba et al., 2005). If individuals with a recent history of an eating disorder desire to become pregnant, it usually is advisable to refer them to a reproductive endocrinologist for discussion of treatment options and to also ensure that they have sufficient psychiatric support to help control their abnormal eating behaviors during pregnancy.

Pregnancy for a patient with an eating disorder is a decision that should be made only after judicious deliberation. Referral to a multidisciplinary team is critical for all these patients so that the health of the mother and her fetus are preserved to promote the best possible outcome. Long term, after a patient recovers from anorexia nervosa and bulimia, there does not appear to be a negative impact on later ability to achieve pregnancy.

Osteoporosis

Osteoporosis is a disease characterized by low bone mass and deterioration of the microarchitectual structure of bone, resulting in bone fragility and the clinical syndrome of nontraumatic fractures as a direct result of this low bone mass. *Osteoporosis* is quantitatively defined by bone densitometry measurements, using dual-energy X-ray absorptiometry (DEXA), as a z-score greater than a [minus]2.5 standard deviation decrement from young bone mass. A loss of bone mass with a z-score from [minus]1 to [minus]2.5 standard deviations is classified as *osteopenia*. Peak bone mass is defined as the highest level of bone mass achieved as a result of normal growth. Most skeletal bone growth occurs during childhood and adolescence. The timing of peak bone mass may vary but generally occurs between ages 17 and 22, a time that unfortunately frequently coincides with the onset of anorexia nervosa. Rapid bone loss, at an annual average rate of 2.5 percent, occurs in young women with osteoporosis. Osteoporosis is present in almost 40 percent of patients with anorexia nervosa, and osteopenia is present in 92 percent of these women (Grinspoon et al., 2000). Trabecular bone, found in the lumbar spine and hips, is more affected than cortical bone.

Achieving an optimal peak bone mass depends on heredity and lifestyle factors. Lifestyle influences causing less than optimal peak bone mass may be nutritional, such as a low-calcium or low-phosphate intake, a diet low in animal protein, excessive intake of carbonated dark soda-type drinks, a high-sodium diet, high caffeine intake, or a strictly vegetarian diet. Other lifestyle influences that have deleterious effects on bone mass include cigarette smoking, a low level of physical activity, and alcohol consumption. Weight-bearing exercise in females usually promotes skeletal development and maintenance. However, when exercise is excessive, as in the athletic amenorrhea syndrome seen in female runners, it may be associated with low bone mass and fractures. Weight-bearing exercise may be protective only if menstruation is preserved.

FACTORS INFLUENCING BONE REMODELING
IN ANOREXIC PATIENTS

Whether an individual achieves peak adult bone mass depends on the time of onset and the duration of the eating disorder, the degree of nutritional depletion, changes in body composition, and the stress associated with anorexia nervosa. Once amenorrhea is present, the estrogen-progesterone deficiency plays a role in arresting bone development and promoting bone resorption. Anorexia nervosa appears to be a low-turnover state characterized by increased bone resorption without concomitant increased bone formation. This imbalance contributes to the significant bone loss that characterizes anorexia nervosa. As noted from our discussion of the hypothalamic hormonal influences accompanying the disorder, there is, in addition to the hypothalamic hypogonadal state, excess hydrocortisone secretion, low IGF-1 levels (somatomedin C), and low androgen levels. Low levels of IGF-1 reduce the levels of osteocalcin and cause abnormalities in the osteoblasts, the bone-building cells. These low levels of IGF-1 have been demonstrated to be the major correlate of bone formation in anorexia nervosa, in contrast to the high levels typically found in normal adolescents. The elevated levels of cortisol mentioned earlier are inversely related to levels of osteocalcin (Misra et al., 2004). All of these factors, in addition to estrogen and androgen deficiency, promote the development of osteoporosis and render the osteoporosis associated with anorexia a different entity from that found in the typical postmenopausal state (Miller et al., 2007). Markers of bone resorption, such as N-teleopeptide and deoxypyrdoline, are higher in patients with anorexia nervosa, while markers of bone formation, such as osteocalcin, are not concomitantly elevated (Lennkh et al., 1999). This pattern is most closely analogous to steroid-induced osteoporosis. However, serum levels of calcium, vitamin D, and parathyroid hormone are all within the normal range. Body weight (especially fat cell mass) and muscle strength are positive predictors of bone mineral density in young women. Patients with anorexia nervosa have altered body composition with depleted fat stores. In addition, in females, the fat cell is capable of independent estrogen synthesis from adrenal androgen precursors. However, a total body fat cell mass of at least 10 percent is needed for normal menstrual function.

Individuals with anorexia nervosa may be intensively involved in rigorous exercise programs, which contribute to the secondary amenorrhea. Secondary amenorrhea is common in many young women who continually pursue high levels of physical activities, such as running, ballet dancing, cycling, and swimming. The "female triad" seen in competitive female athletes is characterized by disordered eating, menstrual irregularity, and osteoporosis (Nativ et al., 1994). Osteoporosis and a tendency to stress fractures are associated with menstrual irregularity in these women. The estrogen deficiency state found in some competitive athletes causes lower bone density and places these women at risk for stress fractures (Cobb et al., 2003). Young estrogen-deficient women may lose bone mass at 3–5 percent per year.

THE DIAGNOSIS OF OSTEOPOROSIS

With the advent of single- and dual-photon bone densitometry, it has been observed that osteoporosis is a highly prevalent complication of anorexia nervosa. The assessment of bone mineral density is easily obtained with a dual-energy X-ray absorptiometry (DEXA) scan, which allows for a reliable and highly precise measurement of skeletal bone mineral content in the lumbar spine and hip (Fig. 8.1). For every one standard deviation decrement in bone mineral content of the lumbar spine, the fracture risk of an individual is increased twofold. Likewise for the hip, for every decrement in bone mineral content by one standard deviation, the attributable fracture risk is elevated 2.5 times. Currently, DEXA is the gold standard for assessing bone mineral content in both a screening mode as well as for monitoring bone density in patients undergoing therapy for established osteoporosis. The quantitative ultrasound measurement is a newly endorsed diagnostic tool for the assessment of osteoporosis; although it is still in its infancy, it does appear to be easier to perform and may be a more efficient test than DEXA. The Food and Drug Administration (FDA) has approved peripheral assessment of bone density in the hand by DEXA and the achilles with the use of quantitative ultrasound. While peripheral measurements of bone density by ultrasound are about 25 percent of the cost of the DEXA, at the current time they do not definitively exclude or confirm DEXA-determined osteoporosis. The indications for bone density measurements are listed in Table 8.1.

FACTORS PREDICTIVE OF BONE MINERAL DENSITY

Two of the most characteristic manifestations of anorexia nervosa are low body weight and the absence of menses. Longitudinal studies have demonstrated that low body weight is a consistent predictor of reduced bone mineral density (Wong et al., 2004). Similarly, duration of amenor-

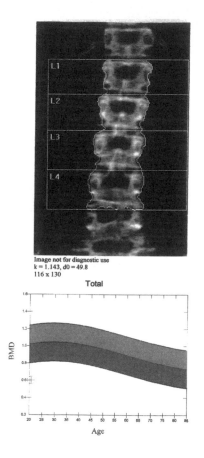

Scan Information:

Scan Date: March 21, 2007
Scan Type: f Lumbar Spine
Analysis: March 21, 2007 13:42 Version 12.6:7
Lumbar Spine
Operator: FCR
Model: Discovery W (S/N 82608)
Comment:

DXA Results Summary:

Region	Area (cm²)	BMC (g)	BMD (g/cm²)	T-score	Z-score
L1	11.16	5.64	0.506	-3.8	-3.6
L2	11.73	7.53	0.642	-3.5	-3.3
L3	13.44	8.85	0.659	-3.9	-3.6
L4	14.87	8.78	0.591	-4.8	-4.5
Total	51.20	30.81	0.602	-4.0	-3.8

Total BMD CV 1.0%, ACF = 1.034, BCF = 1.005, TH = 4.612
WHO Classification: Osteoporosis
Fracture Risk: High

Physician's Comment:

Total

T-score vs. White Female; Z-score vs. White Female. Source: Hologic

HOLOGIC

FIGURE 8.1. DEXA scan.

rhea is a significant predictor of reduced bone mineral density (Baker, Roberts, and Towell, 2000). As a corollary, age at menarche has also emerged as an important predictor of bone density, with an inverse correlation between age at menarche and the patient's bone density. The specific correlations between low body weight or amenorrhea and anorexia nervosa are not yet definitively clarified, but a BMI less than 15 kg/m² and 6 months of amenorrhea are generally accepted as being predictive of loss of bone mineral density in anorexia nervosa. Increased vigilance regarding the presence of the major risk factors for low bone

TABLE 8.1 Indications for bone-density measurements in patients with anorexia nervosa

Patient group	Indicator for measurement
Amenorrheic women	To make a decision about the need for therapy
Patients with vertebral abnormalities and/or osteopenia on plain radiography	To confirm or exclude osteoporosis
Patients undergoing active osteoporotic intervention therapy	To follow the course of therapy

density in these patients may better allow for intervention to improve bone density, thus reducing the long-term risk of osteoporosis and fragility fractures later in life. Males with anorexia nervosa are also at increased risk for loss of bone density and this risk needs to be considered when treating this less common population of patients (Mehler, Sabel, and Andersen, 2008).

THE ONSET OF BONE DISEASE

Owing to the previously held assumption that anorexic adolescents and young adults will not have a problem with osteoporosis, this area has been somewhat neglected until recently. However, emerging evidence suggests that loss of bone mineral density appears to be rapid and occurs relatively early in the disease. Some studies suggest that an illness duration longer than 12 months predicts significant loss of bone mineral (Wong et al., 2001), but a severe degree of demineralization has been reported in adolescents with just a brief illness. In a study of 73 anorexic women with a mean age of 17.2 years, 20 months of amenorrhea was found to be the threshold above which the most severe osteopenia was seen (Audi et al., 2002).

Increased risk for future fracture is a major concern in these young patients, especially because fracture risk is known to double with each decrease of one standard deviation in bone mineral density. Therefore, DEXA should be established as an important screening tool for all anorexia nervosa patients with disease duration greater than 6–12 months to determine the degree of reduction of bone mineral density. Moreover, there may be a psychotherapeutic benefit in providing patients their DEXA results as graphic visual evidence that they are at risk for serious medical problems due to their bone loss. Positive changes in unhealthy eating behaviors can perhaps be obtained through the leverage garnered by showing these patients that they have the same bone density as very old individuals, thus motivating them to more fully engage in treatment (Stoffman et al., 2005). Finally, although the value of repeating DEXA measurements two years after the initial one in postmenopausal osteoporosis has recently been challenged, for individual patients with anorexia nervosa, a repeat scan should be performed 2 years later, especially if the illness is ongoing and a therapeutic intervention for the bone density loss has been initiated (Hillier et al., 2007).

TREATMENT

Hormonal Therapy

Supplemental estrogen in the form of hormone replacement therapy or oral contraceptives is often prescribed in routine practice for people with anorexia nervosa in an effort to minimize or ameliorate osteopenia or osteoporosis. Recent surveys indicate that this inappropriate practice is followed 75–80 percent of the time by practitioners caring for females with anorexia nervosa. In reality, however, there is a distinct paucity of credible evidence supporting this practice (Mehler and MacKenzie, 2009). Early and small retrospective studies seemed to imply that oral contraceptives may attenuate loss of bone mineral density in anorexia nervosa, presumably by impeding osteoclast-mediated resorption of bone. However, there have been only two randomized controlled trials of estrogen therapy in anorexia nervosa. The first, a widely cited study, demonstrated that estrogen treatment did not prevent a reduction in trabecular bone mineral density (Klibanski et al., 1995). A more recent prospective observational trial was performed in 50 adolescents with anorexia nervosa. After two years of treatment, the group who received 35 mg of ethinyl estradiol, in addition to calcium supplementation, did not show any increase in bone mineral density compared with those who received standard treatment. In this study, osteopenia was persistent, and in some cases it was progressive despite estrogen therapy (Golden et al., 2002).

This lack of a beneficial effect from hormone therapy on bone mineral density in anorexia nervosa has been confirmed in other studies as well. An analytic survey of 130 women with anorexia nervosa examined four patient subgroups: (1) estrogen use in the past or the present, (2) estrogen never used, (3) current estrogen use, and (4) estrogen use in the past but not currently. Spine and hip bone density was similar in all four subsets of women despite the differences in estrogen therapy (Grinspoon et al., 2000). An additional practical reason to refrain from using hormonal therapy is that it may cause resumption of menses, which may in turn give the patient a false sense of being cured and reinforce denial in women who are still at a low weight. Of note in the initial hormonal study mentioned above (Klibanski et al., 1995), a subgroup of the estrogen-treated patients who were the most severely underweight, at less than 70 percent of their ideal body weight, had a 4 percent increase in spinal bone mass This limited benefit has not been demonstrated in other studies.

Although there is clear evidence that hormonal therapy is effective in maintaining bone density in postmenopausal women by impairing osteo-clast-mediated bone resorption, it is now increasingly becoming appreciated that health care providers should not continue to extrapolate from this therapeutic success to patients with anorexia nervosa, in whom estrogen's effect on bone density have been disappointing. In actuality, the two states are very different with regard to loss of bone density. The low estrogen levels that characterize the menopausal state and cause bone resorption can be effectively mitigated by the potent antiresorptive effects of estrogen replacement therapy. In contrast, the unique uncoupling of osteoblastic and osteoclastic functions in anorexia nervosa, which results in reduced bone formation concurrent with increased resorption, cannot be successfully treated with estrogen. Thus, the question of whether estrogen replacement therapy slows or reverses bone mineral loss in anorexia nervosa should be considered inconclusive, and estrogen-replacement therapy should not be viewed as evidence-based treatment at this time. Estrogen therapy may be necessary but seems to be insufficient to reverse the profound osteopenia or to promote adequate bone accretion when there is also malnutrition, low levels of circulating bone trophic factors such as IGF-I, cortisol excess, and decreased androgen production.

Most approved therapies for osteoporosis inhibit bone resorption. Another approach is anabolic therapy, in which bone formation is directly stimulated. This seems prudent in anorexia nervosa because this illness is also characterized by decreased bone formation. DHEA has not been shown to be effective in improving bone mineral density, even though it is thought to function as an anabolic factor for bone by increasing levels of IGF-1 and by stimulating osteoblast function. Similarly, transdermal testosterone has not demonstrated to significantly increase markers of bone formation such as osteoclacin and bone-specific alkaline phosphatase in women with anorexia nervosa. There are currently no data from rigorous scientific trials regarding other anabolic agents such as fluoride or the recently released parathyroid hormone medication, teriparatide.

Bisphosphonates

In view of the less-than-favorable effects of commonly used therapeutic modalities for the bone disease of anorexia nervosa, there has recently been interest in the use of bisphosphonates. Past reticence to use these agents was predicated on concerns about their safety in women of reproductive age. Bisphosphonates carry a category C rating for safety in pregnancy because they can persist in the body for many years after the discontinuation of treatment, and there is only anecdotal information about their safety during fetal development; thus, the long-term implications for women of childbearing age are of concern. There is little information concerning infants born to mothers who regularly took bisphosphonates before pregnancy. On the other hand, given the known effectiveness of bisphosphonates in decreasing bone resorption and increasing bone mineral density in osteopenic postmenopausal women, interest in bisphosphonates has been increasing for patients with anorexia nervosa.

The first study to demonstrate their potential effectiveness was a closely monitored study of 10 women with anorexia nervosa who received 5 mg of risedronate and then had bone mineral density measurements at 6 and 9 months. Bone mineral density increased substantially in the spines of those patients who received risedronate (4.1% at 6 months) in contrast with bone loss in the controls despite weight gain (Miller et al., 2004a). A 5 percent increase in bone mass over a 3-year period is generally deemed clinically significant and is associated with a 25 percent reduction in fracture risk. There were no significant side effects reported with its use. The following year a randomized, double-blind, placebo-controlled pilot study of alendronate in 32 osteopenic anorexia nervosa patients was completed. While mineral density in the spine and hip bone increased in both the treatment and the control groups, percentage increase did not differ significantly between groups (Golden et al., 2005). Markers of bone resorption and formation did not undergo significant change. Once again the bisphosphonate was well tolerated. In fact, bisphosphonates have been used for years in adolescent patients with osteogenesis imperfecta to increase bone density without significant adverse events reported.

Currently, bisphosphonates should not be used routinely in patients with anorexia nervosa until further research defines their long-term safety and efficacy. However, they should be considered for severe osteoporosis, especially when the disease is unlikely to revert in the near future. They may also have a role with males with anorexia nervosa, given their known efficacy in male osteoporosis, without the concern about teratogenesis (Ebeling, 2008). There are also no credible studies using calcitonin or raloxifene in anorexia nervosa.

Weight Gain

The cornerstone of treatment for individuals who have anorexia nervosa is weight restoration. Unfortunately, anorexia nervosa is often a protracted illness with a less than favorable outcome. Factors that have been found to be predictive of a poor prognosis include a longer duration of illness, older age at onset, and weight loss that is persistent and is a higher percentage below ideal body weight (Winston, Alwazeer, and Bankart, 2008). The direct effect of weight gain on bone density is not as clearly beneficial. Studies have yielded conflicting results regarding the reversibility of the demineralization. Some previous reports about recovery suggest that restoration of normal bone mass occurs with recovery from anorexia nervosa (Wentz et al., 2003). An annualized rate of increase of 3–4 percent in bone mineral density, attributed solely to weight gain, was demonstrated in different studies of fully recovered anorexia nervosa patients (Zipfel et al., 2001). Many studies, however, demonstrate that bone density may not be fully recoverable (Ward, Brown, and Treasure, 1997). A recent study similarly confirms that despite weight gain, bone mineral density did not increase back to baseline after one year (Misra et al., 2004). In a previously cited randomized controlled study of a bis-phosphonates in anorexic patients, only 17 percent of subjects had a normal bone mineral density despite weight restoration and recovery from their illness (Miller et al., 2004a). This abnormal bone mineral accrual in patients who have recovered from anorexia nervosa may persist despite normalization of bone turnover markers and an increase in IGF-I (Soyka et al., 2002).

Calcium

The American Academy of Pediatrics recommends that adolescents ingest between 1200 and 1500 mg of calcium a day with 400 IU of vitamin D to achieve peak bone mass. Calcium requirements are known to increase during periods of rapid growth. Dietary calcium and vitamin D deficiency are prevalent even in normal adolescent girls. Recently, the requirement for vitamin D was increased to 800 IU. Although necessary, however, calcium may not be sufficient by itself to prevent osteopenia in anorexia nervosa. There have been only a few small studies of calcium in anorexia nervosa, and no correlation was found between calcium intake and bone mineral density in anorexic adolescents. Thus, although calcium and vitamin D are important determinants of developing bone density, they do not appear to be major contributing factors to restitution of bone mineral content in anorexia nervosa.

Summary

Significant bone loss occurs among young patients with anorexia nervosa. Because body weight is the most important determinant of bone density, the optimal intervention is one that promotes weight restoration early in the course of the illness before bone mineral loss has occurred. Once bone mineral is lost, the effect of weight restoration on bone density is variable. Moreover, most tested treatments for osteoporosis, including those that are undeniably effective for postmenopausal women, such as estrogen therapy, have been ineffective for individuals with anorexia nervosa. Because so few studies have been done on bisphosphonates, the possibility of effectiveness has not been excluded. More randomized clinical trials are needed, to focus on combined anabolic/antiresorptive strategies, drugs able to increase osteoblast function, including teriparatide, and bisphosphonates to prevent bone loss in young women with anorexia nervosa. Because of the long-term increased risk of fracture in this young population of patients, there is a compelling need to define an effective and safe treatment to both prevent and reverse bone loss in anorexia nervosa. Prevention, however, remains a key intervention. Therefore, identification of the patient who has anorexia and effective treatment before the patient has suffered irreparable loss of bone density are of utmost importance.

REFERENCES

Audi L, Vargas DM, Gussinye M, Yeste D, Marti G, and Carrascosa A. 2002. Clinical and biochemical determinants of bone metabolism and bone mass in adolescent female patients with anorexia nervosa. *Pediatric Research* 51:497–504.

Baker D, Roberts R, and Towell T. 2000. Factors predictive of bone mineral density in eating disordered women: A longitudinal study. *International Journal of Eating Disorders* 27:29–35.

Cobb KL, Bachrach LK, Greendale G, et al. 2005. Disordered eating, menstrual irregularity, and bone mineral density in female runners. *Medicine and Science in Sports and Exercise* 35:711–19.

Crow SJ, Argas WJ, Crosby R, Halmi K, and Mitchell JE. 2008. Eating disorder symptoms in pregnancy: A prospective study. *International Journal of Eating Disorders* 41:277–79.

Doufas AG and Mastorakos G. 2000. The hypothalamic-pituitary-thyroid axis and the female reproductive system. *Annals of the New York Academy of Science* 960:65–76.

Ebeling PR. 2008. Osteoporosis in men. *New England Journal of Medicine* 358:1474–82.

Frisch RE and McArthur JW. 1974. Menstrual cycle: Fatness as a determinant of minimum weight for height necessary for maintenance or onset. *Science* 185:949–51.

Gendall KA, Bulik CM, Joyce PR, McIntosh VV, and Carter FA. 2000. Menstrual cycle irregularity in bulimia nervosa. *Journal of Psychosomatic Research* 49:409–15.

Gendall KA, Joyce PR, Carter FA, McIntosh VV, Jordan J, and Bulik CM. 2006. The psychobiology and diagnostic significance of amenorrhea in patients with anorexia nervosa. *Fertility and Sterility* 85:1531–35.

Golden NH, Jacobson MS, Schebendach J, Solanto MV, Hertz SM, and Shenker

IR. 1997. Resumption of menses in anorexia nervosa. *Archives of Pediatrics and Adolescent Medicine* 151:16–21.

Golden NH, Lanzkowsky L, Schebendach J, Palestro CJ, Jacobson MS, and Shenker IR. 2002. The effect of estrogen-progestin treatment on bone mineral density in anorexia nervosa. *Journal of Pediatric and Adolescent Gynecology* 15:135–43.

Golden NH, Iglesias EA, Jacobson MS, et al. 2005. Alendronate for the treatment of osteopenia in anorexia nervosa: A randomized, double-blind, placebo-controlled trial. *Journal of Clinical Endocrinology and Metabolism* 90:3179–85.

Golden NH, Jacobson MS, Sterling WM, and Hertz J. 2008. Treatment goal weight in adolescents with anorexia nervosa: Use of BMI percentiles. *International Journal of Eating Disorders* 41:301–6.

Grinspoon S, Thomas E, Pitts S, et al. 2000. Prevalence and predictive factors for regional osteopenia in women with anorexia nervosa. *Annals of Internal Medicine* 133:790–94.

Hillier TZ, Stone KL, Bauer DC, et al. 2007. Evaluating the value of repeat bone mineral density measurement and prediction of fracture in older women. *Archives of Internal Medicine* 167:155–60.

Katz M and Volenhowen B. 2000. The reproductive consequences of anorexia nervosa. *British Journal of Obstetrics and Gynaecology* 107:707–13.

Klibanski A, Biller BMK, Schoenfeld DA, Herzog DB, and Saxe VC. 1995. The effects of estrogen administration on trabecular bone loss in young women with anorexia nervosa. *Journal of Clinical Endocrinology and Metabolism* 80:898–904.

Kouba S, Hallstrom T, Lindholm C, and Hirschbert AL. 2005. Pregnancy and neonatal outcomes in women with eating disorders. *Obstetrics and Gynecology* 105:255–60.

Lennkh C, deZwaan M, Barker U, et al. 1999. Osteopenia in anorexia nervosa: Specific mechanism of bone loss. *Journal of Psychiatric Research* 33:349–56.

Mehler PS and MacKenzie TD. 2009. Treatment of osteopenia and osteoporosis in anorexia nervosa: A systematic review of the literature. *International Journal of Eating Disorders* 42:195–201.

Mehler PS, Sabel A, and Andersen AE. 2008. Male osteoporosis in anorexia nervosa. *International Journal of Eating Disorders* 41:666–72.

Miller K, Grieco KA, Mulder J, et al. 2004a. Effects of risedronate on bone density in anorexia nervosa. *Journal of Clinical Endocrinology Metabolism* 89:3903–6.

Miller K, Grinspoon S, Gleysteen S, Grieco K, Ciampa J, and Breur J. 2004b.

Preservation of neuroendocrine control of reproductive function despite severe under-nutrition. *Journal of Clinical Endocrinology and Metabolism* 89:4434–38.

Miller K, Lawson EA, Mathur V, et al. 2007. Androgens in women with anorexia nervosa and normal-weight women with hypothalamic amenorrhea. *Journal of Clinical Endocrinology and Metabolism* 92:1334–39.

Misra M, Miller K, Almazan C, et al. 2004. Alterations in cortisol secretory dynamics in adolescent girls with anorexia nervosa. *Journal of Clinical Endocrinology and Metabolism* 89:4972–80.

Nativ A, Agostini DR, Drinkwater B, and Yeager KK. 1994. The female athlete triad. *Clinical Journal of Sports Medicine* 13:405–18.

Norre J, Vandereycken W, and Gordts S. 2001. The management of eating disorders in a fertility clinic. *Journal of Psychosomatic Obstetrics and Gynecology* 22:77–81.

Pinheiro AP, Thornton LM, Plotonicov KH, et al. 2007. Patterns of menstrual disturbance in eating disorders. *International Journal of Eating Disorders* 40:427–34.

Soyka LA, Misra M, Frenchman A, et al. 2002. Abnormal bone mineral accrual in adolescent girls with anorexia nervosa. *Journal of Clinical Endocrinology and Metabolism* 87:4177–85.

Stoffman N, Schwartz B, Austin SB, Grace E, and Gordon CM. 2005. Influence of bone density results on adolescents with anorexia nervosa. *International Journal of Eating Disorders* 37:250–55.

Swenne I. 2004. Weight requirements for return of menstruation in teenage girls with eating disorders, weight loss and secondary amenorrhea. *Acta Paediatrica* 93:1449–55.

Ward A, Brown N, and Treasure J. 1997. Persistent osteopenia after recovery from anorexia nervosa. *International Journal of Eating Disorders* 22:-71–75.

Warren MP, Brooks-Gunn J, Jox RP, Holderness CC, Hyle EP, and Hamilton WG. 2002. Osteopenia in exercise-induced amenorrhea using ballet dancers as a model: A longitudinal study. *Journal of Clinical Endocrinology and Metabolism* 87:3162–68.

Wentz E, Mellstrom D, Gillberg C, Sundh V, Gillberg IC, and Rastam M. 2003. Bone density 11 years after anorexia nervosa onset in a controlled study of 39 cases. *International Journal of Eating Disorders* 34:314–18.

Winston AP, Alwazeer AEF, and Bankart MJG. 2008. Screening for osteoporosis in anorexia nervosa: Prevalence and predictors of reduced bone density. *International Journal of Eating Disorders* 41:284–87.

Wong JC, Lewindon P, Mortimer R, and Shepherd R. 2001. Bone mineral density in adolescent females with recently diagnosed anorexia nervosa. *International Journal of Eating Disorders* 29:11–16.

Wong S, Au B, Lau E, Lee Y, Sham A, and Lee S. 2004. Osteoporosis in Chinese patients with anorexia nervosa. *International Journal of Eating Disorders* 36:104–8.

Zipfel S, Seibel MJ, Lowe B, Beumont PJ, Kasperk C, and Herzog W. 2001. Osteoporosis in eating disorders: A follow-up study of patients with anorexia and bulimia nervosa. *Journal of Clinical Endocrinology and Metabolism* 86:5227–33.

CHAPTER NINE

General Endocrinology

COMMON QUESTIONS

What symptoms of patients with eating disorders are suggestive
of endocrine dysfunction?

Are there routine endocrine tests that should be used in the initial
assessment of patients with eating disorders?

Why are some thyroid hormone levels often low in patients with
anorexia nervosa?

What is the significance of a low fasting blood sugar in anorexic
patients?

What is the etiology and significance of hypercortisolism (elevated
cortisol levels) in patients with anorexia nervosa?

Is there a role for growth hormone (GH) in the treatment of anorexia
nervosa?

Are adolescents with insulin-dependent diabetes mellitus (IDDM)
at risk for eating disorders?

What level of blood sugar control should patients with IDDM and
eating disorders strive for?

Case

L.L. was a 24-year-old female admitted for bulimia nervosa not responsive to outpatient treatment, type I diabetes mellitus, and depression
with suicidal ideation. She had had insulin-dependent diabetes mellitus
(type 1 diabetes) since age 11, when, following a viral illness, she presented with polyuria and polydipsia (excessive urination and thirst), a

15-pound weight loss, and a blood sugar of 600 mg/dL (normal 60–110). By age 13, she perceived herself as fat and began episodic dieting. Her blood sugar control was consistently poor. She was never able to lose a significant amount of weight and experienced binge episodes followed by purging, leading to a diagnosis of bulimia nervosa by age 15. L.L. also learned to frequently omit her insulin, which would raise her blood sugar and cause her to lose weight rapidly. This had caused multiple admissions to an acute-care hospital for diabetic ketoacidosis. She was aware of the relationship between insulin, blood sugar, and weight loss, saying, "I stopped using my insulin to produce ketones, and that made me lose weight."

L.L. attempted suicide at age 16 by insulin overdose. She was subsequently treated with a sequence of fluoxetine (Prozac), sertraline (Zoloft), paroxetine (Paxil), venlafaxine (Effexor), buproprion (Wellbutrin), and fluvoxamine (Luvox), all without substantial improvement in her mood. She had an unstable relationship with her boyfriend, which increased her binge-purge behavior. Her ophthalmic retinopathy disease required bilateral surgical vitrectomy. Despite this procedure, her vision progressively diminished. She had also experienced decreased sensation in her feet (diabetic neuropathy) for the preceding 5 years. Gastric emptying studies demonstrated gastric atony and slowed gastric emptying.

Her last acute care hospital admission followed a period of relationship difficulties with her boyfriend, during which she neglected her regular diabetic care. Physical examination showed that deep tendon reflexes were absent in her ankles, and she had decreased pain and vibratory sensation in both feet. She now had developed proteinuria, probably because of her previous history of poor glucose control. Treatment included restoration of regular meals and management of her brittle diabetes, directed by frequent medical consultation with the diabetes consultation service. Occasional middle-of-the-night episodes of symptomatic hypoglycemia were treated with a late-evening protein snack and adjustment of insulin. Her mood stabilized with cognitive-behavioral therapy and couples therapy. She was discharged on calcium 1200 mg per day, vitamin D 800 IU per day, lisinopril 10 mg per day, lantus insulin 15 units q AM, and humalog insulin 6 units before meals. She has not required repeat admission for her eating disorder, diabetes, depressive illness, or borderline personality traits. Her case illustrates the complexity of an eating disorder plus diabetes mellitus and the need for joint medical-psychiatric care in its treatment.

Background

People with anorexia nervosa have a number of abnormalities in neuroendocrine function. The hypothalamic amenorrhea that almost uni versally accompanies this disorder (see Chap. 8) represents one manifestation of hypothalamic dysfunction that is probably also responsible for the elevated urine and serum cortisol levels seen in anorexia nervosa.

Secretion rates of cortisol (an adrenal gland steroid) in anorexia are generally normal, although some studies suggest an increased cortisol production rate. Metabolic clearance rates are decreased, with the result that the half-life of cortisol may be prolonged in malnourished individuals. The normal circadian rhythm of cortisol and adrenocorticotropic hormone (ACTH) secretion is not disrupted in anorexia, but serum cortisol levels are not suppressed after the administration of dexamethasone. Recent studies suggest that hypercortisolism develops in anorexic individuals because of hypersecretion of corticotrophin-releasing hormone (CRH) from the hypothalamus. People with anorexia have elevated cerebrospinal fluid levels of CRH; ACTH responses after the administration of CRH are also elevated despite elevated serum cortisol. The pituitary also appears to respond normally to regular feedback from glucocorticoids. Rather, after the administration of a glucocorticoid antagonist to anorexic patients, there is prominent stimulation of cortisol and ACTH, suggesting a defect at or above the hypothalamus. The clinical significance of this elevated cortisol level is unknown.

Hormone Abnormalities
GROWTH HORMONE

Alterations in growth hormone (GH), insulin-like growth factor 1 (IGF-1), and growth hormone binding protein (GHBP) are not as well understood as the abnormalities in the hypothalamic-pituitary-adrenal (HPA) axis. Levels of IGF-1 are decreased in anorexia and improve with weight recovery (Golden et al., 1994). Fasting growth hormone levels in anorexia may be normal or elevated, while serum GHBP is low. Serum GHBP levels correlate well with body mass index (BMI), suggesting that nutritional deprivation may downregulate the GH receptor and that this effect is reversible with refeeding. Administration of IGF-1 to patients with anorexia has been shown to increase markers of bone turnover, but the effect of chronic administration on weight gain or bone metabolism has not been tested (Grinspoon et al., 1996). Thus, IGF-1 does not currently have a role in the treatment of anorexia nervosa.

THYROID

The thyroid abnormalities in individuals with anorexia nervosa resemble those of the euthyroid sick syndrome, in which total thyroxine (T4) and triiodothyronine (T3) levels are low. The key, however, is that thyroid-stimulating hormone (TSH) usually remains in the normal range (Mehler, 2001). Levels of T3 usually decrease in proportion to the degree of weight loss. Total T4 levels are low because T4 is preferentially converted to a biologically inactive reverse T3. As is true in the euthyroid sick syndrome, thyroid hormone replacement is not beneficial and is not indicated. Only when a high TSH and a low T4 persist after several weeks of weight restoration should thyroid replacement hormone be prescribed. It is important to avoid unnecessary and potentially dangerous thyroid hormone for low-weight anorexic patients because of the starvation-related alterations in thyroid function tests, which usually normalize with nutritional rehabilitation. The risk of unnecessary thyroid hormone is especially prominent because of its deleterious effect on bone mineral density in a population of patients who are already at risk for severe osteoporosis. For a summary of general endocrine changes in anorexia nervosa, see Table 9.1.

GLUCOSE AND OTHER HORMONES

Dietary restriction accompanied by weight loss and excessive exercise lead to depletion of hepatic glycogen stores and disruption of hepatic gluconeogenesis, resulting in abnormalities of glucose metabolism. In early, milder cases of anorexia, hypoglycemia rarely causes symptoms. In contrast, individuals with advanced anorexia nervosa and persistent severe hypoglycemia have a poor prognosis; severe hypoglycemia has been

TABLE 9.1   A summary of endocrine changes in anorexia nervosa

Hormonal or metabolic change	Alteration	Cause
Cortisol (hypothalamic-pituitary-adrenal axis)	Increased plasma	Increased CRH from cortiso hypothalamus; decreased metabolic clearance; normal pituitary response
Growth hormone	Decreased IGF-1; increased or normal fasting GH; decreased serum GHBP	Downregulation of GH receptor by nutritional deprivation
Thyroid	"Euthyroid sick syndrome": 1. Low or low normal T4 and T3 2. Normal TSH 3. Increased reverse T3	T4 decreased due to conversion to inactive reverse T3
Glucose	Fasting hypoglycemia present with severe anorexia nervosa	Depleted liver glycogen stores; disrupted gluconeogenesis
Serum leptin	Decreased	Unknown, possibly low fat mass
Cholesterol (total)	May be increased due to increased HDL	Possible changes in thyroid, estrogen, and glucocorticoids
Gonadal hormones	Decreased estrogen in females; decreased testosterone in males	Central hypothalamic hypogonadism from low weight associated with inappropriately low pituitary LH and FSH levels

associated with sudden death because it indicates liver failure and a depletion of substrate to maintain safe blood glucose levels (Rich et al., 1990). In the presence of hypoglycemia, insulin levels are appropriately decreased, and insulin sensitivity is normal in most individuals with eating disorders. A frequent finding is a flat glucose response during a glucose tolerance test or a glucose response suggestive of diabetes. A glucose tolerance test should therefore not be part of the evaluation of anorexia nervosa-related hypoglycemia, as this test may also be affected by decreased gastrointestinal motility. Rather, documented hypoglycemia should simply imply an urgent need for weight restoration.

Adrenal androgens in women with eating disorders are usually normal to low-normal, while men with eating disorders usually have low testosterone levels. These low testosterone levels may be associated with the osteoporosis seen in males with anorexia nervosa, although there is no known therapeutic role for testosterone replacement therapy for anorectic bone disease (Miller, Grieco, and Klibanski, 2005). Serum prolactin is generally normal.

Leptin levels are reduced in subjects with anorexia and correlate well with weight, percentage of body fat, and IGF-1 (Mehler, Eckel, and Donahoo, 1999). The clinical significance of this is unknown. Although some reports suggest abnormalities of vasopressin secretion, polyuria and diabetes insipidus are uncommon.

As many as 50 percent of patients with anorexia have been reported to have hypercholesterolemia. It is often due to a high level of cardioprotective HDL but insignificant elevations in LDL levels (Mehler, Lezotte, and Eckel, 1998). The reason for the elevated HDL is not well understood, but presumably it reflects excessive exercise and weight loss. Abnormalities in estrogen, thyroid hormone, and glucocorticoids may explain the mildly elevated LDL levels lipids, which in general should not be treated with lipid-lowering agents.

Changes in sex hormone-binding globulin (SHBG) may serve as an index of nutritional status in patients with anorexia. Patients with anorexia have elevated SHBG concentrations before treatment, but levels return to normal after weight restoration. This condition is reflective of the low protein stores found in anorexia nervosa and thus a low level of binding capacity.

Symptoms and Signs of Endocrine Disorders

Abnormalities on physical examination that suggest endocrine dysfunction in patients with eating disorders include hypotension (low blood pressure), cold intolerance, and hypothermia. Only rarely will the hypotension represent adrenal hypofunction, and the characteristic findings of primary adrenal insufficiency (decreased serum sodium levels, increased serum potassium levels, and hyperpigmentation) will generally be absent. Cold intolerance, low heart rate, and hypothermia are all consistent with hypothyroidism, while weight loss could be exacerbated by overactive thyroid function. Other findings that suggest endocrine dysfunction are hair loss, easy bruisability, light-headedness, and dizziness. It is not surprising that the patient with symptoms of anorexia nervosa, especially occult anorexia with denial of dieting, may be referred to an endocrinologist.

Despite the high serum and urine cortisol levels that may accompany anorexia nervosa, the striae, hyperglycemia, hypertension, and skin atrophy seen with cortisol excess (Cushing's syndrome) are not common. The lack of symptoms related to cortisol excess suggests that tissues may be resistant to glucocorticoids. However, studies with glucocorticoid antagonists have shown that the hypercortisolism is a manifestation of hypothalamic excess CRH secretion, not tissue resistance (Kling et al., 1993). It is widely assumed that the hypercortisolism contributes to the osteopenia of anorexia, although patients with eating disorders do not have elevated urine calcium excretion, which should occur in the presence of hypercortisolemia.

Endocrine Testing

With anorexic patients it may at times be necessary to obtain a large battery of endocrine tests to define the accurate diagnosis (Table 9.2). On initial evaluation, thyroid function should be tested and is best assessed with a free T4 and TSH. It is not necessary to measure T3 and reverse T3 to confirm the diagnosis of euthyroid sick syndrome because the diagnosis can be made clinically and neither measurement will affect therapy.

TABLE 9.2 Suggested hormone and hormone-related metabolic testing in patients with eating disorders

1. TSH and free T4 (anorexia nervosa)
2. Fasting glucose
3. Testosterone (anorexic males)

When the free T4 and TSH levels are normal, thyroid hormone replacement is not indicated. Very low or suppressed levels of TSH suggest hyperthyroidism, hypopituitarism, or the effects of malnutrition and need to be interpreted carefully in conjunction with measurements of free T4 and T3 in the setting of the clinical picture. However, a patient with an eating disorder who has a low free T4 and an elevated TSH has primary hypothyroidism and should receive replacement doses of thyroid hormone. A dose of 0.05–0.075 mg of levothyroxine is a good starting point. A TSH level should be repeated three months after therapy begins with a goal level of 0.4–4.5 mg/dL.

There is little advantage in measuring GH or IGF-1 levels in individuals with anorexia, as replacement therapy is not widely available. Stimulation tests of pituitary function are also rarely helpful. In an individual who has anorexia and an expected low T4, but an unexpected low TSH level and symptoms of pituitary dysfunction, a thyroid-releasing factor (TRF) stimulation test could be employed, but it will be difficult to interpret as malnutrition, and depressive illness may affect THS responsiveness to TRF. Referral to an endocrinologist may be prudent for some of these more complicated scenarios. Growth hormone and IGF-1 remain experimental therapy and are not available or recommended for routine treatment of endocrine dysfunction seen with anorexia nervosa. Both require parenteral administration, and growth hormone, in particular, may cause significant edema and weight gain. There are some preliminary data using growth hormone for the treatment of osteoporosis in individuals who have anorexia nervosa (Grinspoon et al., 2002).

Eating Disorders and Insulin-Dependent Diabetes

It has not been clearly established whether there is a specific association between eating disorders and insulin-dependent diabetes mellitus (IDDM), type 1 diabetes. Studies applying stringent diagnostic procedures and matching criteria do not show an increased prevalence of eating disorder symptoms in type 1 diabetes. There are, however, some important clinical problems when the two syndromes occur together, a not uncommon challenge that may be diagnosed only after multiple visits to the emergency room for unexplained diabetic ketoacidosis (Table 9.3) (Rodin and Daneman, 1992).

TABLE 9.3   Eating disorders and insulin-dependent diabetes mellitus (IDDM)

Suspect an eating disorder if there are multiple unexplained episodes of diabetic ketoacidosis.

Recognize that insulin may be misused by

- omitting doses to lose weight secondary to high blood glucose exceeding renal threshold and causing an osmotic diuresis
- increasing dose to compensate for binges

Recognize that individuals who have eating disorders with uncontrolled IDDM experience

- increased retinopathy
- increased nephropathy
- increased neuropathy

Patients who have eating disorders and type 1 diabetes mellitus are likely to be characterized as having "brittle diabetes" and may have repeated episodes of symptomatic hypoglycemia associated with insulin misuse and excessive dieting, falsely attributed to the diabetes alone if misuse of insulin is not uncovered. These patients quickly realize that if they omit their insulin, and thus allow their blood sugar levels to rise, there is resultant excessive urination and weight loss (Crow, Keel, and Kendall, 1998). Hemoglobin A1C levels are often higher in patients with type 1 diabetes who have eating disorders, especially those who have bulimia. The elevation in hemoglobin A1C and poor control is in part related to erratic food intake and to poor compliance with an insulin regimen. In patients with combined anorexia nervosa and type 1 diabetes mellitus, mortality rates are much higher (Nielsen, Emborg, and Molbak, 2002).

It has been demonstrated that there is a high incidence of retinopathy (eye disease), nephropathy (kidney disease), and neuropathy (nerve damage) in insulin-dependent diabetic women with clinically apparent eating disorders, especially those with bulimia. While the causation associating type 1 diabetes mellitus and eating disorders is debatable, there is incontrovertible evidence that patients who have both illnesses do develop the more severe complications and at an earlier stage of their diabetes versus diabetics who do not also have an eating disorder (Rydall et al., 1997).

Summary

People who have eating disorders may present to endocrinologists with symptoms suggestive of adrenal, pituitary, thyroid, pancreatic, or reproductive hormone abnormalities. Most endocrine changes are secondary to weight loss, nutritional alteration, and purging behavior. It is best to diagnose an eating disorder by history and mental status examination, not by "ruling out" all possible medical causes. Of note, most of the endocrine complications of eating disorders revert to normal with early diagnosis and successful treatment of the eating disorder.

Consider treating hypothyroidism in anorexic patients only if free or total T4 is decreased and TSH is also increased. Further evaluation of pituitary function should also be considered if atypical, non-starvation-related endocrine findings are present. Suspect an eating disorder for unexplained frequent ketoacidosis in adolescents with IDDM. It is prudent to aim for moderate rather than rigid glucose control in eating disorder patients with type 1 diabetes mellitus, at least until weight and exercise patterns are both stable and the eating disorder is quiescent.

REFERENCES

Crow SJ, Keel PK, and Kendall D. 1998. Eating disorders and insulin-dependent diabetes mellitus. *Psychosomatics* 39:233–43.

Golden NH, Kreitzer P, Jacobson MS, et al. 1994. Disturbances in growth hormone secretion and action in adolescents with anorexia nervosa. *Journal of Pediatrics* 125:655–60.

Grinspoon S, Bau H, Lee K, Anderson E, Herzog D, and Klibanski A. 1996. Effects of short-term recombinant human insulin-like growth factor I administration on bone turnover in osteopenic women with anorexia nervosa. *Journal of Clinical Endocrinology and Metabolism* 81:3864–70.

Grinspoon S, Thomas L, Miller K, Herzog D, and Klibanski A. 2002. Effects of recombinant human IGF-1 and oral contraceptive administration on bone density in anorexia nervosa. *Journal of Clinical Endocrinology and Metabolism* 87: 2883–91.

Kling MA, Demitrack MA, Whitfield HJJ, et al. 1993. Effects of the glucocorticoid antagonist RU 486 on pituitary-adrenal functioning patients with anorexia nervosa and health volunteers: Enhancement of plasma ACTH and cortisol secretion in underweight patients. *Neuroendocrinology* 57:-1082–91.

Mehler PS. 2001. Anorexia nervosa in primary care. *Annals of Internal Medicine* 134:1048–59.

Mehler PS, Lezotte D, and Eckel R. 1998. Lipid levels in anorexia nervosa. *International Journal of Eating Disorders* 24:217–21.

Mehler PS, Eckel R, and Donahoo WT. 1999. Leptin levels in restricting and purging anorectics. *International Journal of Eating Disorders* 26:189–94.

Miller KK, Grieco KA, and Klibanski A. 2005. Testosterone administration in women with anorexia nervosa. *Journal of Clinical Endocrinology and Metabolism* 90:428–33.

Nielsen S, Emborg C, and Molbak AG. 2002. Mortality in concurrent type 1 diabetes and anorexia nervosa. *Diabetes Care* 25:309–12.

Rich LM, Caine MR, Findling JW, and Shaker JL. 1990. Hypoglycemic coma in anorexia nervosa. *Archives of Internal Medicine* 150:894–95.

Rodin GM and Daneman D. 1992. Eating disorders and IDDM: A problematic association. *Diabetes Care* 15:1402–12.

Rydall AC, Rodin GM, Olmstead MP, Devenyl RG, and Daneman D. 1997. Disordered eating behavior and microvascular complications in young women with insulin-dependent diabetes mellitus. *New England Journal of Medicine* 336:1849–54.

CHAPTER TEN

Oral and Dental Complications

COMMON QUESTIONS

What oral findings are consistent with purging through self-induced vomiting?

What effect does bulimia have on the salivary glands, and when does it usually occur?

What are the treatment options for swelling of the salivary glands (sialadenosis)?

What should you recommend as mouth care for a patient who has bulimia and engages in self-induced vomiting?

What is the significance of the amylase level in a patient who has bulimia and purges?

Case

S.B. was a 25-year-old female with a 5-year history of bulimia and admitted to intermittently vomiting five to seven times per day. She presented to her internist complaining of painless swelling on both sides of her face in the area of her jaws. Although she was working with a therapist, she admitted that she had had a binge and purge episode 4 days before the visit to her internist.

On physical examination, S.B. had obvious enlargement of her parotid glands bilaterally, which were soft and not tender to palpation. Oral examination revealed erosion of the enamel on the lingual surfaces of her maxillary teeth and a reddened posterior pharynx. Laboratory examination demonstrated a total serum amylase of 220 U/L (normal, 16–90 U/L). Her serum lipase, bicarbonate, and potassium levels were normal, however.

The internist recommended that S.B. suck on tart candies to induce excessive salivation, apply warm compresses to the swollen area multiple times per day, and increase her visits with her therapist. On a follow-up visit 2 weeks later, she reported no further purging episodes, and the parotid swelling had completely resolved.

Six months later, S.B. returned with more severe bilateral parotid swelling, as well as submandibular gland enlargement. She had not seen her therapist in more than 2 months and reported numerous self-induced vomiting episodes, but none in the last 2 weeks. Although she had tried warm compresses and tart candies, there was no decrease in the size of her glands. She was frustrated that the swelling seemed to develop a few days after she had decided to stop purging but was not present during her bouts of excessive vomiting.

She was advised to see her therapist and was given a prescription for pilocarpine hydrochloride tablets to be taken three times daily. Blood was drawn to check electrolytes. On follow-up in one week, the parotid swelling had completely resolved. She did not complain of any serious side effects except for flushing after taking this medication. The pilocarpine was discontinued.

Over the next 2 years, S.B. had four episodes of parotid swelling, which once required the use of pilocarpine, but which generally resolved with conservative care. She had a job as a receptionist in a large firm and was concerned about the cosmetic appearance of the swollen glands. The option of having a surgical procedure to remove her parotid glands was raised, but given the potential morbidity and facial scarring, S.B. opted to continue to use the standard treatments of warm compresses and tart candies and, if needed, intermittent pilocarpine while trying to cease her purging behaviors.

Background

Oral complications are common among individuals who have bulimia. These complications are primarily related to the chronic regurgitation of acidic gastric contents with self-induced vomiting. Oral complications may be the first and only clue to an underlying eating disorder. The main complications of self-induced vomiting include angular cheilosis (sores in the angles of the lips), loss of enamel and dentin on the lingual surface of the teeth (perimolysis), dental caries, pharyngeal soreness, gingivitis, and hypertrophy of the salivary glands (sialadenosis) (Table 10.1). Focusing the history and physical examination of these possible complications can alert a health care provider to an underlying eating disorder. Dentists and dental hygienists can play a crucial role in the secondary prevention of bulimia nervosa through timely identification of the oral and physical manifestations of this disorder and referral of the individual to an eating disorder professional (DeBate, Tedesco, and Kerschbaum, 2005). Early identification is especially useful with individuals with bulimia, who often maintain normal body weight and are better able to hide the severity of their illness than individuals who have anorexia.

Cheilosis

Angular cheilosis is a form of stomatitis characterized by pallor and maceration of the mucosal lining at the corners of the mouth. The lesions

TABLE 10.1   Oral complications associated with bulimia nervosa and self-induced vomiting

Oral finding	History and physical findings	Proportion of patients
Cheilosis	Erythematous, dry, painful fissures at angles of lips	Uncommon (<10%)
Erosion of the enamel (perimolysis)	Erosion primarily of the lingual and occlusal surfaces of the maxillary teeth; sensitivity to hot and cold foods	Up to 40%
Gingivitis	Painful, erythematous gums	Uncommon (<10%)
Salivary gland enlargement (sialadenosis)	Bilateral enlargement of the parotid (less often submandibular) glands; generally painless	10%–50%
Hyperamylasemia	None	10%–66% of patients with sialadenosis

TABLE 10.2   Treatment of oral complications associated with bulimia nervosa

Oral finding	Treatment
Cheilosis	B complex multivitamins; topical petroleum jelly
Enamel erosion (perimolysis)	Dental consultation; rinsing of mouth with baking soda solution (1 tsp in 1 qt water) and brushing gently after vomiting
Gingivitis	Mouth rinses; flossing
Salivary gland enlargement (sialadenosis)	Hot compresses, sialagogues (tart candies), and pilocarpine (5.0 mg twice a day in recalcitrant cases)

Note: The primary goal of treatment is the cessation of self-induced vomiting.

are mainly due to the direct caustic effects of the acidic content of the vomitus. In severe cases, linear fissures can leave scars upon healing. The lesions are typically painful and should be distinguished from herpes simplex vesicles, which are more often unilateral and in the middle of the lips and away from the corners of the mouth. Herpetic lesions are also different in that they have a prodrome of mild pain and itching a few days before the lesions appear. Cheilosis may also represent an independent underlying vitamin deficiency, which is usually a lack of riboflavin (B2) and possibly pyridoxine (B6). It may be prudent to check a serum B12 level and to recommend B complex multivitamins to these patients. Topical petroleum jelly following gently washing with warm water can assist in healing of these sores. Keeping the area clean and dry is the main modality to hasten resolution (Table 10.2).

Erosion of the Enamel (Perimolysis)

Perimolysis is the most obvious manifestation of bulimia and has been reported to occur in up to 38 percent of people who have bulimia (Woodmansey, 2000). Chronic contact with acidic gastric contents leads to loss of dentin and tooth enamel. The areas affected first are the lingual, palatal, and posterior occlusal surfaces of the maxillary teeth. By contrast, other causes of enamel erosion, such as eating a highly acidic diet (i.e., lemons), first affect the facial surfaces and spare the lingual surfaces. The teeth appear shortened in length and have dull enamel surfaces with irregular incisal edges. In severe cases, there may be loss of enamel on incisal edges of the anterior teeth and, finally, involvement of the posterior teeth. If a tooth with a previous restoration is involved, a characteristic prominence is created when the loss of enamel leads to the amalgam restoration's projecting above the tooth's surface.

If destruction of the enamel is visible, the care provider can assume that the patient has experienced at least two years of regular and excessive vomiting. Other factors that influence the severity and rate of enamel loss include the types of food consumed, the quality of tooth structure, and oral hygiene. Patients with severe cases will complain of excessive sensitivity to hot and cold food due to exposed dentin, along with chipping of the edges of the teeth.

Treatment involves cessation of vomiting along with attention to oral hygiene. Although brushing after purging was previously not recommended, current recommendations are to brush gently using fluoride toothpaste. In addition, neutral pH mouthwashes or mouthwashes that have a slightly basic pH can reduce oral acidity and are encouraged. Crowns or restorative dental work may be needed after bulimic behaviors are controlled and recovery is imminent (Christensen, 2002).

Caries

It is unclear whether people with bulimia have an increased incidence of caries. It may be that those people who binge on sweet, high-carbohydrate foods are more likely to develop caries (Little, 2002). On the other hand, some people with eating disorders are fastidious in their dental care and have healthy teeth. Further, other factors are important in the development of caries, such as the use of fluorinated water, oral hygiene, type of diet, and genetic predisposition.

The most beneficial means of preventing and treating dental complications is to stop the self-induced vomiting. As success in this effort takes time, care providers need to counsel patients on what to do if they are still engaging in self-induced vomiting. There has been concern that aggressive brushing with fluoride toothpaste after vomiting episodes may further injure weakened enamel, leading to more rapid erosion. This, however, has never been proven to be true. Thus, a reasonable recommendation is to have patients rinse with a baking soda solution (one teaspoon in one quart of water) to neutralize the acid residue after gently brushing. Finally, patients with any oral complications should be referred for dental care, preferably to a practitioner with experience in working with patients who have eating disorders.

Gingivitis

Gum disease (gingivitis) is a result of the chronic irritation from the low pH (acidic) gastric contents and is associated with pain and erythematous gums. Although patients who have bulimia appear to have an increased incidence of gingivitis, they do not seem to be predisposed to progressive periodontitis. Associated with gingivitis can be throat erythema and soreness (discussed in Chap. 6), which can also be a manifestation of gastroesophageal reflux disease (GERD).

Enlargement of Salivary Glands

Sialadenosis (hypertrophy of salivary glands) is common in patients with bulimia, occurring in up to 50 percent of patients. The diagnosis of bulimia should be considered in any young women with persistent, bilateral enlargement of the parotid glands without another apparent cause (Mignogna, Fedele, and Lo Russo, 2004). Other causes of salivary gland enlargement are obstruction of the ducts, local infection, Sjögren's syndrome, diabetes mellitus, alcoholism, cirrhosis, hypothyroidism, and hypovitaminosis A. In patients who have bulimia, the swelling is usually painless, bilateral, and readily apparent on physical examination, with the parotid salivary glands being enlarged to two to five times their normal size. In some patients, the submandibular glands are also involved. In general, swelling begins two to three days *after* a purging episode, which can be disconcerting for the patient with bulimia who has finally decided to cease purging. The frequency and severity of sialadenosis are directly related to the frequency of vomiting. Further, it appears that patients with parotid swelling are more likely to also have enamel erosion.

The causes of the swelling are multifactorial and include

1. chronic regurgitation of stomach contents, leading to increased cholingergic nerve stimulus;

2. consumption of high-calorie foods over short periods and, thus, repetitive stimulation of the glands (work hypertrophy);

3. chronic metabolic alkalosis, which is the most common electrolyte abnormality found in individuals with bulimia who purge through self-induced vomiting; and

4. increased autonomic stimulation secondary to the stimulation of lingual taste receptors by pancreatic proteolytic enzymes, which come in contact with the oral mucosa during vomiting.

Biopsies of the parotid glands are often normal but may demonstrate increased acinar size and increased amount of secretion granules but no inflammatory cells (Aframian, 2005).

Treatment of sialadenosis depends on the severity of the swelling and the patient's concern over his or her cosmetic appearance. Abstinence from vomiting alone will lead to the resolution of swelling in most cases (Mandel and Abai, 2004). In addition, hot compresses and sialagogues (tart candies) can aid in the resolution of swelling. More severe cases have been successfully treated with pilocarpine tablets (5.0 mg three times per day). This is a cholimimetic parasympathomimetic agent that works by causing increased salivation and resultant decompression of the glands (Mehler and Wallace, 1993). The main side effects of pilocarpine are transient blurring of the vision, lacrimation, sweating, a lowering of the heart rate, and dizziness due to lowering of the blood pressure. Patients with significant cardiovascular disease may be unable to compensate for the transient changes in blood pressure and pulse induced by pilocarpine, and thus it should be used with caution.

Last, recalcitrant cases have been treated with the surgical procedure of parotidectomy. Unfortunately, parotidectomy can lead to facial scarring and disfigurement, which can be particularly troublesome to patients who already are extremely fixated on their self-image. Additional morbidity from the surgery, such as a dry mouth (xerostomia), can also be problematic for patients.

Hyperamylasemia

Associated with sialadenosis is an elevation in the serum amylase blood level, which is seen in 10–66 percent of patients. It is important to order a fractionation of the serum amylase to confirm that it is of salivary and not pancreatic origin and thus does not portend a serious abdominal process. Another way to differentiate bulimia from a pancreatic etiology of the elevated amylase level is to send blood for a concomitant lipase level. Normal lipase in the presence of the elevated amylase level speaks to a salivary gland source, and not a pancreatic source, for the elevated amylase level. As is the case with salivary gland enlargement, elevated amylase levels are more common in patients who have more frequent binge eating and vomiting. If treatment of bulimia is successful, the amylase levels will return to normal within a few days to weeks.

Summary

Individuals with suspected eating disorders should have a thorough examination of the oral cavity. Health care providers need to ask about a history of posterior throat pain, thermal sensitivity of the teeth, problems with the gums, and sores at the angles of the mouth. Likewise, the physical examination should focus on detecting cheilosis, perimolysis, posterior pharyngitis, and swelling of the parotid glands. If the history or physical findings are consistent with an eating disorder, then a more complete general history and physical are warranted to look for some of the other manifestations and complications associated with eating disorders. However, the treatment of oral complications, first and foremost, involves concerted and coordinated efforts directed at resolving or improving the underlying eating disorder.

REFERENCES

Aframian DJ. 2005. Comment on Anorexia/bulimia-related sialadenosis of palatal minor salivary glands. *Journal of Oral Pathology and Medicine* 34:-383–84.
Christensen GJ. 2002. Oral care for patients with bulimia. *Journal of the American Dental Association* 133:1689–91.
DeBate RD, Tedesco LA, and Kerschbaum WE. 2005. Knowledge of oral and physical manifestations of anorexia and bulimia nervosa among dentists and dental hygienists. *Journal of Dental Education* 69:346–54.
Little JW. 2002. Eating disorders: Dental implications. *Oral Surgery, Oral Medicine, Oral Pathology, Oral Radiology and Endodontics* 93:138–43.

Mandel L and Abai S. 2004. Diagnosing bulimia nervosa with parotid gland swelling. *Journal of the American Dental Association* 135:613–16.

Mehler PS and Wallace JA. 1993. Sialadenosis in bulimia: A new treatment. *Archives of Otolaryngology: Head and Neck Surgery* 119:757–88.

Mignogna MD, Fedele S, and Lo Russo L. 2004. Anorexia/bulimia-related sialadenosis of palatal minor salivary glands. *Journal of Oral Pathology and Medicine* 33:441–42.

Woodmansey KF. 2000. Recognition of bulimia nervosa in dental patients: Implications for dental care providers. *General Dentistry* 48:48–52.

CHAPTER ELEVEN

Athletes and Eating Disorders

COMMON QUESTIONS

Do athletics predispose to or protect from eating disorders?

Which sports tend to increase eating disorders in females?

What is the female athletic triad?

Which sports tend to increase eating disorders in males?

What are some vulnerabilities that predispose particular athletes to developing eating disorders?

When does a sport become unhealthy in regard to eating disorder concerns?

What role do coaches play?

How do you approach an athlete about whom you have concerns?

Can athletes who have eating disorders return to sports after treatment?

Do preventive efforts work in sports?

How does muscle/body dysmorphia relate to eating disorders?

How risky are performance-enhancing drugs in relation to the symptomatology of eating disorders?

What role do primary and secondary schools play?

Does losing weight increase performance?

What do overactive, underfed rats teach us?

Case 1

A.B. was a 19-year-old female long-distance runner whose eating disorder began at age 12. Shortly after she entered puberty, she lost weight by dieting because she disliked the changes in her body shape, and menses stopped. She responded to outpatient treatment with limited insight but a 10-pound increase in weight. At age 14, she began to challenge herself with endurance running, a sport in which she excelled, winning many championships. She maintained her weight at an improved, but still low-for-age level, so by 16, she weighed 115 pounds at 5 feet 7 inches tall (BMI 18). Menses never returned due to a combination of low weight and strenuous exercise. In addition to chronic restricted eating, she developed at age 15 a pattern of small binge episodes followed by purging, which led to chronic gastroesophageal reflux; at times unwanted food spontaneously came up into her mouth. At 16, she was placed on metaclopramide one hour before meals, but this was of limited help. In addition to diagnosing and treating her gastroesophageal reflux disease (GERD), her primary care physician referred her to orthopedics for evaluation of chronic knee and hip pain. The more she ran, the more painful her symptoms became, but she had not disclosed her discomfort until her physician found knee pain on palpation.

Orthopedics noted hamstring tendonitis with pes anserine bursitis. Upon examination, A.B. experienced tenderness along the semitendinosus tendon of the pes anserine bursa. With resisted flexion of the knee, she had significant pain. The bursitis was treated with injection into the bursa of 1 percent Xylocaine and 2 cc of Celestone. She obtained complete relief, but would agree to rest for only one day before running 5,000 m the second day after treatment. DEXA scan of bone mineral density showed a deficiency of -2.5 standard deviations in the left hip and -2.0 in the lumbar spine.

Because of significant anxiety, A.B. was started on escitalopram, titrating up to 20 mg/d, with partial relief. She continued to be preoccupied with staying thin and continued to be very competitive. Secondary amenorrhea continued. She was started on Ortho-Novum 1/35 to restore menses artificially. At age 17, she complained of feeling tired, out of energy, and drained. She began falling asleep in classes, a new problem, and started to take naps, something that she previously disdained as a sign of weakness. Lab work revealed total serum iron of 35 mcg/dL (normal 72–130). Iron saturation was 7 percent (normal 27–44). Hemoglobin was 11.0 g/dL (normal 11.9–15). Weight was stable. The night before track competitions, she experienced high anxiety, experienced an increase in regurgitation, and induced vomiting multiple times. For the first time, she had on examination a weepy affect and scratched herself to obtain relief. Escitalopram was increased to 30 mg/d.

At the end of her eighteenth year, she began college. Menses were regular on birth control pills but only 3 days in duration. She took a break from competitive running, working as a library assistant for her freshman year. Her anxiety decreased; she felt "stronger and healthier." Hemoglobin increased to 12.5 g/dL. Weight increased to 120 pounds. She was considered to have improved but to still meet the diagnostic criteria for the female athletic triad because of her continued amenorrhea without oral contraceptive, continued low weight resulting from disordered eating with fear of fatness, and deficient bone mineral density.

At age 19, in the fall of her second year, A.B. resumed running, working up to 60–80 miles per week, with several runs of more than 10 miles. Her gastroesophageal reflux was improved. Anxiety had lessened over her year of abstention from competitive running. She still had joint pain but continued to override it with a "runner's high." Only the future will tell whether she will remain healthy enough to run competitively without serious medical complications. She plans on a career as an orthopedic surgeon.

Case 2

C.D. was a 16-year-old male high school sophomore who was referred by his parents for evaluation of abnormal eating and weight fluctuation. In the eighth grade, at 5 feet 8 inches, he had weighed 185 pounds (BMI 28.2). He became winded running across the football field. When a teammate called him "fat ass," he stopped drinking soda pop and cut out snack food. He reduced his weight to 140 pounds over 18 months, but by then had grown to 6 feet 3 inches tall (BMI 17.5). He became cold compared with others, felt weak, and was mentally preoccupied with his body much of the day.

C.D. then decided to develop his body through body building, eating six meals a day, consisting only of fruits, vegetables, whole grains, chicken, skim milk, and yogurt. He consumed five 2-pound containers of soy protein in short periods of time, causing distress to his parents. He insisted on eating every 90 minutes, consuming a gallon of soy milk and a gallon of water daily. When, on New Year's Day, the fitness club was closed, he went up to the door and pounded on it, then went home and used his weights in the basement. He underwent cycles of weight increase and bulking, followed by cutting weight with running. His goal was to win a body building contest at age 17. He stated, "I don't care what I weigh, as long as I keep getting bigger, get well-defined, and have 'cut' muscles with no body fat."

BMI at the time he was seen in clinic was 22.3 (178.2 pounds, 6 feet 3 inches tall). C.D. looked in every mirror he passed, as well as his reflection in shop windows he passed. He said his self-esteem depended on his body size and shape. He met the criteria for muscle dysmorphic disorder with a past history of anorexia nervosa. His "emergency weights" went with him whenever he left home. He would not answer questions about steroid abuse. He agreed to see a psychologist experienced with athletes for therapy close to his home.

Background

Participation in sports may be a predisposing factor in the development of eating disorders or may be a strongly protective factor. Much depends on the nature of the sport, the gender of the athlete, the motivation and temperament of the athlete, and the actions of the coaching staff, especially for elite athletes. For the majority of the population, sports serve as recreation, as stress release, as a contribution to identity, and as a bonding experience from childhood throughout life, in addition to providing well-documented health benefits, both physical and psychological.

For elite athletes—those on school varsity teams, in competition for the Olympics, and in training for competitive sports like the Boston Marathon, as well as for professionals—the pressures to succeed in sports are greater. Powers and Johnson (1996) described thinness for performance goals and thinness for appearance goals in sports as separate risk factors. The combination, as in girls' gymnastics, appears to pose a greater risk than either separately. Since their delineation of these variables, additional studies have noted the predisposition, primarily in males, to eating disorders when the sport requires substantial muscle development, such as is increasingly common in professional sports (football, baseball) and in competitive nonprofessional sports such as weight lifting and varsity football.

A glance at photos of Joe DiMaggio, a great player in baseball in the past, compared with photos of Barry Bonds or José Conseco in today's game, shows the difference in body bulk that has become almost normative. One report on a university football team defensive line has documented an increase in average body weight of approximately a pound a year for the past 100 years. As with the population in general, female athletes are most liable to develop eating disorders in the context of sports. Compulsive running and working out in gyms by nonathletes who are in the process of developing eating disorders represent secondary overexercise syndromes, rather than predisposing factors.

Table 11.1 suggests, by gender, sports that emphasize thinness or muscle bulk alone (endurance running; weight lifting) versus thinness or muscle bulk plus the added pressure of weight-related appearance norms for adjudicated performances (figure skating; body building).

TABLE 11.1   Body norms or requirements, by gender, of some of the most common sports

Body norm/requirement	Sport by gender	
	Females	Males
Slimness for performance	Cross-country and marathon running	Low-weight crew Cross-country and marathon running Horse racing (jockey) Low-weight wrestling Rock climbing Cycling
Slimness and appearance for adjudicated sports	Ballet Gymnastics Figure skating Diving	Diving Figure skating
Increased muscularity for performance	Sprinting Basketball, softball Weight-lifting	Football, baseball, basketball Hockey Sprinting Weight-lifting
Increased muscularity and appearance for adjudicated sports	Bodybuilding	Gymnastics Bodybuilding

The Prevalence of Eating Disorders in Athletes

The prevalence of eating disorders and eating disordered behaviors among athletes varies greatly from sport to sport. A large study of 1,445 student varsity athletes of all sports surveyed from Division 1 schools found almost 3 percent of females had a clinically significant problem with anorexia nervosa versus 0 percent for males, while 11 percent of females reported binge eating at least weekly versus 13 percent for males (Johnson, Powers, and Dick, 1999). Thirty-one percent of women versus 5 percent of men had BMIs of 20 or lower. Women desired a body with 13 percent fat, while males desired 8.6 percent. Norms for body fat content for women of college age are 19–23 percent and 10–15 percent for men. It was estimated that 34.75 percent of women were at risk for anorexia nervosa, compared to 9.5 percent of males. Regarding bulimic disorders, 38 percent of both females and males were at risk. These were conservative estimates based on the nature of the survey criteria.

Diagnosis and Evaluation of Athletes for Eating Disorders

In sports that encourage thinness for excellence, a number of issues are involved. First, thinness is probably overrated despite the almost unquestioned iconic status given to a skeletal body in some sports. Powers (1999) noted that "athletes think being thinner, no matter what, improves performance. There is good evidence that this is not the case." How much thinness is too much? No easy answer can be given, since the weight-performance relationship varies from sport to sport, but a few guidelines may be helpful. One obvious measure is a decrease in performance. A more subtle measure is present when, despite improved performance, thinness becomes an all-consuming goal. In such cases the athlete is paying excessive attention to limiting calories, weighs frequently, and exhibits the psychological features of starvation, such as decreased mental concentration, lowered mood outside of competitive situations, and obsessive fear of becoming fat. Table 11.2 lists synonyms for anorexia-like syndromes in athletes.

A diagnosis of anorexia nervosa is made, when a clinical interview is possible, with the same criteria noted in Chapter 1. For anorexia nervosa

TABLE 11.2   Other terms for eating and weight disorders in athletes

Obligatory running	Weight cycling
Anorexia athletica	Reverse anorexia
Pathogenic weight control	Exercise dependence
Activity induced anorexia	Cutting weight
Female athletic triad	Manorexia

these criteria are overvaluation of the benefits of thinness, self-induced starvation to a degree producing medical or psychological symptomatology, a morbid fear of becoming fat, and, often, overestimation of body size despite obvious thinness. For bulimia nervosa symptoms are frequent episodes of binge eating that lead to guilt, regret, or medical discomfort followed by compensation by purging (80%) or nonpurging methods (stricter dieting, increased exercise, 20%). Screening questionnaires are useful for identifying eating disorders, but there is a tendency for athletes to "fake normal" to avoid limitations in sports activities. Additionally, less ethical coaches may limit access to athletes, or, more benign in intent but no less damaging in consequence, coaches may simply ignore or be unaware of eating disorders symptomatology in the face of "win at all costs" attitude. Bulimia in athletes is not as obvious as the publicly visible body of anorexic athletes, but bulimic athletes have similar preoccupations with weight at less thin levels. Binge eating disorder is seldom present in sports mandating thinness.

Predisposing Factors

Table 11.3 lists some predisposing factors to the development of eating disorders in athletes. The nature of the sport is a major factor in the probability of developing an eating disorder, but an unresolved question is whether more predisposed individuals are more attracted to certain sports, such as endurance running. Certain sports, like girls' gymnastics, with its requirements of thinness for both performance and appearance standards, appear to try to maintain girls at a prepubertal weight with minimal breast development and continued open epiphyses for longer bones. This stance presents ethical problems that are sometimes over-

TABLE 11.3   Psychological and behavioral characteristics that predispose athletes to eating disorders

Perfectionism	Emotional immaturity relative to age
Low self-esteem	All-or-none reasoning: winning versus
Lack of identity outside of sports	failure seen as only outcomes
Sports injury limiting participation	Excess parental pressure
Rejection sensitivity	External locus of control
History of childhood/	Participation in sports to please others
preadolescent obesity	Body weight dissatisfaction
History of abuse	Chronic dieting, frequent weighing
Body/muscle dysmorphia	Anxious or depressive illness or traits
Social isolation	

looked by trainers and coaches. There are exceptions, thankfully, in the performance of some normal-weight world-class female athletes competing in gymnastics.

Ballet is in many ways an athletic activity, requiring more and more athleticism in modern dance. In preprofessional schools of ballet, a high percentage of girls (50% in one study) have amenorrhea, and there is a sevenfold increase in cases of anorexia nervosa compared with the general population. Anorexia nervosa is as much a correct diagnosis when there is failure to increase in weight proportional to increases in height and age, as when there is a loss of weight through dieting and excess exercise.

Psychological factors play a major role in predisposition to eating disorders in athletes. An external locus of control—jargon for letting self-esteem be based primarily on approval from others—mandates continued winning in athletics at all costs, a fragile basis for self-esteem. An external locus of control predisposes an athlete to be excessively sensitive to comments from coaches and peers. Perfectionism is associated with all-or-none thinking: not winning equals losing and being a failure. An added burden is rejection sensitivity, with the perception that less than first place is assumed to be a rejection. Performance anxiety may be severe enough that an eating disorder comes to be an alternative strategy for relief from anxious participation in sports.

A sports injury may represent an annoyance or a major tragedy in the mind of an athlete. For those with little identity outside of athletics, an injury that requires a time of healing away from sports—or more traumatic, discontinuation of a sport in which the athlete had shown excellence—can be devastating. During time away from sports, an injured athlete may overcompensate for reduced energy output by an excessive restriction of food intake, predisposing the athlete to anorexia nervosa. In addition, for those with an almost exclusive focus on sports for identity, depression, demoralization, and a perception that life has passed them by, may ensue. Overuse injuries represent an imbalance between activity and recuperative forces, fostered by drivenness in athletics.

Risk of Eating Disorders by Gender and Sport

GENDER-NEUTRAL SPORTS

Numerous studies have evaluated symptoms of eating disorders in endurance runners and triathletes. Thompson (2007) found that 19.4 percent of female cross-country runners had previous or current eating disorders, 23 percent had irregular or absent menses, and 29.1 percent had inadequate calcium intake. Low lumbar spine bone mineral density was found in both male and female endurance runners (Hind, Truscott, and Evans, 2006). The majority of female triathletes with a healthy BMI desired to be smaller versus 19.3 percent in males (DiGioacchino DeBate, Wethington, and Sargent, 2001). High dietary restraint, a prelude to eating disorders, has been documented in female adolescent endurance runners (Barrack et al., 2008). A Scandinavian study found a high proportion (46.7%) of athletes in leanness sports had clinical eating disorders versus 19.8 percent in nonleanness sports (Torstveit, Rosenvinge, and Sundgot-Borgen, 2008).

FEMALE-RELATED SPORTS

The *female athletic triad* is a construct referring to a combination of an eating disorder, amenorrhea, and osteoporosis that can develop in young female athletes who have achieved a low body weight (Sundgot-Borgen, 1994). Most amenorrheic distance-running young women had a relative with a mood disorder and/or an eating disorder, while no relatives were affected with an eating disorder or a mood disorder in a comparison group of eumenorrheic runners (Gadpaille, Sanborn, and Wagner, 1987). A family history of mood or eating disorders predisposes female athletes to seek low body weights.

Women's gymnastics contrasts markedly with men's gymnastics. The ideal female performer is often very young, often prepubertal in endocrine development. Pubertal changes may diminish flexibility and competitive performance in complex gymnastic maneuvers. Female gymnasts accepted into college on sports scholarships may find their body development into an adult habitus endangers their performance and their scholarship status. In contrast, male gymnasts often do not reach their peak until the end of college years or shortly thereafter, with developmental body changes along with strenuous training improving their performance.

Only a few female sports require increased muscularity and weight. These sports—for example, female bodybuilding—are somewhat anomalous for most young women. Lean muscularity is more normative in female sprinters. In both of these categories, females may be at risk for anabolic steroid abuse, more common in male athletes.

MALE-RELATED SPORTS

Thinness for performance in males as a risk factor for eating-disordered behavior has been documented in lightweight rowers compared to heavyweight rowers (Pietrowsky and Straub, 2008), with lightweight rowers scoring very high on restrained eating and body dissatisfaction. Thinness for performance as a risk factor has also been documented in low-weight wrestlers (Thiel, Gottfried, and Hesse, 1993), as well as in male racing jockeys (King and Mezey, 1987), young rock climbers (Morrison and Schöffl, 2007), and male cyclists (Riebl et al., 2007).

Many primarily male sports require increased muscle bulk, usually associated with striving for extremely low body fat at the same time. The more professional the level of participation in the major sports (football, baseball, basketball, hockey), the more muscularity is valued, with a few exceptions, such as the quarterback in football, who may maintain slim muscularity in place of bulky muscularity. For male sports requiring both greatly defined muscularity and low body fat, such as body building, the dark side of competitiveness enters with abuse of anabolic steroids, often at heroic doses (Pope and Kanayama, 2004). These athletes may have "reverse anorexia," which is characterized by perceptual distortion of the opposite kind seen in female anorexia nervosa—never being large enough, muscular enough, insufficiently "cut," and too fat, even at very low percentages of body fat. Binge eating is common.

Some of the health hazards of anabolic steroid abuse, in both genders, include excessive weight increase, abnormal liver function tests, increased hemoglobin (predisposing to strokes, blood clots), and abnormal functioning of reproductive hormones. The quest for performance and winning gold, unfortunately, overrides rational consideration of the health hazards of anabolic steroids (see Table 11.4). In males, especially, the judgment centers of the brain, primarily in the prefrontal cortex, develop later, hopefully by the mid-20s, compared with the earlier, less regulated impulsivity centered in the amygdala. The catchphrase "Get big or die" is unfortunately too often promoted. "Get big and live—by healthy means" is a rational choice, in contrast.

TABLE 11.4   Medical and psychological problems associated with abuse of anabolic steroids

Males	Females	Both genders
Atrophy of testes	Facial hair	Acne
Reduced sperm count	Irregular or absent menses	Abnormal liver function, jaundice
Impotence		
Baldness	Clitoral enlargement	Reduced "good" (HDL) cholesterol
Gynecomastia (enlarged breasts)	Deepened voice	
	Reduced breast size	Increased chance of injury to tendons, ligaments
Premature prostate enlargement	Laryngeal enlargement	
		Edema, fluid retention
Increased rage and lack of anger control in predisposed males		Increased body weight
		Increased hemoglobin (clots, strokes)

Treatment Recommendations for Athletes

How can I approach an athlete with a possible eating disorder? is the first question worried peers, teaches, coaches, and parents ask. A nonjudgmental expression of concern is the beginning. When several concerned individuals, such as peers and a coach, together approach the athlete and give a specific recommendation to an expert in eating disorders who is familiar with athletes, the athlete will often accept a confidential referral. A period of absence from a sport until improvement occurs is often necessary, but the long-term goal of coming back as an even better athlete needs to be stressed. Occasionally an athlete is simply not suited to a particular sport. For example, a larger-boned woman who wants to compete with low BMI endurance runners may do better in another sport. Similarly, a larger male who wants to row in lightweight crew is at increased probability for an eating disorder.

The core of eating disorders, of course, has little to do with weight, shape, or food. Eating disorders are strategies for dealing with deeper issues in life, such as peer approval, self-esteem, perfectionism, lack of balance, developmental arrests, mood regulation, and relationship conflicts. Activities therapy experts in an experienced eating disorders team can guide the athlete back into a slowly graded increase in athleticism as the eating disorder improves. Significantly lowered bone density, probably less than -2 standard deviations from norms, suggests that high-impact sports should be avoided. Specific advice about participation in a sport with be geared toward individual differences. Intervention in the female athletic triad early on benefits the long-term health of girls and women (Lebrun, 2007).

The injured athlete presents a challenge, especially when that person's identity is largely centered on excellence in sports. Early intervention in injuries, rather than after repeated trauma to joints, ligaments, and tendons ("Let me complete the season"), is essential.

Inappropriate dietary restraint is unhealthy, whereas abstention from "junk foods" high in transfats or concentrated sweets, is healthy. Excess dietary restriction limits calcium, an essential component of improved bone mineral density. Up to 95 percent of bone density is completed by the late teen years. Lowered calcium intake during those years has long-term consequences in building strong bones that will last a lifetime.

Garner, Rosen, and Barry (1998) summarize recommendations for intervention and treatment in eating-disordered athletes.

Typically, a team approach to treatment of the athlete with an eating disorder (see Chap. 2) works best, with the coach and the trainer being involved in nonconfidential aspects of the treatment. No specific psychopharmacological agents have been shown to be of benefit in the treatment of anorexia nervosa, but specific antidepressants may be individually prescribed, especially for comorbid depression and anxiety. For bulimia nervosa, cognitive-behavioral therapy is still the gold standard, but here too, antidepressants may be of use as minority partners in treatment.

The Role of Coaches in Promoting or Preventing Eating Disorders

Coaches can either promote eating disorders among athletes or be essential partners in their treatment by supporting the clinician and encouraging the athlete to seek full remission of the eating disorder rather than a small amount of improvement. Coaching style clearly affects an athlete's vulnerability to an eating disorder. There are important ethical issues in coaching. Placing the long-term welfare of the athlete first is crucial. The "winning at all cost" philosophy is unethical, certainly from grade school through college. Professional athletes may choose to play when injured and are of reasonable age to make such a choice, even though it is an unwise one. Developing young athletes are not able to make choices against their best interest in good conscience, despite what they think, and may be overly influenced by pressure from coaches to place performance above all else. Good coaches are among the most influential and admired persons in an athlete's life. One study (Sundgot-Borgen, 1994) found that 67 percent of athletes with eating disorders reported that they were dieting on advice by their coach. Sherman et al. (2005) summarized the role of the coach in identifying and managing athletes with disordered eating in 23 sports, noting that "athletic trainers, teammates, and coaches are frequently involved in identification."

Case 3

E.F. was a 21-year-old junior from the University of Kansas who self-referred for continuation of treatment for an eating disorder. She had been diagnosed with an eating disorder her sophomore year in high school. Despite having had surgery on her knee, she decided to lose weight because her coach told her to get thinner. She went from 140 pounds at 5 feet 8 inches tall (BMI 21.2) to 105 pounds (BMI 16.8), eating 300 calories a day. The patient realized she was too thin, decided to increase her lean muscle weight by weight lifting, and restored to 130 pounds (BMI 19.8), with body fat of 13 percent. Her menses stopped. She switched to basketball, again restricted, and began to binge-eat and induce vomiting before each game. A diagnosis of a stress fracture was made when she reported foot pain. At 135 pounds (BMI 20.6) she reported to volleyball summer camp. The coach said she needed to lose "quite a bit of weight" if she wanted a college athletic scholarship. She reduced to 105 pounds again, the weight at which she reported to college.

In college, she could not stop throwing up spontaneously and lost weight to 95 pounds (BMI 14.5). She required treatment in an emergency room for dehydration. A shoulder tear required surgery, and she increased weight during convalescence. At the soonest possible time after surgery, she returned to working out, exercising 8–10 hours per day, and reduced her weight to 93 pounds (BMI 14.2). Her binge-purge cycles, throwing up 20 times a night, required repeated emergency room treatments with IV fluids. She often had EKG abnormalities. The school restricted her athletic training and forbade volleyball practice. When she tried to restore weight using weight lifting, a trainer threw her out of the training room because she did not officially belong to a team anymore.

When she began to work out informally with the tennis team, the coach said he wanted to "break her," and the trainer kept asking her if she had "had enough yet?" She continued to binge and purge 2–3 times a day, with binges now triggered by any "crummy feeling" rather than hunger. She continued to work out 4–5 hours per day, despite stress fractures, engaging in running and weight lifting. She met the criteria for anorexia nervosa, binge-purge subtype, and obsessive compulsive disorder.

A year later she presented herself to clinic weighing 169 pounds (BMI 25.7). By that time her illness had migrated to a diagnosis of bulimia nervosa, purging subtype. She complained of a sore throat and hoarseness and had significant parotid swelling. Despite being at a higher weight, she never regained menses. She used six laxatives a day, felt cold, and was continually preoccupied with thoughts of food and weight. Her mood was low, and the perfectionistic aspects of her temperament were apparent. She agreed to treatment, but having concealed her disorder from her college, she required that they not be told. Her future was unclear. She illustrates the complex course of an eating disorder in an athlete driven to put sports ahead of health.

The Role of Schools in Healthy Athleticism

Schools, by their action or inaction, promote or hinder healthy athleticism. Table 11.5 summarizes some of the school policies and practices that promote healthy sports. The ruthless decimation of sports activities for average students during school years only leads to more obesity and later heart disease, major public health issues. It is said that "World War II was won on the playing fields of Eton" in terms of building character and fitness. Likewise, many of the lifelong hazards of adulthood in modern society may be prevented or lessened by participation of all students in sports of some kind, and certainly in daily physical activity. The contribution of regular participation in aerobic sports, as well as in strength training, to achieve "mens sana in corpore sano"—a healthy mind in a healthy body—is supported by many evidence-based studies. Regular exercise can be as effective as antidepressants in nonpsychotic depression and in anxiety states.

The division of students at about the middle school level into elite athletes for whom facilities are provided while neglecting serious athletics for the large majority is an invidious practice. School board decisions govern these practices of attention and neglect. While political advocacy is not the usual focus of an academic physician, this author strongly supports the use of tax monies for serious daily physical education in schools and the participation of all students in some level of sports, with financial support for these activities as assured as for teaching English and mathematics. Unfortunately, most students cannot afford the expensive preparatory schools that have already implemented this kind of balanced education.

TABLE 11.5 School policies and practices to promote fitness and prevent eating disorders

- Involve all students in athletics: cardiopulmonary, strength, flexibility, team sports.
- Stop limiting athletics to elite athletes, as is currently done beginning in junior high school.
- Regulate the body fat and recent weight loss allowed in wrestlers, cross-country and endurance runners, and gymnasts.
- Identify eating disorders early and refer students for treatment.
- Involve coaches in designing a programmatic balance between promoting competitiveness and preventing eating- and weight-disordered behavior.
- Specially monitor sports requiring leanness and good appearance (girls' gymnastics, cross-country, ballet).
- Involve parents with coaches in programmatic balance with coaches.
- Include judges of adjudicated sports in the loop with health professionals, coaches, and parents for a role in promoting fitness.
- Emphasize fitness in place of thinness.
- Make nutritional education and school lunches fun and healthy at the same time.
- Take out soda machines.
- Provide individualized programs for academic year athletic goals for each student.
- Provide psychological counseling for injured athletes unable to perform.
- Promote a functional view of body in girls and young women versus objectification of body size and shape for critical judging by self and others.
- Emphasize lifetime "carryover" sports and fitness patterns for after school years.

Prevention

Means of preventing eating disorders in athletes vary among nations. Norway, for example, has a nurse clinician in each district who is trained to intervene early with athletes who might have an eating disorder. The United Kingdom and the United States tend to wait until eating disorders are more fully entrenched, or to ignore their existence in the service of winning performances. Powers and Johnson (1996) address "small victories" that are occurring in prevention of eating disorders in athletes. Oppliger et al. (1995) report on states such as Wisconsin that have instituted mandatory standards to limit unhealthy dieting among student wrestlers. Limiting the amount of weight that may be lost to participate in endurance running or ballet will sometimes turn around a potential eating disorder before it reaches the point of having no voluntary component.

More indirect, long-term preventive efforts, include changing the culture whereby women's bodies are objectified. Young women need to learn to view their bodies from a stance of functional instrumentality (i.e., having a healthy body to *do* things), not to be objectified and judged by peers or oneself in terms of thinness norms. Skepticism of the media is healthy, as is replacing magazines that promote thinness with healthy role models. "Normative cultural distress"—giving lip service to the need to diet a little, but having that desert anyway—is healthy; a total unconcern about weight is unrealistic. Building "body armor" by encouraging a balance between sports participation and academics in girls will allow girls to increase in self-esteem by internalizing skills in athletics during developmentally critical years.

Dieting is the crucial behavior that promotes a transition from an athlete with a culturally healthy concern about weight to one with an eating disorder. We are as much an underfit nation as an overfat nation. If every parent required each student to present a sweat-stained T-shirt before allowing the student to use a computer or play video games, there would be less adolescent obesity and less need or desire to diet. "Diet" is, after all, a four-letter word.

Basic Science Research: What Can Rats Teach Us?

Scientists have reproduced in laboratory rats conditions similar to those faced by athletes: unrestricted access to an activity wheel and restricted food intake. This combination of "dieting" plus hyperactivity, very common in athletes, leads to a vicious circle of more weight loss and eating less and less food, despite availability of calories. Activity-based anorexia is facilitated by neuropeptide Y (Nergårdh et al., 2007) and suppressed by leptin (Exner et al., 2000), suggesting that this anorexia nervosa hyperactivity and self-starvation model is regulated in the hypothalamus and other limbic system areas, areas in which neuropeptide Y and leptin interact. The basic science model of anorexia, of course, cannot duplicate the overvaluation of thinness, but it does strongly suggest that biological factors may lock in anorexia nervosa when conditions similar to those under which athletes compete are present. Obligatory runners and other compulsive exercisers will often feel dysphoric when not allowed to run. Eating disorders may be initiated by choice but also may be sustained past a certain point by brain peptides.

Summary

Eating disorders are a major concern in the field of athletics. The emphasis on thinness for performance and appearance increases the probability of developing an eating disorder. The participation of predisposed young athletes with a number of risk factors in these thinness-mandating sports leads to the highest prevalence of eating disorders. Clinicians need to be knowledgeable about the healthy and unhealthy aspects of sports and to work closely with coaches, trainers, and sports educators. Success in detecting eating disorders by having athletes respond to questionnaires is limited by a number of factors, including the athlete's wish to appear healthy and fit and not be excluded from sports participation. A well-educated, ethical coach, as well as a programmatic school-based approach to prevention, can identity and treat or, even better, prevent eating disorders.

REFERENCES

Barrack MT, Rauh MJ, Barkai HS, and Nichols JF. 2008. Dietary restraint and low bone mass in female adolescent endurance runners. *American Journal of Clinical Nutrition* 87(1):36–43.

DiGioacchino DeBate R, Wethington H, and Sargent R. 2002. Body size dissatisfaction among male and female triathletes. *Eating and Weight Disorders* 7:316–23.

Exner C, Hebebrand J, Remschmidt H, et al. 2000. Leptin suppresses semi-starvation induced hyperactivity in rats: Implications for anorexia nervosa. *Molecular Psychiatry* 5(5):476–81.

Gadpaille WJ, Sanborn CF, and Wagner WW. 1987. Athletic amenorrhea, major affective disorders and eating disorders. *American Journal of Psychiatry* 144:939–42.

Garner DM, Rosen LW, and Barry D. 1998. Eating disorders among athletes:

Research and recommendations. *Child and Adolescent Psychiatric Clinics of North America* 7(4):839–57.

Hind K, Truscott JG, and Evans JA. 2006. Low lumbar spine bone mineral density in both male and female endurance runners. *Bone* 39(4):880–85.

Johnson C, Powers PS, and Dick R. 1999. Athletes and eating disorders: The National Collegiate Athletic Association study. *International Journal of Eating Disorders* 26:179–88.

King MB and Mezcy G. 1987. Eating behaviour of male racing jockeys. *Psychological Medicine* 17:249–53.

Lebrun CM. 2007. The female athlete triad: What's a doctor to do? *Current Sports Medicine Reports* 6(6):397–404.

Morrison AB and Schöffl VR. 2007. Physiological responses to rock climbing in young climbers. *British Journal of Sports Medicine* 41(12):852–61; discussion 861.

Nergårdh R, Ammar A, Brodin U, Bergström J, Scheurink A, and Södersten P. 2007. Neuropeptide Y facilitates activity-based-anorexia. *Psychoneuroendocrinology* 32(5):493–502.

Oppliger RA, Harms RD, Herrmann DE, Streich CM, and Clark RR. 1995. Grappling with weight cutting: The Wisconsin wrestling minimum weight project. *The Physician and Sportsmedicine* 23(3):69–78.

Pietrowsky R and Straub K. 2008. Body dissatisfaction and restrained eating in male juvenile and adult athletes. *Eating and Weight Disorders* 13(1):14–21.

Pope HG Jr and Kanayama G. 2004. Bodybuilding's dark side: Clues to anabolic steroid use. *Current Psychiatry* 3(12):12–20.

Powers PS. 1999. Athletes and eating disorders: Some ramifications of the NCAA study. *Eating Disorders Review* 10(6):1–3.

Powers PS and Johnson C. 1996. Small victories: Prevention of eating disorders among athletes. *Eating Disorders* 4(4):364–77

Riebl SK, Subudhi AW, Broker JP, Schenck K, and Berning JR. 2007. The prevalence of subclinical eating disorders among male cyclists. *Journal of the American Dietetic Association* 107(7):1214–17.

Sherman RT, Thompson RA, Dehass D, and Wilfert M. 2005. NCAA coaches survey: The role of the coach in identifying and managing athletes with disordered eating. *Eating Disorders* 13:447–66.

Sundgot-Borgen J. 1994. Risk and trigger factors for the development of eating disorders in female elite athletes. *Medicine and Science in Sports and Exercise* 26:414–19.

Thiel A, Gottfried H, and Hesse FW. 1993. Subclinical eating disorders in male athletes: A study of the low weight category in rowers and wrestlers. *Acta Psychiatrica Scandinavica* 88:259–65.

Thompson SH. 2007. Characteristics of the female athlete triad in collegiate cross-country runners. *Journal of American College Health* 56(2):129–36.

Torstveit MK, Rosenvinge JH, and Sundgot-Borgen J. 2008. Prevalence of eating disorders and the predictive power of risk models in female elite athletes: A controlled study. *Scandinavian Journal of Medicine and Science in Sports* 18(1):108–18.

CHAPTER TWELVE

Males with Eating Disorders

COMMON QUESTIONS

How is the diagnosis of eating disorders different in males and females?

Which males are more likely to develop eating disorders?

What is the prevalence of eating disorders in males?

What are the medical needs of males with eating disorders?

How can males with anorexia nervosa achieve a desired body shape and be less likely to return to dieting after weight restoration?

Do males with eating disorders develop osteoporosis?

What are the most common comorbid disorders in males?

How do you determine a target weight for anorexic males?

How do you treat binge eating disorder in an obese male?

Can an eating-disordered male return to intensive sports activities?

What is the body image most males desire?

How common is a gay orientation in eating disordered males?

Case

C.R. was an 18-year-old male admitted for treatment of anorexia nervosa, binge-purge subtype. As a preteenager, he had been teased for having a "gut." At age 14, at 170 pounds, 5 feet 6 inches tall (BMI 27.5), he dieted to improve his performance in wrestling. In the spring of each year, he dieted more intensively to improve his cross-country running. By age 16, he weighed 115 pounds at 5 feet 8 inches (BMI 17.5) and began to experience regular binge-purge episodes, with purges increasing to three times a day before admission. His weight increased to 125 pounds while he was in outpatient therapy, but his binge-purges did not decrease.

C.R.'s childhood had been marked by his father's verbal abuse of him and his mother when the father was drunk, leading to a divorce when C.R. was 10, and only occasional contact between the patient and his biological father thereafter, unknown to his mother, who was protective of the patient, not allowing contact with the father. In the year before admission, C.R. had experienced depressed mood.

As his weight declined, he was no longer able to participate in sports because of weakness. Testosterone decreased to 200 (normal 340–800 ng/dL). His sexual drive diminished, but he continued to "hang out" with his girlfriend. TSH and T4 were normal. Potassium was slightly low at 3.3 meq/L. During treatment, his weight improved, and he gained skills in cognitive-behavioral therapy to challenge his overvaluation of the benefits of obtaining better athletic performance through dieting. Sertraline, titrated up to 100 mg/d, was added for antidepressant effect. In men's group, the patient began to open up and discuss his emotions and the challenges of response inhibition of his urges to purge. He decided against joining the Marine Corps as a way to "grow up." Instead, he began courses at a community college toward an A.A. degree. Testosterone levels increased to normal range after two months in his target weight range of 143–47 pounds. He gradually returned to recreational sports.

Background

Galen said that men did not withstand fasting as well as women. Western societies have been less preoccupied with promoting thinness in males compared with the brain-washing about weight directed toward females. But men have been vitally concerned about body shape, with half of males wishing to increase weight and half wishing to decrease, in both cases most commonly with the goal of improving body shape rather than of achieving a certain weight. The "holy grail" of body definition for most males is lean muscularity (David Beckham, Brad Pitt), although a minority wish boney thinness (Mick Jagger) or extreme muscle gain without fat (Arnold Schwarzenegger). The media have increasingly presented extreme images of impossibly fit males with "washboard abs" as ideals, resulting in viewers' and readers' making negative self-comparisons (Hobza et al., 2007). The three most common body image ideals in males with eating disorders are shown in Figures 12.1, 12.2, and 12.3: the very thin ideal, the lean muscular ideal, and the extreme muscled body builder.

In the social learning process, boys learn to perceive themselves as fat on the average only at weights slightly above population norms, while

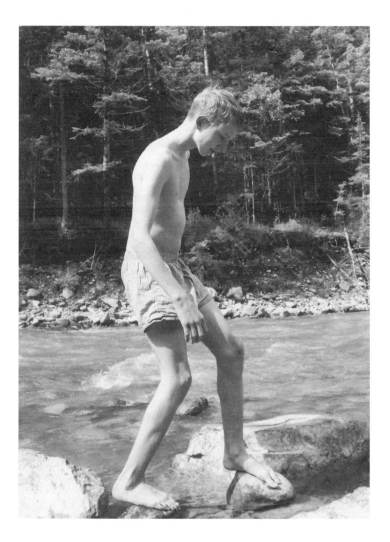

FIGURE 12.1. Thin ideal. (*Source:* istockphoto.com.)

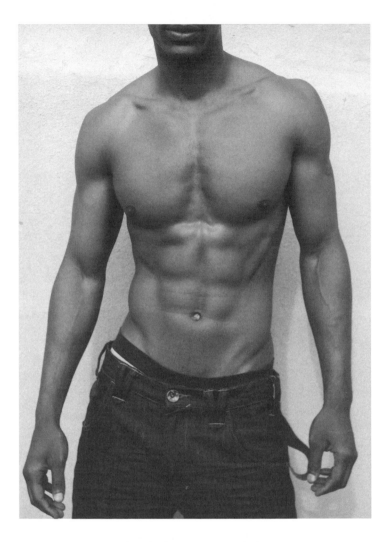

FIGURE 12.2. Lean muscular ideal. *(Source:* istockphoto.com.)

women perceive themselves as fat at more than 15–18 percent below population norms. This early social learning process takes place largely between the first and fifth grades. After that time, there exists a continuing perception of body fatness in 40–75 percent of school-age girls (Schreiber et al., 1996) and in about half as many boys. Actual obesity, even by medical standards, is lower, despite recent increases in average weights.

Because there is less general cultural endorsement for boys to diet, they tend to do so only when they are objectively heavier than average and commonly for four specific reasons: (1) to avoid being teased for childhood obesity; (2) to increase sports performance; (3) to avoid developing weight-related medical illnesses that they have seen in their fathers; and (4) to improve a gay relationship. More than half of our males

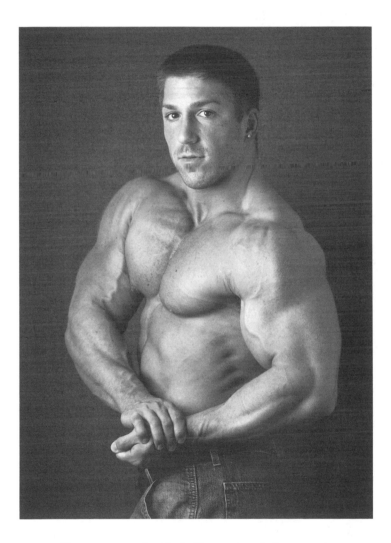

FIGURE 12.3. Extreme muscular ideal. (*Source:* istockphoto.com.)

with eating disorders began dieting for one of these reasons, in contrast to approximately 10 percent of girls. Males with eating disorders fall into three age categories: childhood onset before twelve years of age, an adolescent category up to the early twenties, and young or more mature adults. The issues prompting dieting in these three groups are quite different, with very young boys often expressing family issues; adolescent males struggling with general identity and performance concerns, especially in sports or dating; and older males dealing with workplace advancement, new sexual partners, or health concerns. Eating disorders have been diagnosed in males from 10 to 60, even though onset in the majority of cases is in the teens and early twenties.

About 18 percent of males with eating disorders have a gay orientation, approximately four or five times the population average, but still a minority (Fichter and Dasher, 1987). The reason for this increased sexual orientation appears to be the increased valuation of thinness, especially thin muscularity, in the gay culture rather than any intrinsic consequence of sexual orientation. Bulimic males with gay orientation are at increased risk for HIV infection due to unprotected impulsive sexuality. Many young anorexic males are simply asexual.

Diagnosis of Eating Disorders in Males

The first concern in male patients is simply to think of eating disorders as a diagnostic possibility rather than to overlook abnormal eating and body image preoccupation as "guy behavior." For some time, physicians dismissed the possibility of eating disorders in males because boys and men did not fit within archaic psychoanalytic formulations or because they could not manifest amenorrhea. Yet the first report of anorexia in the English language, in the late 1500s, and the first modern studies in England by Sir William Gull in 1873, included males (Gull, 1873).

Diagnosis of an eating disorder in males is made by criteria similar to those used to diagnose women, with some differences. It is important to state that diagnosis is made simply and accurately by a brief set of questions and responses in the patient's history and interview, and *not by ruling out all conceivable medical possibilities*. Anorexia nervosa requires the presence of (1) self-induced starvation (with or without binge-purge features); (2) a morbid fear of becoming fat and/or a relentless drive for thinness, leading to substantial and sustained weight loss over at least three months; (3) abnormality of reproductive hormones (because amenorrhea is impossible); (4) general medical signs of starvation; and (5), among many, a distorted perception of body image. Abnormality of reproductive hormones (low testosterone, LH, FSH), as with amenorrhea, is probably a simple secondary consequence of weight loss rather than an intrinsic part of the disorder. Many, but not all males have a distorted perception of body image, seeing themselves as fatter than they are or viewing some body part as unacceptably fat, despite overall starvation.

Males with bulimia nervosa in the normal or overweight range experience binge eating, followed in 80 percent of cases by purging, but in 20 percent by other forms of compensation, such as overexercise or additional food restriction. Increasingly recognized is the presence of binge eating disorder (BED), binge eating in males with no purging or any other compensation (Pope et al., 2006). Binge eating disorder occurs primarily in older males, in their 30s to 50s, and is more common than anorexia nervosa or bulimia nervosa. It is often intermixed with mild to severe medical obesity. Bulimic males are more likely than females to have the companion disorders of substance abuse and antisocial personality features. In contrast, most anorexic males with restricting subtype have self-critical, anxious, persevering, perfectionistic, or obsessive-compulsive personality features.

The issue is not settled as to whether the lower number of males with eating disorders is because males are less exposed than females to social pressures promoting thinness, or because they have intrinsic biological protection against eating disorders. The prevalence of eating disorders in males is somewhat controversial, but it is much more common that the previous estimates of 1:10–20 male-to-female ratio. Most recent community-based studies support a ratio of 1:2–3 of males to females with some form of eating disorder (Woodside et al., 2001; Hudson et al., 2007). The much lower ratio of male to female patients that are seen in eating disorder clinics means that many males are overlooked in diagnosis or inhibited from coming for help.

Males who participate in sports, hobbies, or vocations requiring thinness for appearance or performance, or both, develop eating-disordered behaviors more commonly than other males (Thiel, Gottfried, and Hesse, 1993). About 18 percent of high school males who wrestle show some form of eating-disordered behavior and thinking during the wrestling season (Oppliger et al., 1993), although most of them improve spontaneously when the season is over. A high percentage of males in wrestling, gymnastics, swimming, track, horse racing, and football are vulnerable to eating disorders, with the direction of weight change desired determined by the nature of the sport. Before stricter regulations were put in place in some states recently, many wrestlers attempted to wrestle in artificially low weight categories. The recent deaths of the three wrestlers noted in the media have highlighted the dangers of rapid and excessive weight loss. Other sports in which males participate extensively, such as bodybuilding and football, may require artificial gains in weight. The jury is out on whether the common use of creatinine supplements to increase muscle mass is unhealthy. Male weightlifters are especially subject to muscle dysmorphia (Olivardia, Pope, and Hudson, 2000) and eating disorders (Ruffolo et al., 2006).

Some forms of eating disorder occur relatively exclusively in males. Males who think of themselves as never being big enough, never muscular enough, even though large and "cut," may suffer from "reverse anorexia," a form of body dysmorphia. Adolescent males with gynecomastia are very sensitive about chest shape and may initiate dieting to get rid of their breasts (Fisher and Fornari, 1990). Surgical reduction is very successful.

The very starved male and female patients are similar medically with the exception that the male starts with a lower reserve percentage of body fat and a higher lean muscle mass, allowing him less weight loss before the onset of ketosis from protein breakdown. Males appear to be less attentive to taking vitamins while dieting and may also suffer more vitamin deficiency syndromes. In contrast to the occurrence of amenorrhea in females, males have no comparable "signal" that alerts a family and others to the medical consequences of weight loss. In addition, boys and men who suspect they may have an eating disorder often perceive, accurately, stigma from society, from eating-disordered females, and from peers, and thus may be hesitant to discuss this possibility with clinicians. Unfortunately, many professionals also fail to recognize eating disorders in males, either through theoretical bias or lack of diagnostic training. Not uncommonly, we treat males whose eating disorders were only belatedly recognized because of denial of illness or stigma, or who were refused treatment in other programs simply because they are male.

TABLE 12.1   Clinical features of males with eating disorders

---

1. Feeling of increased stigma from self, from society, and from female peers with eating disorders

2. Less recognition from professionals of the possibility of an eating disorder. Increased probability among participants in sports requiring weight loss for performance or appearance, and among persons with vulnerable personality, childhood obesity, gay orientation

4. High probability of comorbid substance abuse as well as presence of OCD, depression

5. Anorexia nervosa usually associated with low plasma testosterone, low LH and FSH

6. Preoccupation with stomach, chest, shoulders, arms, upper body

7. Binge eating disorder as common in males as in females, often associated with obesity

---

Men in general are more dissatisfied with their bodies waist-up, while women are predominantly dissatisfied waist-down (see Table 12.1). Most anorexic men and boys find that relentless self-starving does not produce the shape change they desire despite drastic weight change and become morbidly afraid of being fat, despite evident thinness, if some body part, especially the stomach, has not been visibly reduced. There is a strong possibility that the cultural pattern of valuing thinness in women has not been followed by men because, in the early to mid-1980s, the thin, cachectic male became socially identified with possible AIDS.

Because males, compared with females, develop within a different social learning experience regarding ideal body weight and shape, have a different hormonal milieu, value different goals in sports, diet for different and more personal reasons, may have different comorbid disorders, and will be returning to a different gender role in society, it is of great importance for the clinician to recognize and treat males with eating disorders, respecting the male-specific components in diagnosis and treatment.

Medical Evaluation

In the history-taking part of the evaluation, unless the patient has been initially referred with a diagnosis of an eating disorder, the physician, physician's assistant, or advanced registered nurse practitioner (ARNP)

will make the diagnosis in a straightforward manner by appropriate questions as described in Chapter 3. It is helpful to have a short set of diagnostic screening questions for each common behavioral disorder and age group, comparable to the CAGE questionnaire for alcohol abuse. A comparable set of screening questions regarding eating disorders is the SCOFF questionnaire (see Table 1.3) (Morgan, Reid, and Lacey, 1999).

Participation by the patient in higher-risk sports that emphasize thinness for appearance or shape will alert the physician to pose diagnostic questions even in a routine physical of a young male, as will unexplained low potassium, weight loss of more than 15 pounds, parotid gland swelling (from purging), or nonspecific gastrointestinal discomfort. The primary care physician will ask about changes in eating and exercise history and in the results of the physical examination compared with previous visits. Once the diagnosis of an eating disorder has been made, or if the patient has been referred to the primary care clinician with a diagnosis of an eating disorder, then the circumstances around the patient's onset of weight loss or binge-purge activities should be explored, especially the reason for weight or shape change and the methods of weight loss. It is interesting to note that with mixed-gender twins, the male twin may be at increased risk of anorexia nervosa from the intrauterine hormonal milieu due to hormonal production by the female twin (Procopio and Marriott, 2007), suggesting that gender effects begin as early as *in utero*.

Eating disorders almost always come as "package deals," with one to several comorbid psychiatric diagnoses separate from the eating disorder. Depression is seen in 50–70 percent of males with eating disorders, a number comparable to the occurrence in eating-disordered females. Other diagnoses are more likely in males than in females. At times the comorbid condition—such as substance abuse, OCD, and impulsive, antisocial personality traits—will determine the long-term prognosis more than the eating disorder itself. If street drugs have been used, their relationship to the eating disorder should be explored; for example, it is not uncommon to snort a line of cocaine to inhibit an urge to binge or to promote further weight loss. The presence and medical consequences of compulsive exercising, including march hemoglobinuria (blood in the urine) and stress fractures, should be noted.

The history will include changes in sexual desire and functioning, including decrease in sexual drive, sexual fantasies, and masturbation frequency, in proportion to weight loss. Sexual orientation should be determined because of the health implications of unprotected sex, either heterosexual or homosexual. Physical exam will note the general degree of emaciation and decline in lean muscle mass, as well as general medical findings including vital signs. Bulimia nervosa is less obvious on physical examination, and patients may be secretive about binge-purge behaviors. With obese males, screening questions should be asked to determine if binge eating disorder is present.

Laboratory studies in the male, in addition to the general evaluation noted in Chapter 2, will include serum testosterone level (both total testosterone and free testosterone) if weight loss is present. Normal absolute testosterone varies typically from 340 to 800 ng/dL, while free testosterone is usually in the range of 1.8 to 6.8 (ages 20–49). Testosterone declines in proportion to weight loss (Andersen, Wirth, and Strahlman, 1982). LH and FSH will be correspondingly diminished in anorexia nervosa because the changes in gonadotropins are due to central hypo thalamic hypogonadism secondary to starvation, rather than increasing as would be expected with a failing gonad. Testicular examination will often reveal testes that are decreased in size in anorexic males, comparable to testicular volume of prepubertal males. If unprotected sex or intravenous drug use is disclosed in the history, then a request for HIV testing is appropriate (Ramsay, Catalan, and Gazzard, 1992).

For males with binge eating disorder, the medical complications of the commonly associated obesity should be evaluated through lipid panel testing, with attention to the presence of type II diabetes mellitus and hypertension. Any male with anorexic levels of weight loss for more than 6 months will generally be referred for a DEXA scan to determine loss of bone mineral density. Osteoporosis and osteopenia are common in chronic eating disorders (anorexia nervosa and bulimia nervosa). Males, somewhat surprisingly, have even worse deficiencies in bone mineral density than females with eating disorders (Mehler et al., 2008).

Treatment

The treatment of low-weight anorexic males is similar to that of under-weight females, with a few additional male-specific concerns (Andersen, 1990). The general goals of all eating disorder treatments are as follows:

1. To normalize weight, with a healthy goal weight or a healthy weight range of about 4 pounds (for example, 143–47 pounds for the case described at the beginning of this chapter). A subset of bulimia nervosa patients will be mildly underweight, and this contributes to binge urges if not corrected.

2. To normalize eating behavior by teaching patients how to choose balanced adequate meals anywhere, anytime, whether by oneself, in a school cafeteria, at a family meal, or at a celebration.

3. To challenge and change the patient's overvaluation of the benefits of weight loss or shape change. This is the core of lasting treatment benefits and involves helping the individual learn to deal with fundamental issues in living, such as identity formation, mood regulation, and harassment, and gain a sense of control.

4. To reach a decision about whether the comorbid medical and psychiatric diagnoses are secondary (in which case, these conditions—for example, hypothermia—improve on their own) or primary, perhaps predisposing the patient to the disorder (for example, preexisting depressive disorder), and whether they are long lasting, as in the case of osteoporosis caused by the eating disorder.

5. To provide treatment that prepares males for return to their gender-specific social roles as well as to work out issues in sexuality. Males especially need work to accurately identify and express feelings.

There is merit to the consideration of physiological replacement of testosterone in adolescent males and adult males who have reached all or most of their axial height. In the case of anorexic males with documented low levels of testosterone, there are no definitive studies regarding the specific benefits of testosterone replacement versus allowing hormone levels to return naturally. If testosterone replacement is chosen during the weight restoration phase, the typical mode used currently is topical gel, with a 5 mg/d dose. Once full weight restoration has been attained, supplemental testosterone is discontinued (see Table 12.2).

TABLE 12.2 Testosterone replacement therapy during weight restoration in anorexic males at full height

1. Assess serum testosterone.
2. If low, consider supplementation with topical gel testosterone until body weight is restored.
3. After weight restoration, discontinue testosterone for one month and retest testosterone level.
4. Normal testosterone one month after weight restoration may help confirm the presence of healthy body weight; low testosterone may indicate a need for more weight restoration.
5. Consider the possibility of testicular defect in some males with eating disorders who have low testosterone despite return to normal weight.

Testosterone level is reassessed one month later to determine if an adequate weight has been reached for normal hormone production in the patient. Because virtually all late adolescent and adult males of normal weight should be producing normal amounts of testosterone, a continued low level usually indicates inadequate weight or persisting testicular disorder independent of weight. The therapeutic use of testosterone in anorectic males is based on an extension of testosterone use in underweight AIDS patients or burn patients. Caution would be indicated in males who are not close to full height and maximal bone growth because testosterone can cause premature closure of the bony growth plate. The eventual benefits versus risks of this short-term anabolic hormone need to be rigorously studied.

We recommend the inclusion of graduated resistance exercises along with weight restoration for all patients, but especially for males, who generally express more interest. Ideally, these exercises will be guided by a team member trained in exercise physiology, starting "low and slow," building up to moderate levels of resistance, and emphasizing good form to enhance lean muscle development and decrease the tendency for early weight restoration to be in the abdominal area. When restored weight is concentrated in the abdomen, it provokes fears of becoming fat and concerns about repeating the body weight distribution that may have prompted the dieting originally.

Monitoring of liver function tests, hemoglobin, and other laboratory tests typically continues during testosterone replacement. There is some concern about long-term testicular deficiency in males who have had an eating disorder, a result noted in a study that showed that two out of eleven males who returned to a healthy weight remained oligospermic or azoospermic. The physician should ask the patient about the return of normal sexual drive, fantasy, and sexual function during the weight restoration process. Often the male patient's social behavior and spontaneous discussion of sexually related topics will indicate a return to more normal hormone production. Flirting with the nurses and signs of masturbatory activity are signals of improved weight and testosterone production.

What Is a Healthy Weight for Recovering Anorexic Males?

In determining a healthy weight, the rule of thumb is to ask the body for the answer, rather than an insurance table, although "ideal body weights" from standard tables may be used for the short-term goal within acute treatment. If the patient had been at a stable weight and height for some time prior to the eating disorder and this was not an obese weight, then the pre-illness weight may be a good target in fully grown males. When an individual has grown taller during an illness of several years, the goal weight may not be obvious. Here, the Metropolitan Life "Ideal Body Weight" scales or the mean matched population weight chart may be reasonable initial choices, but final weight range should be modified according to the body's messages that it is functioning in a stable range. Specific signs of a return to a healthy body weight are present when

- the patient has achieved full normalization of temperature control with no signs of hypothermia;
- there is a return of normal patterns of hunger before meals and satiety afterward;
- tests show normal LH, FSH, and testosterone;
- normal TSH if low when the individual is ill; and
- there is a lack of mental preoccupation with food due to the psychobiology of starvation.

Continued mental preoccupation with weight and shape is a different issue, not yielding to the simpler measures of weight restoration, but usually requiring expert psychotherapy, most clearly accomplished with CBT. As with return of estrogen, normal testosterone is a necessary but not sufficient guideline for determination of a normal weight range. It is important for patients to understand that body functioning may not be fully normal until healthy behaviors have continued and weight has been stable in a healthy range for six to nine or more months after acute weight restoration. A final weight appropriate for age, height, and individual physiology will be worked out during the year after initial treatment is concluded, a year of intensive relapse prevention. The patient needs to be reassured that the disproportionate concentration of some weight in the abdominal area during weight restoration is a natural occurrence; this weight will be redistributed during the year of relapse prevention and psychological growth after acute care.

The bulimic male suffers medical consequences similar to those of the bulimic female, with medical symptoms divided between the consequences of weight loss and the specific problems associated with the particular purging behaviors used. Binges themselves are uncomfortable physically and psychologically, triggering urges to purge or otherwise compensate for the excessive calories ingested, but have fewer medical complications generally than the purges, except for the rare gastric rupture. Hypokalemia with resulting arrhythmias is the most common serious medical complication of purging. Tender, enlarged parotid glands may be the most obvious medical sign. If a bulimic male is HIV positive (usually from comorbid IV substance abuse or unprotected sex, often due to an impulsive personality or bipolar II mood disorder), then appropriate treatment should be offered according to the best recent studies.

When binge eating disorder is diagnosed in an obese male, the physician's treatments are directed first toward improvement of the binge eating disorder, through a combination of nutritional guidance, cognitive-behavioral therapy, and often an SSRI, typically fluoxetine, sertraline, or escitalopram. Once the binge eating behaviors are improved, second-phase treatment involves directing attention to the overweight or obesity, deciding whether it should be treated at all because of medical complications, or whether the patient should be encouraged to develop overall cardiovascular fitness and attain greater lean muscle mass, accepting a weight up to a BMI of 28 or so. Evidence is good that a BMI from 25 to

28, along with good cardiovascular fitness, low body fat, and no hypertension, may be compatible with excellent health, and accepted, rather than being fought by relentless and ineffective dieting. Interestingly, older males with a BMI of less than 22.7 had the highest mortality (Breeze et al., 2006). Simply telling a patient in the weight range of a BMI of 26–30 to lose weight is easy for physicians to recommend, much harder to carry out, and sometimes not necessary if fitness goals are defined.

If weight loss is sought, one runs into all the problems of trying to trick the body into attaining, and more importantly, maintaining, a lower weight than the weight during the active binge eating disorder. It is sometimes possible to obtain moderate, long-lasting changes in the "set point" of an individual's weight through improved choices of healthy foods, with the emphasis on choosing food groups rather than limiting calories; moderate regular exercise; and improved stress management. The role of alcohol use, either solitary drinking or in a social context, in disinhibiting eating behavior in males must be explored and discussed. The increased eating associated with alcohol binges (the latter present in 60%-70% of first-year college students) is often passed off as normal behavior but may be a substantial contributor to undesired weight increase.

Finally, males with eating disorders who have had any sustained underweight for six months or more should be tested for bone mineral density with a DEXA scan. Anorexic males experience more osteoporosis than do anorexic females (Andersen, Watson, and Schlechte, 2000). There is less likelihood the clinician will think of osteoporosis in association with a male. The contributing factors to the pathogenesis of osteoporosis in a male appear to include low testosterone as well as the factors shared with females of diminished calcium intake, lowered body weight, elevated cortisol, and the like. The best current treatments for osteoporosis in males include moderate exercise through low-impact weight-bearing activities (avoiding high-impact sports, which increase fracture risk), prompt restoration to normal body weight, restoration of natural production of testosterone, fully adequate calcium intake (1,500 mg/d), and vitamin D (800–1,000 IU/d). (Use of bisphosphonates for osteoporosis in men is not yet validated but may be considered.) A return to normal weight, involvement in low-impact weight-bearing activities, and normal testosterone production are the major contributing factors to improved bone mineral density.

The prognosis for males with anorexia nervosa is equal to or better than that for females (Strober et al., 2006). Any beliefs that maleness is by itself an adverse risk factor for recovery in eating disorders need to be updated by evidence-based studies supporting the fact that males have an excellent prognosis if treated promptly and fully. Individuals with eating disorders can be better off after remission through successful treatment than if they never had the disorder (although it's a tough way to go) because they will have learned to deal more effectively with the sociocultural forces that overvalue weight and shape changes. A book accessible to the general public, *Making Weight* (Andersen, Cohn, and Holbrook, 2000), offers more details about men's issues with food, weight, shape, and appearance.

Some "pearls" and tips about diagnosis and treatment of eating disorders in males are listed in Table 12.3.

TABLE 12.3   Clinical "pearls" for the diagnosis and treatment of eating disorders in males

- Boys and men tend to feel fat at weights above population normal, whereas women often feel fat even when objectively thin.
- Males tend to be more concerned with shape than with weight and predominantly want to change the body waist-up rather than waist-down. The most frequently desired body image is lean muscularity.
- Males more often diet for very specific, personal reasons rather than because of a general cultural endorsement of thinness.
- Males with eating disorders are less well recognized by clinicians, who may not think of the diagnosis. They also are under-recognized because of the perception of stigma on their part and a resulting reluctance to seek either diagnosis or treatment.
- While not a proven therapy, there is merit to considering short-term replacement of testosterone during the weight-restoration phase of anorexic males, especially in those at or close to maximal height attainment.
- Although being gay increases the risk for an eating disorder because of stringent sociocultural body image ideals, the majority of males with eating disorders are not gay or bisexual. Many young anorexic males are asexual.
- Males with eating disorders develop osteoporosis as frequently as and with even more severity than women, most likely tied to the gender-specific contributing factor of low testosterone, as well as the gender-shared contribution of low calcium intake, low body weight, elevated cortisol, and probably excessive consumption of diet sodas.

(continued)

TABLE 12.3 *(continued)*

- Males especially often benefit from resistance exercises during weight restoration: these exercises improve morale, provide a sense that the individual is making a personal contribution toward a desired body shape, result in an increased percentage of lean muscle mass, help to decrease relapse, and provide a setting in which to work out with other males.

- Males, rarely females, may have "reverse anorexia," in which they exercise relentlessly and attempt to increase their body weight because of the perception that they are never large enough, even though they may objectively be very muscular with extreme muscle definition. In contrast to the more common "drive for thinness," these males experience a "drive for bigness."

- Males with "reverse anorexia nervosa," are liable to use anabolic steroids to attain the "bigness" they desire: extreme muscularity with little body fat.

- Males with diminished bone density should avoid high-impact sports activities until there is an improvement in bone strength. After a healthy weight, freedom from binge-purge behaviors, and a healthy attitude toward food, weight, and shape have been attained and maintained for several months, they can return to their chosen sports activities. Some males need to stay away from wrestling, figure skating, modeling, or other activities that promote weight loss when they continue to have a high drive for thinness.

- Wherever possible, it is beneficial to have some male-specific components within the eating disorders program. These components include "guys-only" groups (comparable to females-only rape survivor groups), consideration of testosterone replacement, strength training programs, and individual therapy that addresses issues of gender orientation, decisions about sports and vocational goals, and especially, improved relationships with fathers and peers.

Summary

Males develop eating disorders more frequently than was previously believed, in a ratio of approximately one male to three females. Many fewer seek medical care, however, indicating multiple roadblocks for males, especially shame, clinicians' failure to recognize this order in males, nonacceptance in treatment facilities, assumptions on the part of caregivers of sexual orientation, and fear of being treated like females. Males with eating disorders have a plurality of body image choices compared with females: very thin, mesomorphic, or overdeveloped. The common factor to all is lean muscularity, with minimal body fat, favoring upper body development. The media have increasingly presented body image ideals for males that are as impossible to achieve as the starved images for females. Males are more likely to develop eating disorders for specific personal reasons rather than because of sociocultural endorsement of slimness for all males. Some of the more common reasons are to avoid being teased for childhood obesity, to improve sports performance, to avoid medical illnesses, and to improve a gay relationship. Males are often more concerned with shape than weight.

Screening tests are used to identify males with eating disorders. Diagnosis is similar for males and females with anorexia nervosa or bulimia nervosa, but only males develop "reverse anorexia," a condition in which fear of smallness dominates despite huge muscular development, predisposing these patients to use of anabolic steroids. Treatment needs to appreciate male concerns, including establishing support groups for males, striving for improved relationships with fathers, implementing strength training, and occasionally using testosterone supplementation. Gay males are about five times more likely to develop an eating disorder than the general population, but still constitute a minority of cases. Males have a prognosis as good as or better than that for females.

REFERENCES

Andersen AE (ed.). 1990. *Males with Eating Disorders*. New York: Brunner/ Mazel.

Andersen A, Cohn L, and Holbrook T. 2000. *Making Weight: Men's Conflicts with Food, Weight, Shape, and Appearance*. Carlsbad, CA: Gurze Books.

Andersen AE, Watson T, and Schlechte J. 2000. Osteoporosis and osteopenia in men with eating disorders. *Lancet* 355:1967–68.

Andersen AE, Wirth JB, and Strahlman ER. 1982. Reversible weight-related increase in plasma testosterone during treatment of male and female patients with anorexia nervosa. *International Journal of Eating Disorders* 1:74–83.

Breeze E, Clarke R, Shipley MJ, Marmot MG, and Fletcher AE. 2006. Cause-specific mortality in old age in relation to body mass index in middle age and in old age. *International Journal of Epidemiology* 35:169–78.

Fichter MM and Dasher C. 1987. Symptomatology, psychosexual development, and gender identity in 42 anorexic males. *Psychological Medicine* 17:-409–18.

Fisher M and Fornari V. 1990. Gynecomastia as a precipitant of eating disorders in adolescent males. *International Journal of Eating Disorders* 9:115–19.

Gull WW. 1873. Anorexia nervosa (apepsia hysterica). *British Medical Journal* 2:527–28.

Hobza CL, Walker KE, Yakushko O, and Peugh JL. 2007. What about men? Social comparison and the effects of media images on body and self-esteem. *Psychology of Men and Masculinity* 8:161–72.

Hudson JI, Hiripi E, Pope HG Jr., and Kessler RC. 2007. The prevalence and correlates of eating disorders in the National Comorbidity Survey Replication. *Biological Psychiatry* 61:348–58.

Mehler PS, Sabel AL, Watson T, and Andersen AE. 2008. High risk of osteoporosis in male eating disordered patients. *International Journal of Eating Disorders* 41:666–72.

Morgan JF, Reid F, and Lacey JH. 1999. The SCOFF questionnaire: Assessment of a new screening tool for eating disorders. *British Medical Journal* 319: 1467–68.

Olivardia R, Pope HG, and Hudson JI. 2000. Muscle dysmorphia in male weightlifters: A case-control study. *American Journal of Psychiatry* 157:1291–96.

Oppliger RA, Landry GL, Foster SW, and Lambrecht AC. 1993. Bulimic behaviors among interscholastic wrestlers: A statewide survey. *Pediatrics* 91:-826–31.

Pope HG, Lalonde JK, Pindyck LJ, et al. 2006. Binge eating disorder: A stable syndrome. 2006. *American Journal of Psychiatry* 163: 2181–83.

Procopio M and Marriott P. 2007. Intrauterine hormonal environment and risk of developing anorexia nervosa. *Archives of General Psychiatry* 64:1402–8.

Ramsay N, Catalan J, and Gazzard B. 1992. Eating disorders in men with HIV infection. *British Journal of Psychiatry* 160:404–7.

Ruffolo JS, Phillips KA, Menard W, Fay C, and Weisberg RB. 2006. Comorbidity of body dysmorphic disorder and eating disorders: Severity of psychopathology and body image disturbance. *International Journal of Eating Disorders* 39:11–19.

Schrieber GB, Robins M, Striegel-Moore R, Obarzanek RD, Morrison JH, and Wright DJ. 1996. Weight modification efforts reported by black and white preadolescent girls. *Pediatrics* 98:63–70.

Strober M, Freeman R, Lampert C, Diamond J, Teplinsky C, and DeAntonio M. 2006. Are there gender differences in core symptoms, temperament, and short-term prospective outcome in anorexia nervosa? *International Journal of Eating Disorders* 39:570–75.

Thiel A, Gottfried H, and Hesse FW 1993. Subclinical eating disorders in male athletes: A study of the low weight category in rowers and wrestlers. *Acta Psychiatrica Scandinavica* 88:259–65.

Woodside BD, Garfinkel PE, Lin E, Goering P, Kaplan AS, Goldbloom DS, and Kennedy SH. 2001. Comparison of men with full or partial eating disorders, men without eating disorders, and women with eating disorders in the community. *American Journal of Psychiatry* 158:570–74.

CHAPTER THIRTEEN

Using Medical Information Psychotherapeutically

COMMON QUESTIONS

What is psychoeducation?

How can clinicians use medical information psychotherapeutically with patients who have eating disorders?

Can you scare patients into healthy behavior?

Will medical information, if accurately presented, demoralize patients who have eating disorders?

Which medical tests offer the best possibility for psychotherapeutic use?

When is medical information not appropriate for psychotherapeutic feedback?

What information is helpful to families?

Case 1

C.Y. was a 47-year-old surgeon whose wife persuaded him to come for evaluation for an eating disorder because of compulsive exercising and weight loss. The patient insisted that he was overweight at 185 pounds at 5 feet 10 inches tall. Three years before evaluation, the patient began a strenuous exercise program of long-distance running, swimming, and bicycling. His father's death at about that time had caused him to fear that he might, like his father, be at risk of death from cardiac disease. Also, his older daughter was preparing to leave for college. His weight decreased to 130 pounds. He counted calories and limited fat grams to 10 grams a day, including monosaturated lipids. Despite feeling cold, becoming irritable at suggestions to decrease his several hours a day of exercise, and suffering two ankle sprains and knee pain, he continued his program.

At evaluation, the surgeon insisted he was only practicing healthy behaviors. He met criteria for anorexia nervosa in a male but would not accept the diagnosis until his DEXA scan and testosterone blood levels were shared with him. He met the criteria for osteoporosis with a femoral neck bone mineral density of -2.7 standard deviations below normal and an L1-5 finding of -2.3 standard deviations. His testosterone was 180 ng/dL (normal 340–800). Gentle confrontation with these data allowed him to accept treatment, which included vigorous exercise but at a much more reasonable level, a gradual increase in weight to 165 pounds, coming to terms with his fears of mortality, and establishing a more adult-to-adult relationship with his daughter, including acceptance of her transition to becoming a college student. His marriage improved. Providing him with reading information about bone density loss in males (Andersen, Watson, and Schlechte, 2000) was helpful, as he was a clinical researcher as well as surgeon.

Case 2

S.J. was a 20-year-old engineering student at the top of her class. In the course of her eating disorder, in addition to restricting her food intake, she began to abuse laxatives. She developed significant electrolyte problems, which were corrected in treatment. She was presented with information in a published study that 80 percent of calories ingested are absorbed despite laxative use excessive enough to lose 6 L of diarrhea fluid a day (Bo-Linn et al., 1983). When she saw this information, she said, "It doesn't make sense to do things that don't work," and stopped using laxatives. She went on to recover her weight and cease all purging behavior, as well as to change her core beliefs that thinness was essential to her sense of control and effectiveness. Medical information produced a helpful psychotherapeutic response.

Background

Eating disorders are characterized, according to Hilde Bruch (1979), by denial of thinness, denial of illness, and denial of sexuality. Patients with eating disorders, especially anorexia nervosa, often live an intellectualized life, from the neck up, with little attention to the reality of what is happening to their bodies. They often appear to produce "insightful" responses in psychotherapy but then show no change in illness behaviors or illness-based abnormal thinking. Clinicians can use medical tests that document significant changes in body function in a number of different ways while interacting with patients who have eating disorders. First, medical information may simply be screened from the patient and never presented (the paternalistic style). Second, information may be presented in a neutral manner with neither psychotherapeutic discussion nor blame (the *Dragnet* style: "Just the facts, ma'am"). Third, information may, unfortunately, be used to blame or scare patients (club the victim). Scaring patients does not last for long, certainly not long enough for motivation and engagement in successful treatment. Last, and preferably, information can be used psychotherapeutically (the ideal use). Psychoeducation means the use of information about the nature of the disorder and medical testing results in a manner that respects the patient, empowers her or him to become a partner in decision making, and helps draw out the implications of accepting versus refusing treatment.

Using Medical Tests Psychotherapeutically

The goal of using medical information psychotherapeutically is to form a therapeutic alliance with the healthy side of the patient to overcome the patient's denial of illness or denial of the seriousness of the illness. It is an attempt to form a working partnership with patients to help them interrupt the belief that they do not have an illness or that it has no significant consequences. Blaming patients for medical consequences is inappropriate because they often already have significant self-blame. Scaring patients doesn't work; at best, it produces a short-term alteration in behavior.

The following are suggestions for possible use of medical information based on experience but not on any established studies with statistical confirmation. A good background reading for the clinician is the chapter on psychoeducation in Garner et al. (1985), which has stood the test of time. Presenting accurate medical information, both from current medical testing and from expected symptoms during the course of recovery, will reassure the anxious, fearful patient. It will also increase respect for the staff through patient awareness that this illness is understandable and predictable to the staff, as well as treatable. The following examples of medical information can be used therapeutically (Yager and Andersen, 2005).

VITAL SIGNS AND ACUTE MEDICAL INSTABILITY

When a patient is seen for a diagnostic evaluation or first admitted and has electrolyte disturbances with associated EKG changes, information about these test results may help the patient either accept the diagnosis and the need to begin treatment or, if already admitted, accept the need for staff-directed treatment instead of self-directed efforts. This information generally is best presented by using the laboratory reports themselves, which show the normal levels as well as the patient's results. Along with the presentation of the medical information, an explanation of their significance and cause is helpful so that the prescribed treatment will make sense. Unfortunately, many restricting anorexic patients have normal laboratory values despite marked cachexia. Fairburn (1995) reviewed the physiology of anorexia nervosa.

BONE MINERAL DENSITY BY DEXA SCAN

A dual-energy X-ray aborptiometry scan often provides graphic visual evidence that the patient has a serious medical problem. This information is usually first received by the clinician in the form of the patient's findings on a graph that compares the patient's results with those of normal, same-gender individuals at different ages. (See Fig. 13.1.) It is easy to show patients with anorexia nervosa, when their findings are traced across the graph, that they have the same bone density as 80- to 90-year-old individuals. A typical response is, "Oh, my goodness. I never realized that this was happening," or, "I didn't know it was this serious." The patient can be reassured that the problem, while not completely understood, will be treated as effectively as possible. Here facts are also presented: because the lifetime maximum bone density is usually reached, at the latest, by the 20s (some recent studies suggest by age 15 or 16), with the maximum rate of accumulation in the midteens, there is an

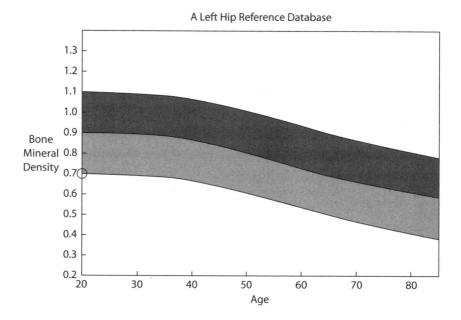

FIGURE 13.1. Visual information about bone density in a typical patient with an eating disorder can be used psychotherapeutically. The clinician can explain that the middle line is the average bone density for age; the results here show that the patient's bone density is equal to that of a 70-year-old woman.

urgency in attempting to build a healthy "bone bank for retirement." Active research is now taking place to address the problem, and most patients with deficient bone mineral density have a number of years to correct the deficiency, which responds slowly to treatment. Incidentally, recent studies have demonstrated that estrogens are relatively ineffective in the starved anorexic patient (Mehler and MacKenzie, 2009), another reason for restoration of full body weight. The DEXA scan, as noted in previous chapters, is widely available, moderate in cost, accurate (Winston, Alwazeer, and Bankhart, 2008), and low in radiation (a tenth that of a chest X-ray).

MAGNETIC RESONANCE IMAGING

While a brain MRI scan is not indicated in all patients, patients with atypical features or a history of seizure or brain injury require an MRI for differential diagnosis and to assess the contribution of structural brain change to mental functioning. When an MRI is obtained for an anorexic patient, it often shows enlarged ventricles and decreased brain volume. Patients may be astounded to see that their MRI is similar to that of a patient who has Alzheimer's disease, which also has enlarged ventricles and decreased brain substance. Assurance can be given that most recent studies demonstrate recovery of brain size in anorexia nervosa with effective treatment and weight restoration, but it is not certain that all brain abnormalities are eventually improved (Swayze et al., 2003).

GASTROINTESTINAL CHANGES

Patients can be shown published studies (Waldholtz and Andersen, 1990, for example) showing that abdominal distress is improved with renutrition and supportive medical care in most patients with anorexia nervosa without medication or GI studies. It is hard to concentrate during therapy when there is significant abdominal distress. Published information about the return to normal gastric emptying, decreased bloating, and normalization of the speed of GI transit time helps the patient tolerate the temporary refeeding symptomatology affecting the GI tract because of the knowledge that it is temporary, will improve, and is a consequence of the illness. Anorexia nervosa doubles the transit time of the gastrointestinal tract.

SIGNS OF MEDICAL STARVATION

Discussion of the signs and symptoms of medical starvation may help the patient accept the fact he or she is medically starved and not simply healthy in a way of which others should be envious. Demonstrations of low T_3, the presence of increased reverse T_3, signs of acrocyanosis, and small, shrunken ovaries on sonogram are all evidence that the body is truly starved. It may help to refer to the studies of Keys, Brozek, and Hemscheo in *The Biology of Human Starvation,* showing that many of the psychological changes and much of the social isolation and altered eating behavior come from starvation, not the core anorexia nervosa psychopathology. "Marcie, that slowness of thinking and the difficulty in finishing the journaling assignment come from the effects of starvation on the brain. They will improve soon." Most of the medical symptoms in anorexia nervosa are understandable as the biology of starvation.

STATUS OF REPRODUCTIVE HORMONES

The presentation of information documenting low estrogen in the female or low testosterone in the male and comparing these results to normal values may help individuals accept the fact they have an illness. Even though patients with anorexia nervosa often avoid discussions about sexuality, a number of them want to have families in the future. Information about their low reproductive hormone levels may help them accept necessary weight restoration. The subsequent demonstration that these values become normal with return to healthy weight will often reassure patients and especially parents that no permanent damage has occurred. "There is nothing broken. Your reproductive hormones have gone back to a prepubertal state, and they will return to normal when your weight is fully normal, your eating pattern is normal, your stress levels are lower. The body has mechanisms for dealing with famine from humankind's long experience with shortages of food. The body thinks it is in a famine. When you let it know that the 'famine' is over, the hormones will return to normal over several months." It is important for women who anticipate being sexually active to know that they may become pregnant before their first period because the ovum is shed before that time, and that they therefore should take appropriate precautions.

ALLERGIES AND COMPLAINTS OF LACTOSE INTOLERANCE

Nutritional rehabilitation is substantially interfered with if patients have significant food allergies and/or lactose intolerance. Some patients complain that virtually all foods they eat cause allergic responses. Other individuals complain of GI symptoms after eating dairy products, denying themselves their beneficial protein and calcium content. Refeeding will often be greatly assisted by requesting a formal consultation early in treatment from a specialist or referral for breath hydrogen testing to confirm or rule out lactose intolerance and allergies to specific foods. About 80 percent of patients complaining of lactose intolerance do not have confirmation on objective testing of lactose intolerance. Similarly, many fears of a generalized allergic response to foods or additives are also not sustained on medical testing. Normal responses on these tests will allow nutritional rehabilitation to proceed with as few limitations as possible and will generally decrease the phobic quality of these foods in the patient's mind.

ABUSE OF LAXATIVES

As noted in the second case study in this chapter, information about the ineffectiveness of laxatives may help patients undergo a program of cessation or tapering of laxatives by recognizing its ineffectiveness in producing the desired goal. (See Bo-Linn et al., 1983.)

NIGHT SWEATS

The first patient in whom night sweats were noted was a pathologist whose occupation brought her in contact with a variety of fungal disorders causing death. An extensive evaluation was undertaken for TB and other fungi, and all results were negative. There was no evidence of any medical disorder besides the medical starvation of anorexia nervosa. When this pattern was inquired about in subsequent anorexia nervosa patients undergoing weight restoration, they all acknowledged "night sweats" as a phenomenon.

Night sweats should be discussed with patients because when its normality as a phenomenon is not recognized, it can worry patients or families, cause iatrogenic unnecessary tests to be ordered, or be considered psychosomatic. Patients can be alerted in advance to expect, usually within a week or two of being hospitalized for anorexia nervosa, that their feelings of coldness and objective hypothermia will usually improve in a sequence: first, they will experience night sweats, sometimes drenching and requiring a change of night clothing, within a week or two into treatment; then there will be a leveling off of the sweating gradually over the next two weeks; and, finally, there will be a return to a state of normal temperature control without subjective coldness. Patients sometimes give an increased respect to staff instead of skepticism when the prediction of night sweats is confirmed by experience. Interestingly, this phenomenon is observed in males as well as females, so estrogen return may not be involved but, rather, some aspect of hypothalamic regulation in the setting of increased nutrition, including change in thyroid hormones or receptors.

When Is It Not Helpful to Give Medical Information to a Person with an Eating Disorder?

Clinical experience suggests that in several situations, sharing of medical information is not appropriate. Very young patients may simply not be able to understand the nature of medical data. If they are too young or too starved, or have substantial deficits in intellect, making it difficult to form a working therapeutic relationship especially for cognitive-behavioral work, then medical information may produce only fear and no therapeutic response, or a negative preoccupation. Some patients with vulnerable personality traits may internalize medical information to increase self-blame, but this can be anticipated and prevented by the manner of sharing information. Information sharing with patients who are self-critical or depressed at the time the medical information is available may need to wait until the depression is improved and/or a psychotherapeutic relationship has been under way for a while. The goal of sharing medical information is not to frighten patients or increase their self-blame but to form an alliance with the patient against the illness.

One form of medical information, in our experience, is not helpful to most patients with anorexia nervosa: daily information about the patient's weight during intensive inpatient programs, and sometimes not even in full-day (partial hospital) or outpatient programs. A preoccupation with daily weight, or learning to "eat your way out of hospital" by complying with the behavioral goals but not changing core beliefs, is not therapy. Not everyone agrees with this advice, but in our experience, daily sharing of the patient's body weight, which is more like daily confrontation, has more drawbacks than benefits. A focus on weight obscures the fact that eating disorders have essentially nothing to do with food, weight, or shape, but are instead strategies to deal with issues in living, mood regulation, relationships, an adequate sense of control in life, and self-esteem.

Obviously, a time comes when patients need to know their weight. We usually tell them their weight and their goal weight range when they are in a healthy target range, or have transitioned from inpatient treatment to partial hospital at 85–90 percent healthy weight. At that time, they are taught the rationale for a 4- to 5-pound range, rather than a single number—for example, 120–25 pounds for a 25-year-old woman who is 5 feet 31/2 inches tall. They are told that it is normal to experience fluctuation within that 4- to 5-pound range. They are asked before that time to concentrate on understanding themselves and changing the thinking and behaviors that form the core of their eating disorders while they trust us to prescribe nutrition as medication. We promise them, based on more than 20 years of experience, that we will not let them become overweight. At times a patient with a personal and family history of obesity may need to have a target weight 10–15 pounds above the ideal weight. Weight, like height, is a bell-shaped curve, and someone has to hold down the upper standard deviation from the average, although few women accept this fact. It is an important therapeutic goal to persuade the patient that the true goal weight will be determined in the year after intensive treatment when the patient and therapist will both ask the body where it functions well, using information on labs, absence of hypothermia, return of normal hunger and satiety, regular menses, and sexual drive and function.

The Role of Parents

Appropriate medical information may also reassure parents that the physical symptoms of the eating disorder are being addressed and that their daughter or son will not die. Parents often fear the worst. If the situation is desperate medically, certainly the possibility of a fatal outcome should not be withheld, but often parents' fears are greater than the situation warrants. Parents appreciate learning the difference between starvation-induced, reversible symptoms versus serious, short-term or long-term complications that need to be separately addressed with specific medical treatments. They may need the medical information if they, too, are doubtful of the need for treatment and have their own form of denial of illness. Parents are often reassured to know that few, if any, medical consequences are permanent.

The Method of Presenting Medical Information

Medical information is psychotherapeutic when it is presented as part of a planned approach aimed at forming a therapeutic alliance to defeat the denial of illness that is characteristic of eating disorders. Information is most convincing when it is shown on a formal report in which the patient herself or himself can see the results and, especially, when she or he can compare her or his results to normal values. Visual appreciation by the patient tends to break down the intellectual denial of illness. It may also help patients understand why they have difficulties with mental concentration and abdominal discomfort, or why the treatment team or clinician has prescribed limitations on high-impact activities and so on. Information on the reversibility of reproductive hormone abnormalities may reassure patients who wish to have a family later. Medical information presented therapeutically rather than in a critical or even neutral manner may allow patients to give themselves permission to accept the refeeding process rather than being fearful or hostile recipients of the nutritional rehabilitation.

Accurate medical information also increases respect for staff knowledge when the patient is told about upcoming symptoms that probably will occur during the course of treatment, how they will be treated, and their transient nature. This includes information about possible "night sweats" during the refeeding process, gastrointestinal discomfort, refeeding edema, changes in mental concentration, and progressive increases in energy, to name but a few.

Summary

Conveying medical information about the physical consequences of the eating disorders to the patient is important so that the treatment team can give good care. In certain situations, or if the information is not presented with due care, some vulnerable patients may perceive the information critically, with negative effects on the clinician-patient relationship. But if the information is presented as we recommend, psychotherapeutically, it can be used to form an alliance with the patient, to establish the reality of illness, and to diminish denial of the illness or the seriousness of the illness.

REFERENCES

Andersen AE, Watson T, and Schlechte J. 2000. Osteoporosis and osteopenia in men with eating disorders. *Lancet* 355:1967–68.

Bo-Linn GW, Santana CA, Morawski SG, and Fordtran JS. 1983. Purging and caloric absorption in bulimic patients and normal women. *Annals of Internal Medicine* 99:14.

Bruch H. 1979. *The Golden Cage.* New York: Vintage Press.

Fairburn CG. 1995. Physiology of anorexia nervosa. In: Brownell KD, Fairburn CG, eds. *Eating Disorders and Obesity.* New York: Guilford Press, pp. 251–54.

Garner D, Rockert W, Olmsted M, Johnson C, and Coscina D. 1985. Psychoeducational principles in the treatment of bulimia and anorexia nervosa. In: Garner D, Garfinkel P, eds. *Handbook of Psychotherapy for Anorexia Nervosa and Bulimia.* New York: Guilford Press, pp. 513–72.

Keys A, Brozek J, and Henscheo A. 1950. *The Biology of Human Starvation.* Minneapolis: University of Minnesota Press.

Mehler PS and MacKenzie TD. 2009. Treatment of osteopenia and osteoporosis in anorexia nervosa: A systematic review of the literature. *International Journal of Eating Disorders* 42:195–201.

Swayze VW, Andersen AE, Andreasen NC, Arndt S, Sato Y, and Ziebell S. 2003. Brain tissue volume segmentation in patients with anorexia nervosa before and after weight normalization. *International Journal of Eating Disorders* 33:33–44.

Waldholtz BD and Andersen AE. 1990. Gastrointestinal symptoms in anorexia nervosa: A prospective study. *Gastroenterology* 98:1415–14.

Winston AP, Alwazeer AEF, and Bankhart MJG. 2008. Screening for osteoporosis in anorexia nervosa: Prevalence and predictors of reduced bone mineral density. *International Journal of Eating Disorders* 41:284–87.

Yager J and Andersen AE. 2005. Clinical practice: Anorexia nervosa. *New England Journal of Medicine* 353:1481–82.

CHAPTER FOURTEEN

Ethical Conflicts in the Care of Anorexia Nervosa Patients

COMMON QUESTIONS

What are the bioethical principles guiding modern medical practice?
When does deciding for the patient trump an individual's autonomy?
How can a clinician avoid doing harm and respect the principle of
   primum non nocere?
Are economic factors of concern in ethical practice?
How do you decide between individual and societal benefits?
What are the ethical benefits of a good relationship between patient
   and physician?

The Principles of Modern Biomedical Ethics

Four guiding principles form the basis of modern biomedical ethics (Beauchamp and Childress, 2001). These principles balance Emmanuel Kant's *categorical imperative* (which could be paraphrased "You gotta do the right thing, no matter what it takes") with John Stuart Mill's and Jeremy Bentham's *utilitarianism* ("Make the best decision for everyone all around"). The resulting principles, often called as a group *principalism*, are

1. respect for *autonomy* (the patient's informed choices take priority);

2. *nonmaleficence* (do no harm, *primum non nocere*);

3. *beneficence* (doing what is best for patients, not always with their consent); and

4. *justice* (balancing individual and social costs, benefits, risks).

Implied in the above is the assumption that practicing these ethical principles takes precedence over self-interest.

Nonmaleficence and beneficence have historically been honored. Only in recent decades has respect for autonomy and (social) justice become emphasized prominently in medical practice, resulting substantially from the growing distrust of all institutions in general, manifested by the social conflict during the Vietnam War.

These four guiding principles are generally applicable in most situations, but none is without exceptions in specific cases. There are conflicts within and between these principles that are relatively specific for anorexia nervosa because of the unique features of this eating disorder:

1. the intermix of medical starvation signs and symptoms with the mental and behavioral consequences of the overvalued beliefs underlying the disorder;

2. the common perception that anorexia nervosa is a voluntary disorder responsive to self-determination in both the development of the illness and the process of regaining health;

3. the moralizing of disorders of eating behavior and weight as disorders of personal failure;

4. the common stereotype of anorexia nervosa limiting the perception of illness to teenage Caucasian females;

5. the multifactorial concept of etiology that generates competing approaches to treatment; and

6. the relatively robust appearance and behavior of many patients even with serious anorexia nervosa.

The following sections weigh these guiding principles against the reality of treating eating disorders.

Respect for Autonomy versus Beneficence

Individuals who have severe anorexia nervosa often look more competent than they are. Deciding when a patient is too ill to make an informed decision about the need for treatment requires placing a *category* ("too sick to be autonomous; make the decision for her") on a linear *dimension* (gradually decreasing weight and mental function). Carefully delineated respect for both autonomy and beneficence combined with experienced assessment of mental and behavioral functioning in anorexia nervosa will determine when beneficence trumps autonomy. The situation is analogous to determining that a deluded, depressed person with suicidal plans or a person with schizophrenia experiencing command hallucinations has to be committed involuntarily for safety and treatment despite protestations. Patients with severe anorexia nervosa give the illusion of sanity even when they are driven by deadly irrationality, failing to appreciate that anorexia nervosa has the highest death rate in psychiatry, approximately 19 percent.

Guarda and others (Guarda et al., 2007; Andersen, 2007) have shown that shortly after patients feel coerced to receive inpatient treatment, they change their minds and come to appreciate the need for treatment. At discharge, they say, in so many words, "thank you," rather than "I'll sue you."

Nonmaleficence versus (Unintended) Maleficence

In nonmaleficence versus maleficence, the issue is not about intended maleficence, which is beyond the pale, but about more subtle forms of maleficence in practice, either active (albeit unintended and even good-willed) or passive. Both forms may occur in a number of ways, illustrated by the following specifics.

ACTIVE HARM

1. Inappropriate refeeding. Inappropriate refeeding may be deadly. Empirical literature documents ways to minimize refeeding problems that should alert clinicians to avoid fluid overload, excess caloric content, or premature use of central lines. Studies have documented that severe medical complications as a result of refeeding include death, cerebrovascular accidents, pneumothorax, and severe metabolic shifts. Some peripheral edema and nonspecific GI complaints from refeeding are common and expected, but repeated severe medical consequences from refeeding suggest a review of methods used.

2. Endless work-ups looking for medical causation, using a "rule-out" approach of discovering medical etiology rather than a "rule-in" approach based on a competent mental status examination. Until relatively recently, the diagnosis of anorexia nervosa was delayed, often by years (Andersen, 2004), by endless medical examinations, such as gastrointestinal scooping, organ biopsies, and excessive laboratory tests— leading to increased morbidity. At times, the medical consequences of starvation are mistaken for causation, resulting, for example, in the prescription of thyroid replacement for starvation-related adaptive low lab values.

3. Abandonment of the anorexic patient because of failure to recognize counter-transference that is stirring up feelings and behaviors of rejection, especially in clinicians with narcissistic features and lack of capacity for empathy.

4. The physician's consent to euthanasia or passive agreement to no treatment in some cases of anorexia nervosa. These practices, thankfully, have been of limited current implementation, but have nonetheless been bruited about, primarily in European medical circles (Draper, 2000).

PASSIVE HARM

1. Failure to refer a patient with anorexia nervosa for either diagnostic confirmation or a more experienced level of care when the clinician's personal skills are not matched to the seriousness or complexity of the illness.

2. Failure to develop a biopsychosocial formulation with integrative treatment, relying instead on single modalities determined to be insufficient by themselves, such as medications alone or a psychodynamic approach without attention to weight restoration.

3. Failure to request administrative colleagues to apply for use of third-party medical insurance benefits for the medical starvation component of anorexia, relying only on the generally much more limited psychiatric benefits. Federal courts have

determined that starvation is a medical diagnosis appropriate for medical benefits, and anorexia nervosa is a medical disorder up to return to 85 percent of healthy weight (*Manheim v. Travelers Insurance Company*, 1995). Treatment costs for anorexia nervosa may be huge, but not larger than transplant surgery or treatment of leukemia, and every effort should be made to secure full coverage of treatment costs. Not to act on the patient's benefit when such action would be in his or her best interest and is a reasonable part of the professional role can be seen as passive neglect.

Authentic Beneficence versus Authoritarian or Pseudobeneficence

True beneficence is at the heart of patient care. It does not imply a patronizing or an authoritarian approach but can veer in those directions. On the one hand, an out-of-date beneficence fails to discuss with the patient the diagnosis, treatment options, prognosis, benefits, and risks from treatment options or from no treatment at all. In this category would fall "doctor knows best" attitudes and behavior (authoritarian beneficence). It would also include limiting the treatment options presented to an overly narrow category consisting only of the skill-set of the clinician, even if not best suited to the needs of the patient. On the other hand, a false view of updated beneficence presents treatment options via a "cafeteria approach," with no guidance or recommendations, but an unguided list of all possible approaches. "Whatever the patient wants" is pseudobeneficence and not in the best interest of the patient.

The ethical clinician will give the patient a clear understanding of the diagnosis, treatment, and prognosis of anorexia nervosa and will offer recommendations based on his or her experience and evidence from sound studies. True informed consent is based on the physician's guidance and opinion as to the course of treatment most likely to lead to lasting improvement. The clinician will also acknowledge limitations in his or her training and will accede to a request for a second opinion or a referral when appropriate. Not every clinician who can competently diagnose eating disorders can treat all forms of eating disorder at every level of severity. Any significant conflicts of interest should be disclosed.

Authentic beneficence grows out of a warm, nonpossessive empathy that appreciates the patient's struggles with giving up the perceived benefits of illness (anorexia is often ego-syntonic) for what seems to be perceived as a loss of control resulting from becoming healthy. It is crucial to listen with the "third ear" and try to reach out to the healthy part of the patient's mind and heart, the healthy side always constituting a larger part of the patient's being than the ill side. Beneficence will appreciate that although the patient's concerns (hair falling out, dry skin) may seem to be clinically less important than the threat of death or chronic illness, these concerns need to be incorporated into a treatment plan. The view of illness from within the illness overlaps only partially with a textbook description of the disease. Authentic beneficence always includes a biopsychosocial formulation that integrates palpable concern for patient suffering with the best available interventions treating the medical, intrapsychic, and interpersonal aspects of the disorder.

Social Justice versus Business as Usual

Social justice views the patient's disorder within a systems approach, as a tapestry in which individual and societal costs, needs, and benefits are interwoven. The patient is *de facto* part of a broad social network of family members, caregivers, communities, governmental regulators, third-party payers, legislators, and judges. While each component in theory has the patient's welfare at its center, in practice each "planet" in the solar system of care has its own orbit, its own self-serving goals, and, at times, its own counter-therapeutic practices.

Legislatures have given lip service to parity, but seldom has this resulted in an impartial approach to all illnesses as worthy of comparable levels of care based on intensity of illness. So-called mental disorders have been carved out for more limited health care benefits than "medical disorders," and eating disorders specifically have seen the most ruthless reductions in coverage limitations. Many psychiatric disorders have 30 days at best of inpatient care coverage, a small number of outpatient visits, and large co-payments. In contrast, "medical disorders" may have almost unlimited benefits. The result has been shorter and shorter inpatient treatments for anorexia nervosa despite evidence-based studies documenting that inpatient treatment short of an attempt at acute full remission leads to more relapses and more frequent rehospitalization (Baran, Weltzin, and Kaye, 1995). Repeat hospitalizations are considered "business as usual," while adequate length of stay is considered a money-losing proposition, although the latter over the course of illness costs less.

True social justice does not tolerate discrepancies in service based on race, gender, or sexual orientation. The exclusion of males from many inpatient or residential care programs represents an injustice, as does failure to reach out to diverse ethnic and racial communities, which data increasingly demonstrate have a high and increasing prevalence of eating disorders.

The health care training system may teach the importance of evidence-based treatment yet fail to provide training for psychiatrists in the most evidence-based psychotherapy for eating disorders, cognitive-behavioral therapy. In many hospital training programs the task of preparing psychiatrists for the multiple therapeutic skills necessary for comprehensive treatment has been abandoned by neglecting supervised experience in evidence-based psychotherapies.

Advocacy for social justice includes, besides a call for comprehensive treatment programs and adequate reimbursement of care, a call for funding of both clinical and translational research studies. An increased knowledge of anorexia nervosa will lead to clinical advances, an end to gender discrimination in eating-treatment programs, community education programs, screening for early diagnosis, and preventive intervention in demonstrated areas of effectiveness. Social justice advocacy also calls for an end to stigma regarding eating disorders in particular, interaction with legislative bodies for actualizing parity, and a willingness to appear before administrative justices and other personnel within the justice system to plead the patient's case for funding. States that currently do not admit patients with severe anorexia nervosa for involuntary treatment, even when clearly necessary in life-threatening cases, need to remediate this deficit in view of evidence that selective involuntary admission and treatment can be life saving.

Summary

There is increasing concern that ethical principles guide modern medical practice. Nowhere is this more evident than in the treatment of persons with anorexia nervosa, a complex biopsychosocial disorder. Historically, physicians and other clinicians have honored the principle to do no harm, but the application of this principle is subtle in the treatment of anorexia nervosa. Respect for the decision-making autonomy of ill persons has become more important as a first principle in current medical care, but even this principle is not absolute. The nature of a disorder like anorexia nervosa, which includes a spectrum of decision-making capacities from intact to absent, may require involuntary care, albeit for as short a period of time as necessary. Continuing refinement of the balance between the needs of ill persons and society is required as these biomedical principles evolve.

Guiding one's practice within the boundaries of the four principles presented in this chapter not only does not stifle vigorous treatment or compassionate clinician interaction with patients, but also broadens historic guidelines to accentuate an appropriate increased appreciation of patient autonomy as a therapeutic partner and widens the horizon of concern to a comprehensive advocacy for social justice within and between all the components of the care system.

REFERENCES

Andersen AE. 2004. Unmasking a current medical pretender: Anorexia nervosa in gastrointestinal practice. *European Journal of Gastroenterology and Hepatology* 16(11):1123–25.

Andersen AE. 2007. Eating disorders and coercion (editorial). *American Journal of Psychiatry* 164(1):9–11.

Baran SA, Weltzin TE, and Kaye WH. 1995. Low discharge weight and outcome in anorexia nervosa. *American Journal of Psychiatry* 152(7):1070–72.

Beauchamp TL and Childress JF. 2001. *Principles of Biomedical Ethics*, 5th ed. Oxford: Oxford University Press.

Draper H. 2000. Anorexia nervosa and respecting a refusal of life-prolonging therapy: A limited justification. *Bioethics* 14(2):120–33.

Guarda AS, Pinto AM, Coughlin JW, Hussain S, Haug NA, and Heinberg LJ. 2007. Perceived coercion and change in perceived need for admission in patients hospitalized for eating disorders. *American Journal of Psychiatry* 164(1):-108–14.

Manheim A v. Travelers Insurance Company. 92–CV-5466 (JG). Sept. 15, 1995.

CHAPTER FIFTEEN

Medical Information for Nonmedical Clinicians and Educators

COMMON QUESTIONS

What background medical knowledge is needed for health and educational experts (psychotherapists, experiential therapists, social workers, nutritionists, educators, coaches) who play a role in identifying, treating, or preventing eating disorders?

How do you approach a student, athlete, or friend you are concerned may have an eating disorder?

When do you refer a person with a possible eating disorder to a physician?

What medical information does a nonmedical health professional (psychologist, nutritionist, social worker) need to know in accepting an eating-disordered person for treatment?

What medical components of care may non-medically trained health professionals or educators carry out?

What are some safeguards against legal consequences for an adverse medical outcome while treating or advising a client or student with an eating disorder?

What ethical concerns are present for nonmedical clinicians and educators interacting with eating-disordered clients or students?

What role does the educator play in the course of eating disorders?

Case 1

Mr. B was a coach for a university cheerleading club that performed at major sports events. Chad, a third-year cheerleader, was 5 feet 10 inches tall and weighed 160 pounds. He complained that he could not lift Jill, who was 5 feet 5 inches and 125 pounds, over his head in a complicated, show-stopping half-time program for the basketball season. Chad asked Mr. B to suggest to Jill that she lose 10–15 pounds of weight. After listening to Chad's concerns, Mr. B suggested that Chad would benefit from a trainer-guided program to increase lean muscle mass, especially increasing strength in the shoulders, back, and quadriceps, so that he could lift Jill in the routines required. He explained that Jill ate normally and was in a healthy, thin-normal range of body fat at 18 percent. He expressed concern that he might provoke eating-disordered behavior in an otherwise healthy young woman by suggesting weight loss. Mr. B recognized the ethical aspects of this gender disparity in completing cheerleader routines, and rather than suggesting the usual change of having the young woman lose weight, suggested instead that the young man gain more strength in a fitness program so that both concerned could benefit with this "win-win" philosophy. Chad's frame would carry extra muscle mass well, as did many male gymnasts his height.

What Do Non-Medically Trained Clinicians and Educators Need to Know about Eating Disorders in Clients or Students?

THE EFFECTS OF OUT-OF-CONTROL DIETING AND EXCESSIVE WEIGHT LOSS

The most common abnormal eating pattern in high school and college students is to skip breakfast, eat a light lunch, and then have to fight hunger later in the day. Sometimes this restrained eating or chronic dieting pattern results in desired thinness through perseverance, but many times it leads to binge behavior later in the day. Most people self-regulate body weight in a narrow 4- to 5-pound range, called the "set point." This range of weight is not fixed in stone but tends to be fairly consistent in each individual. Significant lowering of weight below this point often leads to involuntary preoccupation with thoughts of food, decreased mental attention, becoming more isolative or irritable, feeling colder than peers, and manifesting changed eating behavior toward either eating slowly and in small bites or gulping food ravenously. The studies by Keys and others in the 1940s on volunteers who underwent experimental starvation to help prepare us to take care of prisoners of war documented these changes as being effects of starvation (Keys, Brozek, and Henscheo, 1950). Many of the signs and symptoms of what is called anorexia nervosa are in fact the mental and physical changes of starvation. The component that is truly at the core of the eating-disordered illness is the internalized over-valuation of the benefits of slimness or shape change, and the resulting driven behaviors that are employed to achieve these ends.

THE EFFECTS OF BINGE AND PURGE BEHAVIOR

Binge behavior is driven by three factors: hunger, distressed moods, and habit patterns related to time of day or place. Initially, binges simply start as a response to food restriction, weight loss, and hunger. Gradually, binges become triggered by distressed moods, such as anxiety about a test, a low mood from a relationship upset, anger at perceived unfairness, or feelings of boredom and emptiness. Binge behavior is not an ineffective or "dumb" behavior; it helps the triggering situations, temporarily, somewhat like a drug fix—but then creates more problems than it solves.

Most binge behavior initially represents an attempt at anorexic weights that didn't work because the body has refused to accept this degree of deprivation, allowing hunger to break through despite will power. Anorexia nervosa of the restricting type is possible only in individuals with the genetic endowment of strong perseverance. The diagnosis of bulimia requires binge episodes, even though people often mislabel purging behavior as bulimia. The term *bulimia* comes from the words for "ox-hunger." However, purging behavior takes place in 80 percent of individuals who experience regular binge behavior; it is initiated because of the fear of fatness from the unwanted binge calories, as well as from gastric medical distress from the binge. The 20 percent of individuals who binge but do not purge compensate in other ways: through heroic exercise or through even more severe restriction of food intake. While binges are uncomfortable, the purging usually produces the more dangerous medical symptoms, including a low serum potassium level that can cause heart irregularity, dehydration from loss of fluids, bleeding from the esophagus, chest pain, loss of dental enamel, and enlarged parotid glands (the ones that swell in front of the ears during mumps), to name but a few.

HEALTHY NUTRITION

Educators, coaches, nutritionists, psychotherapists, and experiential therapists are often asked to describe good nutritional patterns There are so many fads and fallacies in the area of nutrition that informal though sincere psychoeducation or guidance in nutritional selection is commonly loaded with personal misinformation, bias, and economically driven misinformation about food choices. Registered dietitians are the most qualified to give accurate advice. In some states, it is illegal for anyone but a physician or a registered dietician to prescribe nutrition.

Many students and athletes count fat grams as much as calories. The preoccupation with fat grams, not distinguishing healthy lipids (mono-unsaturates, such as olive oil, fish, nuts) from unhealthy lipids (trans-fats, saturated fats), is a completely unscientific holdover from recent decades when all fats were considered bad. From the 1970s through the 1990s, the average weight of U.S. citizens increased while fat consumption dropped. The average student who is counting fat grams tries to live on 0–10 fat grams a day. A truly prudent program of nutrition would allow 25–30 percent of daily energy intake as healthy fats. Attempts at 0, 5, or 10 grams of fat are unnecessary, unpalatable, and usually unsuccessful.

For male students and athletes who are wanting to bulk up with lean muscle, carbohydrates have become the recent phobia. Magazines touting muscle development hype low-carb diets as the secret to success. Here again, there is a vast difference between unrefined carbohydrates (grains, fruits, vegetables) and highly refined carbohydrates (white bread, sugar). Avoiding highly refined carbohydrates is reasonable, while avoiding unrefined carbohydrates is unhealthy. There is increasing evidence that the brain connections between the prefrontal cortex, where executive judgment is centered, and the amygdala, where emotions and impulses are primarily experienced, do not have fully formed connections until about age 25 in males. While this is an oversimplification of a profound neuro-developmental process, the basic finding is supported by research. The implication is that many strongly desired but unwise activities during adolescence and early adulthood (driving drunk with a sense of immunity from crashes, going to war, engaging in extreme nutritional programs to bulk up) are pursued without a recognition of their dangers.

Multiple studies support the finding that dieting rarely works. The usual meaning of the word *diet* refers to an attempt to reduce weight quickly by a program that is overly low in calories and poor in nutritional balance. The only weight change plan that works in the long run is a lifetime nutritional plan: eating every day to stay in a healthy range, or, if some weight change is medically indicated or a reasonable personal goal, eating for the desired "set point," so that the program does not need to be changed when the goal weight range is reached. For example, a young woman who is 5 feet 4 inches tall and weighs 140 pounds, with visible excess abdominal obesity, and wants to weigh 125 pounds, should eat the number of calories (with a balance in nutrition) that would maintain a young woman at 125 pounds, so that when she has achieved that weight, she does not have to change. Most diet programs that advertise "40 pounds lost in 10 weeks," for example, never give follow-up at 1, 2, or 5 years to state how many dieters have maintained their weight loss. The behind-the-scenes answer is almost none.

Educators, nonmedical clinicians, nutritionists, and coaches should encourage students to think of "diet" as a bad four-letter word and instead advocate a small cluster of healthy behaviors: good balanced nutrition, regular exercise, and good stress management, along with adequate sleep. Inadequate sleep has been shown to increase snacking and overeating, only recently recognized as an important contributor to abnormal eating patterns.

Evidence is accumulating that there is no benefit from taking vitamins if you are eating a balanced nutritional program (evidence that will be disputed by economic interests). A major factor in helping students to eat nutritionally is to have available attractive, tasty, healthy snacks and meals and to remove all soft drink machines from schools and sports facilities. An occasional soda pop won't hurt most people, but it is too easy to become accustomed to the taste and mouth texture of concentrated sweets and trans-fats (in the form of doughnuts, for example). The best defense nutritionally is a good offense. Studies in Norway have shown that simply having bowls of fruit in a classroom will increase students' likelihood of choosing fruits for the day.

Normal body weight is distributed in a bell curve just like height. Most media promote an unhealthy thinness or impossibly lean muscularity (McCabe and Ricciardelli, 2005). The narrow ranges suggested by insurance company tables or other charts for individual weights are often used inaccurately. These weights are averages, not norms. The real measures of health include a percentage of body fat that is appropriate for age and gender, the location of fat distribution (pear shape vs. apple shape), the resting heart rate, absence of signs of starvation, normal patterns of hunger and satiety, and abandonment of the idea that there are any bad foods or foods that should be phobically avoided. Too many physicians tell patients what to weigh too narrowly, basing their recommendations on average insurance table numbers for longest life span—for example, stating that a 5 foot 4 inch woman should weigh 120 pounds. Instead, the appropriate approach is to take a full personal and family history, use multiple measures of fitness, and identify a range of healthy weight for the patient. Studies have shown that patients with anorexia nervosa will in general pursue low weight to a greater degree than profound religious goals. For example, Roman Catholic girls may skip going to mass because of the calories in the wafer (Graham, Spencer, and Andersen, 1991).

EXERCISE

We are as much an underfit nation as an overfat nation, as well as a nation that has irrationally invested moral and emotional meaning in artificially thin or muscular ideals. With only a few exceptions, the body will self-regulate weight in a narrow range when eating is driven by normal cycles of hunger and satiety (rather than in response to emotional needs) and when daily life includes moderate energy output in any form of exercise or physical activity. In general, we encourage "couch potatoes" to get moving and do three to five moderate exercise periods a week of 30–40 minutes, such as walking; at the same time we guide compulsive exercisers to choose moderate, prudent exercise rather than driven, inappropriate exercise. (See Chapter 11, on athletes and eating disorders.)

DIAGNOSTIC APPROACHES

There is nothing sacred or limited to health professionals about asking screening questions to sort out whether a person may have an eating disorder. Educators, therapists, coaches, and others can use the same SCOFF questionnaire that primary care physicians use (see Chap. 1 and Table 1.3), as well as add their own questions. These questions should cover the following general areas: Are you extremely concerned about your weight? Does attaining a different weight or shape dominate your life? Are you dieting? Have you lost significant weight? Do you experience binge eating or other eating out of control? Do you purge after meals? Do you exercise compulsively? Is there an overvaluation of the benefits of slimness or shape change that overrides normal concerns? Some school systems have used the EAT-26 for screening for eating disorders (D'Souza, Forman, and Austin, 2005).

RISK FACTORS FOR DEVELOPING EATING DISORDERS

Eating disorders usually occur in individuals with known risk factors (see Chap. 1). The more risk factors and the more severe these risk factors, the higher the probability of a person's developing an eating disorder. These risk factors include participation in sports or interest groups that encourage weight loss; a family history of obesity, anxiety, eating disorder, or depression; sensitive, self-critical, persevering personality traits; excess weight gain during childhood or during early puberty; gay orientation in males; and comments from influential individuals (teachers, coaches, and educators) promoting weight loss. Teachers may influence students in unhealthy or healthy habits. See section below on educators for more information.

Case 2

L.M., a 12-year-old female, developed pubertal changes slightly earlier than her peers. In a health class in the fifth grade, she, like every other student in the class, was weighed in front of the class, with the teacher commenting on the weight status of each student. She was told that she was about 10 pounds overweight and should lose some weight. She felt ashamed and criticized. She started a program of severe dietary restriction, cutting out sweets and fats, adding exercise, and becoming preoccupied with the calorie and fat content of foods. Within 6 months she met the criteria for anorexia nervosa, including loss of menstrual periods. For the next 6 years she required continued regular care for her low weight, her morbid fear of fatness, the development of binge-purge behaviors, and overexercising. She avoided social events involving food. When she went to Europe on a student exchange program, she was referred to an experienced clinician who helped to stabilize her weight, change her core psychological overvalued beliefs in the necessity of extreme thinness, and begin a pattern of healthier weight and eating. She still remains preoccupied with weight but has had return of menstrual periods and continues in psychotherapy.

When Should a Client or Student Be Referred to a Physician for Evaluation of an Eating Disorder?

It is good practice at the beginning of psychotherapy for any client with an eating disorder to have a medical evaluation (see Table 15.1). This procedure may disclose hidden medical complications from the eating

TABLE 15.1   When to refer a client or student to a primary care physician

- At the beginning of psychotherapy treatment, for evaluation and to establish liaison relationship
- When the client or student has any of the following symptoms:
  - Severe or rapid weight loss
  - Dizziness, lightheadedness, fainting (hypotension)
  - Uncontrolled binge-purge behavior (electrolytes often abnormal; cardiogram may be abnormal)
  - Constant coldness
  - Medical distress, such as chest pain (often from purging behavior) or abdominal pain
- For psychopharmacology augmentation (preferably by a psychiatrist) to psychotherapy
- Periodic check-ups or weighing (often may be performed by physician's assistant or nurse)

disorder, but at a minimum it offers a baseline of medical evaluation so that future medical symptoms can be compared with this baseline. It is helpful to have an established relationship with a primary care physician with special expertise about eating-disordered young people. This eliminates an inexperienced medical approach to individuals you may refer for evaluation and avoids unnecessary, excessive testing. Subjective complaints that should lead to prompt referral to a primary care physician include constant coldness, faintness or lightheadedness, heart palpitations or chest pain, shortness of breath, abdominal pain, or frequent purging behavior as evidenced by a client's saying that she or he uses many diuretics or laxatives a day, and certainly if Ipecac, an over-the-counter medicine to induce vomiting in kids who have eaten poison, is used. (Ipecac is no longer recommended for poison response.) Common sense and professional judgment will also guide clinicians and educators to refer clients or students when they note significant weight loss; a thin, bony appearance; bluish hands; a cold handshake; or an overall appearance of bad health. Information from parents or friends about excessive purging behavior should also generally lead to referral.

At times, medical referral is deferred because a patient is developing insight. It is important to realize that while "insight" on the part of the patient is critical, there is a huge difference between intellectual insight and behavior-changing insight. Insight is useless unless it leads to sustained behavioral change. Valuing intellectual insight in the presence of continued, severe weight loss; a failure to restore weight; or lack of change in significant binge-purge behavior, is an illusion. The patient has not made progress when she or he gains and then loses weight, with multiple excuses and promises to do better next session. Behavior is behavior is behavior.

When Should a Client Be Accepted for Therapy on Referral from a Physician?

Accepting a client from a physician should ideally involve sufficient assurance from the physician that the patient is well enough to come for nonmedical treatment, primarily psychotherapy and experiential therapy (see Table 15.2). It is important to record agreements regarding when the patient or client should be referred back to the physician and to set up both

TABLE 15.2   When to accept a patient for therapy from a referring physician

- After medical evaluation is under way
- After establishing frequency-of-contact schedule and conditions for return to see physician
- After decisions are made on frequency of checking body weight and who will weigh patient
- After deciding who will instruct patient on healthy nutrition and prescribe a nutritional program (physician or registered dietitian)

TABLE 15.3   How to collaborate effectively among team members

- Establish a regular, agreed-on communication schedule.
- Set up clear, specific conditions for referrals (for example, to dietitian, social worker).
- Clearly define the roles of the various team members.
- Share techniques guiding the overall treatment.
- Set goals for patient care within each discipline that are specific, time-limited, achievable, and ratable.
- Decide who is "captain of the ship."
- Decide on a single, consistent guiding psychotherapeutic strategy, such as CBT.

regular and as-needed communication patterns between the therapist or coach and the physician. It is also important to establish who performs what roles in regard to shared medical functions such as weighing the person. Thus, it is inappropriate to refer an individual for treatment without specification of who will follow weight or monitor binge-purge behavior. Agreements should be in writing and contacts recorded in the medical record. Table 15.3 summarizes the steps of effective collaboration.

What Medical Responsibilities Can Be Carried Out by Non-Medically Trained Clinicians?

A medical degree or specific training is not required to weigh a patient or to encourage healthy behaviors such as good nutrition. These are commonsense practices that can be carried out by nonmedical clinicians and certainly are done frequently by coaches and educators, as well as formally trained nutritionists and physicians. Coaches often monitor resting heart rate. The key here is to be clear on who does what, and under what conditions the client or student needs to be referred back to the physician. Some psychologically trained therapists do not like the idea of weighing a client, or carry outmoded ideas that weighing a client would somehow interfere with psychotherapy. Sometimes it is simply not practical or is too expensive for a client to return to a doctor's office on a weekly basis for weighing when it can be done in a therapist's or a nutritionist's office. Agreements need to be recorded about a weight minimum or simply the lack of progress in the weight restoration process that will prompt referral to more intensive medical treatments. A psychotherapist can ask a patient to keep a nutritional record to assess whether there is compliance with the nutritional prescription, emotionally based alterations in eating, or the presence of binge-purge behaviors. The patient can use a simple 3 × 5 index card to record each day, in columns, the time of day, food eaten, emotions experienced, and events taking place. This record can form the basis for beginning the psychotherapy session.

How to Avoid Legal Problems

The key to avoiding legal problems for comprehensive care includes good record-keeping, decisions about when to refer a patient to a physician (erring on the side of more rather than fewer referrals), documentation of regular communication with the primary care physician and other team members, and acting with knowledge and common sense. Letting a patient lose weight in front of your eyes because she or he is developing "insight," failure to refer someone who simply looks very ill, perpetuating irrelevant or out-of-date nutritional details about calories or fat grams in place of sound nutrition, failure to document the communications with a primary care physician—all would open one to being included in litigation if adverse medical consequences occur. This does not mean that referral is necessary for mild but improving starvation, occasional binge-purge behavior, and so on. It takes time, knowledge, and the development of professional judgment to balance the intrusiveness of medical referrals versus their necessity after the initial evaluation. Working within your limits of qualified training is essential, as is having a team-oriented approach (see Chap. 2). Litigation is rarely a concern when treatment is sound, adequate records are kept, and good patient-clinician relationships are maintained. When these guidelines are followed, the treatment and education of eating-disordered clients, students, or athletes will be satisfying and effective.

Information for Educators

The most common question asked by educators is how they should approach a student whom they are concerned may have an eating disorder. We provide some guidelines in Table 15.4. Seeing that someone is losing significant weight, passively watching an individual consistently exiting

TABLE 15.4   How to approach a person you are concerned may have an eating disorder

- Educate yourself about eating disorders from accurate sources.
- Be caring but firm in approaching the person.
- Share your concern about the possibility of an eating disorder being present. Share what you have observed kindly as evidence for the presence of a problem.
- Gently but firmly tell the person to schedule an appointment with a qualified health professional or eating disorders clinic for assessment, and then "I'll be off your case."
- Don't oversimplify the issue or assume that time will improve the disorder.
- Don't imply that bulimia nervosa is less serious because there is no obvious emaciation.
- Express your concern privately.
- Don't diagnose.
- Don't become the therapist or savior or offer short-term, oversimplified solutions.
- Do act in an emergency, such as the presence of chest pain, suicidal thinking, or passing out, and get help immediately.
- Assure the person that you will maintain friendship through the process of becoming well.
- Encourage the continuation of spiritual growth without "spiritualizing" or "moralizing" the problem.
- Be direct and nonpunitive.
- Avoid arguing.
- If there is no response, consider sharing your concern with a authority figure, such as a teacher, coach, or parent.

after meals or snacks to use the restroom, or becoming aware of significant mental preoccupation with weight and shape should all be signs that alert the educator to the possibility of an eating disorder. Educators are often approached by friends of a student who tell them about behaviors that the educator may not see directly.

The best approach to a student about whom you are concerned is simply to approach the student and say that you're concerned that an eating disorder may be present and that it is essential for them to see a trained individual or clinic for an evaluation. Depending on the age of the student, the parents may be informed and their help solicited.

Educators have multiple important role. One role is preventive intervention, an ideal that is seldom achieved but increasingly possible (Piran, 2004; Russell-Mayhew, Arthur, and Ewashen, 2007). Educators may attempt to prevent eating disorders by talking with students about eating disorder symptoms, but this approach has a contrary effect of probably increasing tendency to eating disorders. Instead of more information about signs and symptoms, students need to know how to develop skills of healthy thinking and behavior in a media-saturated atmosphere that emphasizes thinness or shape change as the most important achievement in life. Runi Gresko, Norway's leading educational expert on prevention of eating disorders in schools, has taught, "Eating disorders are not prevented by talking about eating disorders" (personal communication, 1993).

Almost certainly, if primary prevention is possible, it will happen through insulating vulnerable individuals from our culture's relentless demands for thinness. That eating disorders can be prevented is only partially and selectively proven, but there are hints that the keys to successful prevention include teaching increased assertiveness to young girls especially, helping individuals to be critical of media claims promoting the value of thinness, increasing body self-esteem, and teaching valuation of the normal diversity of weights while strongly encouraging fitness at every set point. Girls benefit by moving from an observational, judgmental, and objectified view of body to an operational, instrumental, and functional view, seeing the body in terms of what it allows one to do, not primarily how it looks. Setting minimum weights and BMIs below which a person may not participate in a sport or an activity (wrestling, ballet) shows some promise of decreasing the behavioral incentive to slim more.

Certainly, weighing individuals in schools has no purpose except to embarrass, distress, or humiliate young people and leads to psychological distress at a minimum, as well as promoting unhealthy and unnecessary dieting. Spotlighting an individual's weight as being excessive may be the starting point for an eating disorder. Educators are role models who need to take seriously their responsibility to teach fitness behaviors in place of dieting and to stress the normality of a wide range of weights. Their personal examples of fitness behavior and healthy weight ranges, as well as their openness to discussion, are essential.

There is increasing evidence that for mild cases of eating disorders, especially bulimia nervosa, self-help modules through Internet-assisted computer methods may be effective (Ljotsson et al., 2007). The Internet is a medium in which educators are usually effectively up to date, and it may offer young sufferers the most helpful program for their needs. Educators can sensitize students to the perils of "pro-anorexia" Web sites by exploring such sites with students and teaching the students to critique and deglamorize them.

Information for Coaches

There is increasing evidence that setting lowest acceptable weights for participation in sports, and maximum rates for weight loss and body fat loss, helps to decrease the onset or perpetuation of eating disorders, especially in wrestling, ballet, and long-distance running. When there is no advantage to further weight loss in ballet or wrestling ("You will have to leave the program if you lose more weight"), then there is less incentive to keep on losing. In Wisconsin, for example, a legislative action has required high school wrestlers to limit the amount of weight lost for qualification for a wrestling weight category and has set minimum body fat levels for participation eligibility. These efforts, partially a response to a number of deaths in young wrestlers associated with weight loss practices in the 1990s, appear to be effective.

In sports, where weight for achievement of performance goals or appearance judgments may be in conflict with an individual's health needs, ethical and health decisions need to be integrated, with the athlete's best interests being the first concern. An individual whose performance in sports is maximized only when there are signs of abnormal eating behavior, or when there is distressed thinking concerning weight and eating patterns, needs to be counseled about the relative importance of health versus performance. Unfortunately, many young men and women live in a bubble of illusory invulnerability, whereby they fail to appreciate that some performance goals are simply not worth the health costs for them. Elite athletes are often driven internally as well as externally through a narrow focus of interest, relentless perseverance, and self-critique. Reports have documented the presence of the "elite athlete triad" of abnormal eating, weight loss, and osteoporosis in young female athletes (Sundgot-Borgen, 1994). Mild to moderate eating disorder syndromes in athletes are missed or overlooked when these athletes are performing with excellence. The case at the beginning of the chapter suggests that women often carry a disproportionate burden to lose weight in couples' sports such as cheerleading and pairs skating. The male partner could just as well be advised to get strength training. It is a personal opinion that the lower and lower weights and younger ages characteristic of girl gymnasts in recent Olympics represent an ethical concern. Bonci et al. (2008) describe how athletic trainers can help to prevent, detect, and manage eating-disordered athletes.

Information for Parents

Parents play major roles in shaping the course of eating disorders in their children. While too often blamed when they are in fact doing their best, parents may exert excess pressure for girls to be thin and boys to be muscular (McCabe et al., 2007). Only recently appreciated are an understanding of the stress of parents living with a child with anorexia nervosa (Kyriacou, Treasure, and Schmidt, 2008) and the needs of siblings of adolescent girls with anorexia (Honey and Halse, 2007). Treasure (1997) has written a survival guide for families, friends, and sufferers. The role of the parents varies with the age of the child with the eating disorder: the younger the child, the more involved the family must be. Families need support, information, and a sense of realistic optimism about the outcome of treatment for eating disorders. Parents also have a role in monitoring computer usage by their children, allowing appropriate changes as children reach their later teen years. Pro-anorexia sites are abysmally silly and unattractive from the viewpoint of an adult without eating disorders and good self-esteem but may have a strange fascination for a subgroups of teens. Talking about these issues openly from a neutral viewpoint may be helpful. Research is robust that having regular family meals most days of the weeks decreases the probability of a teen developing an eating disorder or drug abuse problem (Ackard and Neumark-Sztainer, 2001; Fulkerson et al., 2006).

Summary

A combination of medical knowledge, common sense, and a good working relationship with medical professionals will allow for the shared treatment of clients and students who have eating disorders, as well as for the possibility of prevention, and, certainly, the early identification of eating disorders. Good record-keeping, documenting regular communication with a medical professional, having a low threshold for referral when appropriate, and recognizing the ethical aspect of weight and shape change versus performance goals will enhance the significant role that nonmedical mental health professionals, educators, coaches, and nutritionists have in the care of young individuals. The recognition, treatment, and prevention of eating disorders involves a "village" or community of caring, concerned individuals who are knowledgeable, thoughtful, and proactive.

REFERENCES

Ackard DM and Neumark-Sztainer D. 2001. Family mealtime while growing up: Associations with symptoms of bulimia nervosa. *Eating Disorders* 9:-239–49.
Bonci CM, Bonci LJ, Granger LR, et al. 2008. National Athletic Trainers' Association position statement: Preventing, detecting, and managing disordered eating in athletes. *Journal of Athletic Training* 43:80–108.
D'Souza CM, Forman SF, and Austin SB. 2005. Follow-up evaluation of a high school eating disorders screening program: Knowledge, awareness and self-referral. *Journal of Adolescent Health* 36:208–13.
Fulkerson JA, Story M, Mellin A, Leffert N, Neumark-Sztainer D, and French SA. 2006. Family dinner meal frequency and adolescent development: Relationships with developmental assets and high-risk behaviors. *Journal of Adolescent Health* 39:337–45.
Honey A and Halse C. 2007. Looking after well siblings of adolescent girls with

anorexia: An important parental role. *Child: Care, Health and Development* 33:52–58.

Graham MA, Spencer W, and Andersen AE. 1991. Altered religious practice in patients with eating disorders. *International Journal of Eating Disorders* 10:239–43.

Keys A, Brozek J, and Henscheo A. 1950. *The Biology of Human Starvation.* Minneapolis: University of Minnesota Press.

Kyriacou O, Treasure J, and Schmidt U. 2008. Understanding how parents cope with living with someone with anorexia nervosa: Modeling the factors that are associated with carer distress. *International Journal of Eating Disorders* 41:233–42.

Ljotsson B, Lundin C, Mitsell K, Carlbring P, Ramklint M, and Ghaderi A. 2007. Remote treatment of bulimia nervosa and binge eating disorder: A randomized trial of Internet-assisted cognitive behavioral therapy. *Behaviour Research and Therapy* 45:649–61.

McCabe MP and Ricciardelli LA. 2005. A prospective study of pressures from parents, peers, and the media on extreme weight change behaviors among adolescent boys and girls. *Behaviour Research and Therapy* 43:653–68.

McCabe MP, Ricciardelli LA, Stanford J, Holt K, Keegan S, and Miller L. 2007. Where is all the pressure coming from? Messages from mothers and teachers about preschool children's appearance, diet and exercise. *European Eating Disorders Review* 15:221–30.

Piran J. 2004. Teachers: On "being" (rather than "doing") prevention. *Eating Disorders* 12:1–9.

Russell-Mayhew S, Arthur N, and Ewashen C. 2007. Targeting students, teachers and parents in a wellness-based prevention program in schools. *Eating Disorders* 15:159–81.

Sundgot-Borgen J. 1994. Risk and trigger factors for the development of eating disorders in female elite athletes. *Medicine and Science in Sports and Exercise* 26:414–19.

Treasure J. 1997. *Anorexia Nervosa: A Survival Guide for Families, Friends and Sufferers.* East Sussex, UK: Psychology Press.

Behavioral Guidelines for Staff to Use with Patients Who Have Eating Disorders

University of Iowa Hospital and Clinics, Behavioral Health Services,
Eating Disorder Program (Revised 12/01/07),
by Eating Disorders Treatment Team Review Panel

These are guidelines, not rules. They allow uniformity in many situations and take much of the uncertainty out of meal supervision. The guiding principle in regard to nutrition is "Normal food eaten normally supervised by nursing staff." When necessary for any individual patient, these guidelines will be modified for optimal case management. Because they are locally derived, but with a history of similar use at Johns Hopkins Hospital when Dr. Andersen was on the faculty there, they may need to be modified in different locales. For new programs, they may represent a starting point.

Appropriate rationale must be given for why the guidelines are used; one needs to be kind but firm when redirecting and above all consistent.

Meals

Meals are 45 minutes in length and snacks are 15 minutes.

1. Patients must be supervised at all times while they are eating. The goal is to create as normal an eating environment as possible. Sit at the table with the patient and socialize between the times you are coaching/encouraging her or him to eat. This is not a time to talk about issues related to weight loss, body image, etc. The comment often comes up that we are asking patients to do things that "normal individuals" would not do; this is because these patients have eating disorders, so it is at times necessary to make sure they take in all their required calories and complete their meal and/or snack.

2. When a patient has visitors (families or others) during meals or snacks, please inform them at the beginning of the visit that the patient will have 15 to 45 minutes during which she or he will be eating with peers. The visitors may wait in the patient's room or the visitation area until the patient is finished. If patients are actively going on passes with their families, they may

have a snack with their family if the treatment team deems this appropriate. During meals, patients are to start and finish the meal/snack together and leave the dining room as a group.

3. The patient must eat everything on the tray. (Potato skins are to be consumed if butter and/or sour cream are used. May remove potato skin, and then apply butter and/or sour cream.) Fruit or vegetable juice in the bottom of the dish does not have to be consumed. May elect not to use ketchup, mustard, and salt or pepper. No extra salt allowed. May have one extra pepper. May have an extra ketchup packet for use on appropriate foods. Syrup for pancakes must be entirely applied; the patient does not have to consume extra syrup from the plate but should use the syrup as directed by staff so that little is left on the plate. (Document any changes on the dietary slip.)

4. Patients must finish their milk, and it is important for the staff to ensure that no milk is left in a straw if the patient is using one.

5. Packets for condiments or dressings must be empty. Au jus for French dip sandwich is an exception. Patients must dip sandwich; however, given the amount of juice, the patients are not required to consume all of it. Use good judgment and see that they are routinely dipping the sandwich.

6. Patients will be allowed to remove (under supervision) fat from the exterior portion of a meat serving.

7. Patients are to remain seated with feet on floor in typical eating position, in front of tray a reasonable distance from the table until everything is eaten or until bedtime, whichever comes first. Patients return to the unit when the 45 minutes are over; social contacts and extra attention from the staff end for patients who have not completed their meal.

8. Offer bathroom visits before meals/snacks. Encourage all patients to use the bathroom even if they elect not to use it before the meal. Be sure that patients are not overusing the bathroom to practice eating disorder behaviors, but do not hesitate to allow use if there is no indication of eating disorder behaviors.

9. Patients need to be monitored to be sure that they are eating normal-sized bites of food. The patients are assessed for fear foods, and they are not allowed to leave these for last or eat them rapidly just to get them down. Monitor the patient for inappropriate eating patterns, and redirect as necessary.

10. Patients are not allowed to smear food, specifically butter. (Monitor for

smearing under the table, on napkin, chair, socks, or skin.) If this happens, replace the food item and give an additional food item for the patient to eat with the item (for example, a cracker for butter).

11. Monitor patients for crumbling food onto the floor, tray, or clothes.

12. Patients are to drink 240 cc with each dosage of Miralax that is given. Patients are to receive a minimum of 1500 cc of fluid per day; this includes water, juice, and milk. (Modifications will be made according to age, weight, and medical status.)

13. Water consumed by the patients is to be room temperature; using ice is a deterrent because this requires the body to use more energy bringing the water to body temperature.

14. Replace food dropped on the floor if the amount is significant. Monitor and document to see if this is an ongoing behavior.

15. Monitor the patients closely for hiding food; replace any hidden food. Staff will need to routinely search patients' rooms, under the table, TV room, couches, and pillow cases.

16. Patients are not allowed to mix foods, as they need to learn to appreciate the flavor of food.

17. Patients are not allowed to exchange items that are on the dietary slip. If the dietary slip does not specify what type of item is to be eaten (for example, pudding or juice), then the staff may use the items that are available.

18. Patients may not blot foods with a napkin or other item. (Watch specifically for bacon, pizza, sausage, and condiments.)

19. Patients are to consume any significant amount of food that is on any of their eating utensils.

20. If any food item was left off the tray by dietary, call dietary communications and the item will be replaced. Staff need to check for the patient's dislikes before requesting a replacement from dietary.

21. Patients may designate three food items as hate foods, and these are written in stone unless the patient decides that she or he would like to try the food item. The chosen hate foods may not include an entire category of food but must be a specific item (for example, the patient cannot choose chocolate as a hate food). If the food item is a part of a mixed serving, then the patient will have to eat the item even though it is included in the serving.

22. Staff need to check trays, eating utensils, and under the plate closely at the end of each meal/snack.

23. Patients are not allowed to have tissues at the table during meal times and need only one napkin.

24. Patients need to be monitored to be sure that they are allowing their eating utensils to touch their lips and that they are not just using their teeth to remove the food from their utensils.

25. Patients are not allowed to chew ice because of the damage to tooth enamel and impact on appetite. (Remember, they are not to have ice at all.)

26. If a patient has reflux, make sure she or he sits upright to decrease reflux and to prevent bringing up food to purge. Do not have the patient lie flat on her or his back after meals/snacks. During the night, the head of the patient's bed needs to be elevated to alleviate reflux.

27. Patients will eat any food served while on activity, in school, or as a celebration even if not part of their prescribed dietary intake. Document any intake on the patient's dietary slip.

28. Staff need to redirect any problem behaviors and document them so that the team can address these issues.

29. Patients on the adult unit may have one Styrofoam cup of fluid off of every snack cart. The patient may use one packet of sugar and one of cream with a cup of coffee or tea. To prevent water loading, no cups are allowed in the adult bathrooms.

30. Monitor patients for the following problems: salt loading, hiding salt and/or sugar packets, getting extra water for fluid loading, hoarding food, sprinkling sugar or salt on table, tray, or floor, hiding Sweet'N Low.

Other Issues

31. Patients are not allowed to engage in extra movement and need to be redirected from leg shaking, extra trips, and excessive standing. Monitor patients for overexercising during scheduled activities. Monitor patients for excessive jumping or impact on activities.

32. Patients are to sit in their chairs with their backs relaxed against the back of the chair. Monitor patients for flexing of muscles, toes, and feet.

33. Patients are to sit with their feet on the floor or crossed at the ankles when they are sitting in chairs because of poor circulation. Children and adolescents may sit on the floor as appropriate to the activity they are engaged in

and as approved by staff. Children and adolescents are not allowed to use the rocking chairs on the unit. Patients who are too short to reach the floor while sitting in a chair will have a box given to them to use.

34. Patients are not allowed to carry backpacks or heavy stacks of items. If these are needed, the staff is to carry them or use a wire basket for transport.

35. Monitor patients for moving all of their materials frequently from one place to another. They should not be making trips to their rooms during the day.

36. Patients are not allowed to know their weight or when they are restoring/losing unless approved by the team. It is up to the treatment team to determine if the parents and significant others are to be informed of this information, as the needs of each patient's parents and significant others are different.

37. Weight ranges will be shared at discharge. Patients in partial day programs will be told their weights and whether or not they are making progress with their restoration.

38. Patients are to be weighed with their backs to the scale, in a hospital gown after voiding (jewelry is to be removed). Undergarments and socks are to be taken off before weighing. Staff need to closely monitor for weights of any type that the patient may be attaching to their bodies. Staff need to be sure that the patient is free standing and not pressing against any item to increase the weight.

39. Patients are not allowed to discuss food, calories, or weight outside of group, individual therapy, or structured discussion.

40. Patients are not allowed to speak in a derogatory manner regarding the program, staff, or peers. Patients are encouraged to speak directly with anyone with whom they are having an issue, or they may ask to speak with the head nurse on their unit.

41. Patients may bathe or shower in the morning after they have been weighed. Adult patients may bathe in the evening as well.

42. If the patient's weight is below 80 percent, she or he is required to use an inflated pillow for sitting, have a foam egg crate mattress on the bed, and shower every other day.

43. If the patient's weight is below 70 percent, she or he is to use a Geri-chair and is allowed to walk around the unit once per shift with a staff member in attendance.

44. Some patients may need assistance with appropriate clothing; staff will

need to redirect inappropriate layering and clothing that is too tight or provocative.

45. Patients may brush their teeth twice daily, and this should not follow a meal unless directed by the patient's dental needs and documented, at which time they may brush their teeth one hour after eating. This guideline is to prevent purging or spitting out of food.

46. Patients are not allowed to chew gum or to use caffeinated beverages on the unit. Patients who have used caffeine excessively before admission will be tapered off the caffeine.

47. Patients will have 1 hour between bathroom trips; emergency trips will be allowed, but the staff need to monitor this to make sure it is not related to the eating disorder. Patients will not be allowed to use the bathroom during meal/snack times unless an emergency or medically indicated.

48. Monitor patients to ensure that they remain on observation. If they are observed walking away, they will be redirected and the information will be documented for the team to discuss appropriate consequences.

49. Staff need to avoid appearance-oriented reinforcement, instead focusing on reinforcing good problem-solving, good thinking, being kind, helpfulness, or using effective coping strategies.

50. Patients will not use excessive amounts of time for grooming in the morning. Staff will cover the bathroom as staffing permits and as is reasonable.

51. Patients must be observed during bathroom usage. This needs to be done discretely to provide the most privacy without allowing the option to practice eating disorder behaviors (water loading, purging, exercise). Staff will need to observe the results of each bathroom use by the patient. Staff will document I and O and bowel movements; please chart specifically (include amount, size, consistency, and any other details that will assist the physicians in determining medical care). Staff will have the patients flush the toilet after the observation is completed.

52. Adult patients will have their bathroom doors unlocked unless the treatment team deems it necessary to lock them for the patient's benefit. This is necessary to provide the least-restrictive environment.

53. Bowel protocol is to be used when the patient has no significant bowel movement for 2 days.

54. Patients are not allowed to have blankets and pillows out on the adult unit. Children and adolescents on the child unit may use blankets and pillows as

appropriate, and if they are cold, they are to be encouraged to dress warmly. Neither group of patients is to bring blankets or pillows to group meetings unless directed to do so by staff.

55. If the patient is on a feeding pump, it needs to be covered so the patient is not able to see the rate or the rate change. Monitor patients on feeding pumps as determined by the treatment team.

56. Weights are measured after voiding and before showering in a hospital gown only every Monday, Wednesday, and Friday by night staff. Daily weights may be ordered if the patient is less than 75 percent, if there is a concern about refeeding syndrome, or if there is an inconsistency in weights.

57. Patients will have orthostatic vitals BID for the first 3 days, then daily until the vitals are normalized. Patients will be asked if they are dizzy, feel their heart racing, or feel as though they may faint. If significant changes in vitals occur, consider fluids because the patient may be dehydrated.

58. Patients will be on I and O if ordered by the physician or nurse. This is not required for every patient but needs to be ordered if there is any concern about hydration or kidney function.

59. Observation levels are protocol-driven and are ordered by the physician; a nurse can increase the level of observation as needed, but a decrease has to be discussed by the team and ordered by the physician.

60. Phone calls, visits, and TLOAs are discussed by the team and ordered by the physician and may not be terminated for noncompliance unless this is determined by the treatment team.

61. Patients will be given the EAT/EDI or EDE within 2 days of admission to the inpatient service and 2 days before discharge from inpatient; the testing will also be administered 2 days before discharge from partial hospitalization. Patients admitted directly from the outside to partial hospitalization will be tested 2 days following admission and 2 days before discharge.

62. Child and adolescent patients routinely have neuropsychological testing. Adult patients will have neuropsychological testing as determined by the physician and the treatment team. Neuropsychological testing is not to be interrupted for any reason other than an emergency.

63. Each patient is required to have a bone densitometry done at admission per physician order unless contraindicated or not indicated, as in normal-weight bulimia nervosa with no history of an anorexic episode.

64. Patients may say to you, "So-and-so told me it was okay to ...." Tell the patient: "At times individuals make different decisions from one another, and the staff do their utmost to be consistent. However, it is not a perfect world, and we all have to learn to deal with differences. The most important thing is that we all are working together to help you overcome your eating disorder behaviors."

65. Patients may ask you why the guideline is in effect, and you may give the patient the rationale for the guideline; if you are unsure, tell the patient that you will check on it and get back to her or him.

66. Staff need to use their best judgment when there is no clear guideline. Monitor counter-transference.

Page numbers in *italics* refer to figures.

dietitians, role of, 42–43, 243
diuretic abuse, 100, 103, 105
dual-energy X-ray (DEXA): criteria for, 33, 76; description of, 147, *148*, 223–24; as screening tool, 149–50; used therapeutically, 224

eating disorders: clues to, 13, 14; conceptions of, 39; as culture-bound, 4–6; myths about, 30–31; natural history of, 6, 8; overview of, 3–4; risk factors for, 5–6, 7–8, 187–89, 246
"eating disorders not otherwise specified" (EDNOS), 11–12
edema, 89, 103–4
educators: information for, 251–53; role of, 40, 44, 193, 194. *See also* medical information, for nonmedical professionals
electrocardiogram (EKG), 73, 101–2, *132*, 132–33
electrolyte function: abnormalities in, 98–99, 106; arrhythmias and, 134; clinical cases, 96–97; clinical manifestations of abnormalities, 99; laboratory tests for, 73–74; normal ranges, 98; pathogenesis, 99–102; refeeding and, 90; treatment of abnormalities in, 102–5
elite athlete triad, 254
enamel of teeth, erosion of, 66, 173–74
endocrinology: AN and, 163; background, 161; clinical cases, 159–61; hormone abnormalities, 161–65; overview of, 168; tests, 165–66. *See also* gynecological endocrinology
enteral feedings, 91–92, 93
ethical issues: authentic beneficence vs. authoritarian or pseudobeneficence, 236–37; autonomy vs. beneficence, 233–34; biomedical, 232–33; in coaching, 191; nonmaleficence vs. (unintended) maleficence, 234–36; overview of, 238–39; social justice vs. business as usual, 237–38
evidence-based treatment, 23, 237–38
exercise, 193–94, 195, 245
external locus of control, 186

family history, as risk factor, 7
family treatment, intensive, 25
fasting for religious holidays, 43
female athletic triad, 187–88, 190
fitness promotion in schools, 194
follow-up care, 32–33
fracture risk, 146–47, 149–50

gastroesophageal reflux, 32–33, 114, 120–121; GERD, 33
gastrointestinal complaints: in AN, 111–20, *112*, *118*; background, 109–11; in BN, 120–23; clinical cases, 108–9; guidelines for care of, 124; information used psychotherapeutically, 225; overview of, 123
gastroparesis, 111–13, *112*
gender: of athletes, 182–83, 184, 187–89; body norms of sports by, 183; perceptions of fatness and, 201–2; risk factors and, 7, 187–89
gingivitis, 175
glucose metabolism, 162–64
goals of treatment, 21
group approaches to treatment, 55, 56–59
growth hormone, 161–62, 166
gymnastics, 185–86, 188, 254
gynecological endocrinology: in AN, 140–42; clinical cases, 138–39; hypothalamic dysfunction, 142; reproduction, 143–44; treatment of amenorrhea, 143. *See also* amenorrhea

Harris-Benedict formula, 85–86
heart rate variability, 130–31
heritability, 7, 16
hormonal therapy for osteoporosis, 150–52
hormone abnormalities: glucose and other hormones, 162–64; growth hormone, 161–62; information used psychotherapeutically, 226; thyroid, 162
hyperamylasemia, 176–77
hypercholesterolemia, 68, 164
hypoglycemia, 90–91, 162–64
hypokalemia, 98, 99, 103, 105, 134

hyponatremia, 66–67, 98, 104–5
hypophosphatemia, 84, 84–85
hypotension, 129, 131
hypothalamic dysfunction, 142, 143, 161

ideal body weight (IBW), 71–72, 82–83, 212
IGF-1 (insulin-like growth factor 1), 142, 146, 161–62, 166
informed consent, 236
injury, athletic, 186–87, 190
inpatient treatment: behavioral guidelines for meals, 257–60; behavioral guidelines for other situations, 260–64; description of, 45, 46; reasons for, 24
instruments to validate treatment, 41–42
insulin-dependent diabetes, 166–67
insulin-like growth factor 1 (IGF-1), 142, 146, 161–62, 166
intensive outpatient (IOP) treatment, 45, 46
interest groups, as risk factor, 7. *See also* athletes
internists, role of, 40, 42
interpersonal therapy (IPT), 23, 25, 48
ipecac, 135, 248
irritable bowel syndrome, 109–10

laboratory tests: for males, 209; mandatory, 73–75; optional, 75–76; results of, 67–68, 69
lactose intolerance, 226–27
laxatives: abuse of, 100–101, 121–23, 221, 227; classification of therapies, 117; education about, 115; stimulant-type, 116
legal issues, avoiding, 250–51
leptin levels, 164
levels of care, 44–47, 47
liver function, 74, 90, 119

magnetic resonance imaging (MRI), 224–25
major depressive illness, 13, 15
maleficence, unintended, 234–36
males, body image ideals in, 201, 202, 203

males with eating disorders: AN and, 204–5; as athletes, risk factors for, 188–89; background, 200–204; BED in, 205, 209, 213–14; BN in, 205, 214; clinical cases, 199–200; clinical features of, 207; diagnosis, 204–7; healthy weight for, 212–16; medical assessment of, 207–9; overview of, 17, 18, 216–17; treatment of, 209–12, 215–16
managed care, interactions with, 50–53, 51
mechanical approach to treatment, 53, 54, 55
media influences, 8
medical assessment: diagnosis, 63–68; differential diagnosis, 68–70, 71; importance of, 13; laboratory tests, 73–76; of males, 207–9; overview of, 62–63; physical examination, 70–73
medical diseases, predisposing, 8
medical information, decision to share, 228–29
medical information, for nonmedical professionals: about binge and purge behavior, 242–43; about diagnostic approaches, 246; about dieting and excessive weight loss, 241–42; about exercise, 245; about healthy nutrition, 243–44; about healthy weight, 245; about referrals for evaluation, 247–48; about risk factors, 246; clinical cases, 240–41, 246–47; coaches, 253–54; educators, 251–53; overview of, 255; parents, 254–55; responsibilities, roles, and, 249–50
medical information, used psychotherapeutically: allergies, and lactose intolerance, 226–27; background, 221–22; bone mineral density, 223–24; clinical cases, 220–21; gastrointestinal changes, 225; laxative abuse, 227; MRI results, 224–25; night sweats, 227–28; overview of, 230; reproductive hormone status, 226; signs of starvation, 225–26; test results, 222–28; vital signs and acute instability, 223
medical management, ongoing, 76–77

medications: antidepressants, 21, 23, 25, 28; metaclopramide, 33, 113; prokinetic agents, 33, 120–21; proton pump inhibitors, 32–33, 114; 120–21

menstrual cycle in anorexia nervosa, 140–42. *See also* amenorrhea

mesenteric artery syndrome, 20

metabolic alkalosis, 99–101, 102–3, 105

metabolic complications of refeeding, 90

metaclopramide, 33, 113

methods of treatment, 21–22

mitral valve prolapse, 133

mortality rate from anorexia nervosa, 25, 63, 127

MRI (magnetic resonance imaging), 224–25

multidisciplinary care: assembling team for, 48; background, 38–39; clinical cases, 36–38; cohesiveness vs burn out, 48, 49, 50; collaboration and, 249; levels of, 44–46, 47; members and function of team, 39, 40–44; overview of, viii, 59–60

muscle dysmorphia, 9

myths about eating disorders, 30–31

night eating syndrome, 12

night sweats, 227–28

nonmaleficence, 234–36

normative cultural distress, 195

nurses, role of, 40, 42

nutrition, healthy, 243–44

nutritional rehabilitation: background, 82–83; clinical cases, 80–82; complications, 89–91; importance of, 79–80; overview of, 93–94; refeeding syndrome and, 83–85, 84. *See also* refeeding

obesity, viii, 19

obsessive-compulsive disorder (OCD), 15, 27

occupational therapists, role of, 40, 43–44

oral and dental complications: angular cheilosis, 172–73; background, 171–72; caries, 174–75; clinical cases, 170–71; enlargement of salivary glands, 66, 175–76; gingivitis, 175; hyperamylasemia, 176–77; overview of, 177; perimolysis, 173–74

oral refeeding. *See* refeeding

organ systems, symptoms related to, 3, 4

osteopenia, 145

osteoporosis: biphosphonates and, 152–53; calcium and, 154; clinical cases, 139; diagnosis of, 147, 148; hormonal therapy for, 150–52; in males, 214; onset of, 149–50; overview of, 144–45, 154–55; screening for, 76; weight gain and, 153–54. *See also* bone mineral density

outpatient treatment, 22

paranoid states, 15

parents: information for, 254–55, role of, 229

parotidectomy, 176

partial hospitalization (PPH), 24, 45, 46

passive harm, 235–36

peak bone mass, 145

pediatricians, role of, 40, 42

perimolysis, 66, 173–74

personality: of athletes, 186; as risk factor, 7; vulnerabilities of, 16

personality disorders, treatment of, 27

physical activity, importance of, 193–94, 195, 245

physical examination, 70–73

physicians: acceptance of client on referral from, 248–49; role of, ix, 39, 40, 41, 42

pilocarpine tablets, 176

potassium deficits, 102–3

potassium repletion, 105

PPH (partial hospitalization), 24, 45, 46

pregnancy, 144

prevention: athletes and, 194–95; of burnout, 48, 49, 50; educators and, 252; of refeeding syndrome, 85; of relapse, 22 primary care medicine: clinical cases, 1–3, 20; communication issues, 29, 32; diagnosis and evaluation, 9–19; follow-up and prognosis, 32–33; in multidisciplinary care, 42; overview of, 33–34; presentation to, 3, 4, 13; referrals to specialists from, 29; therapeutic interventions, 20–26. *See also* physicians

principalism, 232–33

prognosis, 32–33, 153, 215

prokinetic agents, 33, 120–21

protestin challenge test, 143

protocols for changes in level of treatment, 47

proton pump inhibitors, 32–33, 114, 120–21

pseudo-Bartter's syndrome, 104

psychiatric disorders: eating disorders and, 15–16; imitating eating disorders, 13, 15; in males, 208; predisposing, 8; reasons for hospital treatment of, 24; treatment of, 26–28

psychiatrists, role of, 39, 40, 41

psychoeducation, 21, 222. *See also* medical information, used psychotherapeutically

psychologists, role of, 39, 40, 41

purging: definition of, 62; effects of, 242–43; electrolyte abnormalities and, 98, 100–102

QT dispersion and QT interval, 127–28

racial and ethnic groups, as risk factors, 8

record-keeping, 250–51

REE (resting energy expenditure), 86, 88

refeeding: alternative modes of, 91–93; complications of, 89–91, 234; importance of, 79–80; inpatient guidelines for, 257–60; tips for, 85–89

refeeding pancreatitis, 118

refeeding syndrome, 42, 83–85, 84

referrals for evaluation, 247–48

reflux, 32–33, 114, 120–21

relapse prevention, 22

reproduction, 143–44

reproductive hormones, 226

resting energy expenditure (REE), 86, 88

"reverse anorexia," 8–9, 189, 206

"revolving door" approach, viii

risk factors: in athletes, by gender and sport, 187–89; overview of, 5–6, 7–8, 246

"rule-out" approach to diagnosis, 13, 70, 235

salivary glands, swelling of, 66, 175–76

scaring patients with medical information, 222

schools, role of, in healthy athleticism, 193–94

SCOFF Questionnaire, 9, 208, 246

screening questions, 9, 53, 208, 246

selective serotonin reuptake inhibitors (SSRIs), 21, 23

serum amylase levels, 67–68, 176–77

serum bicarbonate level, 67, 73–74, 98, 100

serum potassium levels, 67

"set point" of body weight, 241, 244

sex hormone-binding globulin, 164

sexual orientation: of males, 204, 209; as risk factor, 7

sharing of medical information: appropriateness of, 228–29; with parents, 229; presentation of, 230. *See also* medical information, used psychotherapeutically

signs, 64–67

sleep, and diet, 244

social justice, 237–38

social learning in perceptions of fatness, 201–2

social workers, role of, 40, 43

sports participation: by females, 187–88; gender-neutral, 187; by males, 188–89. *See also* athletes

SSRIs. *See* selective serotonin reuptake inhibitors

starvation, signs of, 225–26

stress reactions, 140

substance abuse, treatment of, 27

sudden death, risk of, 127–28, 131

superior mesenteric artery syndrome, 119–20

symptoms: of eating disorders, 63–64; of endocrine disorders, 164–65; organ systems and, 3, 4

team treatment. *See* multidisciplinary care

TEE. *See* total energy expenditure

teeth enamel, erosion of, 66, 173–74. *See also* dental caries

testosterone levels, 164, 210–12

therapeutic alliance, 53, 55, 222, 230

therapeutic interventions: acceptance of client on referral from physician, 248–49; for amenorrhea, 143; with athletes, 190–91; for constipation, 122–23; in electrolyte abnormalities, 102–5; evidence-based, 23, 237–38; group approaches, 55, 56–59; with males, 209–12, 215–16; mechanical, 53, 54, 55; of oral complications of BN, 173; of osteoporosis, 150–54; primary care medicine, 20–26; for

psychiatric disorders, 26–28; validation of, 41–42. *See also* inpatient treatment; medications; multidisciplinary care

thyroid function, 74–75, 162, 165–66

total energy expenditure (TEE), 86

total parenteral nutrition (TPN), 80–81, 91, 92–93

treatment. *See* therapeutic interventions

validation of treatment, 41–42

vital signs, 89, 223

vomiting, self-induced, complications of, 170–72

weight gain: bone mineral density and, 153–54; for recovering anorexic males, 212–16

weightlifting, 206

weight loss, excessive, 241–42

Wellbutrin (bupropion), 23, 28

wrestling, 205–6, 253

X-ray. *See* dual-energy X-ray

ARNOLD E. ANDERSEN, M.D., is professor of psychiatry at the University of Iowa College of Medicine, where he and colleagues initiated a spectrum of care for eating disorders, including an inpatient unit, a Partial Hospital (Day) Program, an Outpatient Diagnostic and Continuing Care Clinic, and a variety of teaching and research programs. Their program is based on the principles of cognitive-behavioral therapy (CBT), including group, family, and individual therapy, with individualized psychopharmacology.

Dr. Andersen is especially interested in the integration of biomedical and psychosocial therapies, the medical complications of eating disorders, the gender factor in behavioral disorders, the neurobiology of eating disorders, and cross-cultural studies. He and colleagues have published numerous peer-reviewed research studies and clinical teaching chapters in books and have presented outcome and other research studies at local, national, and international meetings. His background includes Cornell Medical College, a medical internship, board certification in psychiatry, 15 years on the faculty of the Johns Hopkins Medical Institutions, and participation in numerous scientific groups. His research at Johns Hopkins Medical Institutions and the University of Iowa has included studies on the outcome of treatment of several thousand patients, the effect of eating disorders on bone density (osteoporosis), concerns of males with eating disorders, and theories of the origin of eating disorders.

PHILIP S. MEHLER, M.D., CEDS, is the chief medical officer of Denver Health Medical Center. A Phi Beta Kappa and honors graduate of the University of Colorado and an Alpha Omega Alpha graduate of the University of Colorado Medical School, Mehler has been at Denver Health since training there as a resident in the early 1980s. He served as chief of internal medicine from 1993 to 2003 and as associate medical director from 2003 to 2008. Dr. Mehler is also a professor of medicine at the University of Colorado Medical School, where he holds the Glassman Endowed Chair of Medicine. He has published more than 200 manuscripts and has won numerous teaching and research awards. His main interest is in the medical complications of anorexia nervosa and bulimia, as well as in the medical stabilization of patients with very severe anorexia nervosa who are 30 percent or more below ideal body weight.

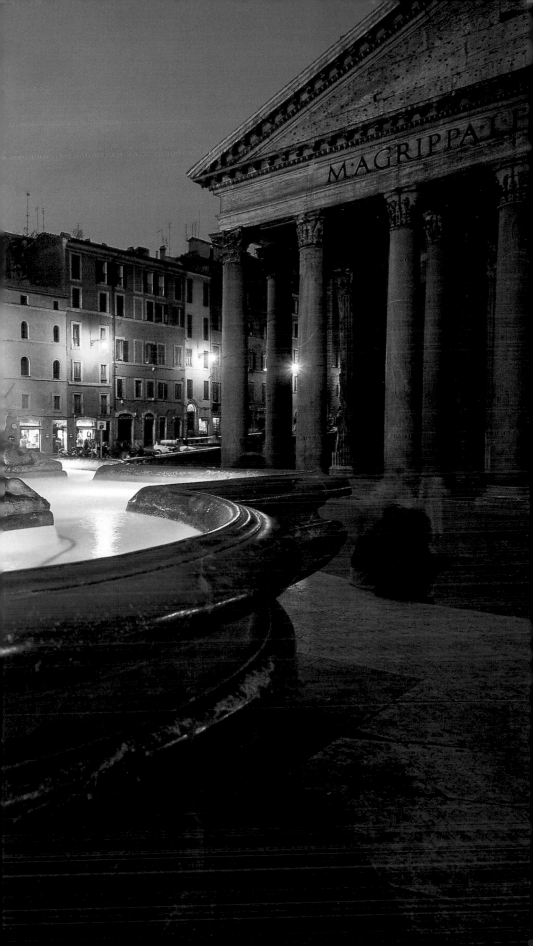

Fodor's Holy Rome

Concept and design: Fabrizio La Rocca
Editorial development: Asterisco s.r.l. – Milano
Project editor: Luca Giannini

Editorial contributors: Emilio Del Gesso, "Rome of
Saints and Martyrs"; Francesco Scoppola and Stella
Diana Vordemann, "Rome's Jubilees: Origins and
Chronology"; Carla Compostella, Holy Rome section;
Donata Chiappori, Artists in Rome biographies.
Translation: Meg Shore
Copyediting: Ellen E. Browne

Photography: Luciano Romano* (with the exception of
those listed on p. 180)
Layout: Tigist Getachew
Photo research: Ornella Marcolongo
Rome Atlas: Cartographic Service of the
Touring Club Italiano
Prepress: Emmegi Multimedia – Milano

The section *Rome, the Year 2000, and the Christian
Jubilee* was prepared by the Rome Agency for Jubilee
Preparations.
Contributors: Francesco Bandarin, Caterina Cardona,
Alberto Cortese, Maurizio d'Amore, Angela Stahl

Fodor's Travel Publications, Inc.
President: Bonnie Ammer
Publisher: Kris Kliemann
Editorial director: Karen Cure
Creative director: Fabrizio La Rocca

Touring Club Italiano
President: Giancarlo Lunati

Touring Editore
Chief executive officer and director general:
Armando Peres
Vice presidents: Marco Ausenda and Radames Trotta
Editorial director: Michele D'Innella

Copyright © 1999 Touring Editore s.r.l. – Milano

Published in the United States by Fodor's Travel
Publications, Inc., a division of Random House, Inc.,
New York, and simultaneously in Canada by Random
House of Canada, Limited, Toronto.
Published in Italy by Touring Editore s.r.l. – Milano
Distributed in the United States by Random House,
Inc., New York.

ISBN 0–679–00454–8
First Edition

Acknowledgments
The Fondo Edifici di Culto (F.E.C.), which is controlled
by the Department of Interior's Central Office for
Religious Affairs, was established by Law N. 222 of May
20, 1985, following the February 18, 1984, agreement
between the Italian State and the Holy See. It oversees
over 600 sacred buildings in the country, as well as the
works of art housed in these structures, an invaluable
documentation of cultural developments in Italy over
the course of centuries. The goal of the F.E.C. is to show
off this patrimony to its greatest advantage, in terms of
both preservation and protection and promotion.

Special Sales
Fodor's Travel Publications are available at special
discounts for bulk purchases for sales promotions or
premiums. Special editions, including personalized
covers, excerpts of existing guides, and corporate
imprints, can be created in large quantities for special
needs. For more information, contact your local
bookseller or write to Special Markets, Fodor's Travel
Publications, 201 East 50th Street, New York, NY 10022.
Inquiries from Canada should be directed to your local
Canadian bookseller or sent to Random House of
Canada, Ltd., Marketing Department, 2775 Matheson
Boulevard East, Mississauga, Ontario L4W 4P7.
Inquiries from the United Kingdom should be sent to
Fodor's Travel Publications, 20 Vauxhall Bridge Road,
London SW1V 2SA, England.

Printed in Italy by Amilcare Pizzi S.p.A., Italy

10 9 8 7 6 5 4 3 2 1

Contents

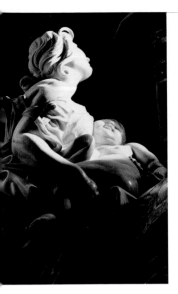

*Gian Lorenzo Bernini
and assistants, Tomb for
Alexander VII Chigi,
detail of the face of the
Bambino della Carità
(Infant Jesus of Charity).*

*Previous page:
Piazza della Rotonda, with
the fountain designed by
Giacomo della Porta and, on
the right, the Pantheon.*

How to Use this Book

A GUIDE TO CHRISTIAN ROME

This book is organized in three sections. The first consists of two essays, dedicated respectively to Rome of the saints and martyrs and to the origins and history of the Jubilee. More than a historical-religious introduction, these essays are a key to the thematic interpretation of Christian Rome. Indeed, the dominant theme of the book is Christianity, experienced through churches, basilicas, tombs of saints and martyrs, catacombs, mausoleums, monasteries, and all the sites that have made Rome a Holy City as well as the Eternal City. Descriptions of these sites make up the entire second section of the book, Holy Rome. The third section contains information of a more practical nature. In 16 pages, the Roman Agency for Jubilee Preparations describes its preparations in the capital for the year 2000 and details the major religious and cultural events. The pages entitled Artists in Rome provide biographical summaries for Rome's most exemplary artists. Finally, the Rome Atlas contains 16 pages of information-filled maps.

Boxes complement the text and provide additional **biographical, historical,** and **artistic** information.

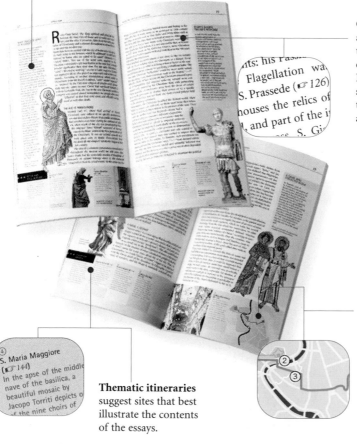

Cross-references allow the reader to move from the essays to the Holy Rome section, where the monuments are described.

Flagellation wa
S. Prassede (☞ 126)
houses the relics of
, and part of the i
S. Gi

Small **maps** at the bottom of essay pages accompany the thematic itineraries, illustrating their stages and placing them within the urban context.

④
S. Maria Maggiore
(☞ 144)
In the apse of the middle
nave of the basilica, a
beautiful mosaic by
Jacopo Torriti depicts o
f the nine choirs of

Thematic itineraries suggest sites that best illustrate the contents of the essays.

②
③

THE GEOGRAPHY OF A CAPITAL

The section Holy Rome consists of 12 chapters listing city monuments most closely linked to the history of Rome as the capital of Christianity. These chapters contain groupings of the 22 *rioni*, or districts, that make up the center of Rome, as defined by the 3rd-century Aurelian Walls that marked the outer limits of the city until the 19th century. The term *rioni* comes from the Latin word *regiones,* which referred to administrative subdivisions of ancient Rome. During the Augustan period there were 14 districts, but the number varied during the Middle Ages. When the municipality was reorganized in 1144, their number changed to 12, then 13 in the early 14th century, and 14 again in 1586. Their boundaries were confirmed in the administrative reorganization of 1743–1744, under Pope Benedict XIV. In 1874 the Monti *rione* was reduced in size and the Esquiline *rione* created. Finally, in 1921, 7 new *rioni* were carved out from the existing ones, raising the number from 16 to 22.

Each of the 12 chapters in the Holy Rome section is cross-referenced to an **area map** that illustrates the *rioni* discussed in the chapter and refers to the Rome Atlas for a more detailed view.

Each area is preceded by a brief **introduction** that illustrates the characteristics of the rioni and quickly summarizes their history and development.

Chiesa Nuova ②
⊞3 E2–F3. In 1575, the little church of Vallicella to the Co the Oratory, which

More than 300 **churches, palazzi, streets, piazzas,** and **monuments**—all closely linked to the history of Christian Rome—are cross-referenced to individual maps marked by ⊞ in the Rome Atlas (⊞**3 E2-F3** indicates map 3, grid coordinates E2 and F3).

The **Rome Atlas,** on a 1:7500 scale, contains eight maps of the city with its most important monuments drawn in 3D. Readers can use this precise, essential tool to get their bearings in the center of the city.

Foreword

I
t is a great pleasure for me to introduce the Italian and international public to this guidebook. The entire publication is dedicated to Rome in the year 2000, when the city will celebrate the Jubilee that marks the passage from the second to the third millennium of the Christian era.

Promoted and developed by the Touring Club Italiano, by Fodor's Travel Publications, and by the Rome Agency for Jubilee Preparation, this guidebook focuses on the exceptional historical significance of the Jubilee, with an understanding that this is an occasion for spiritual reflection that can unite us. This book also conveys the city's pivotal position in a dialogue among peoples, an encounter between different cultures, in the support of peace.

Rome is a special city with unique characteristics. It is the capital of two states. It is also one of the few capital cities in the world that is the product of a millennial history still visible in its archaeological zones, in its streets and piazzas, in its monuments, both civil and religious. Rome is a complex city, and its celebrated beauty and destiny as a great center of international tourism must be compatible with the equally complex workings of a modern metropolis.

This is one of the reasons why, in recent years, Rome has made significant organizational efforts to prepare for this extraordinary event, which will draw millions of pilgrims and visitors. The face of the city has been renovated, new infrastructures have been put in place, and new services for pilgrims and tourists have been made available.

In the year 2000 Rome will be delighted and proud to welcome its guests, who will find a city that is renewed, thoughtful, and ready to receive them, with a yearlong series of events, as well as occasions for spiritual and cultural enrichment. Throughout the Holy Year, those who travel to Rome for religious reasons will be able to experience moments of intense emotion, and the cultural offerings will also be extraordinary. The importance of the passage of the millennium in our city is reflected in exhibitions, theaters, concerts, new installations in the city's great museums, and the renovation of spaces for culture and art.

Giulio Carlo Argan, a great man of culture and an unforgettable mayor of Rome in the 1970s, wrote, "from the 16th to the 18th century, Rome was for European art what Paris was in the 19th century and the first half of the 20th century." He added that "of all the European metropolises, Rome is without doubt the most visited, portrayed and described."

This book is not intended to be yet another guidebook to Rome. Rather it should be viewed as a precious traveling companion on the occasion of the Jubilee. Its originality and scope lie in its inspired mix of holy Rome, historic Rome, and everyday Rome, with all three taken into consideration and presented to the reader as a living and indivisible totality.

Without denying the ancient tradition of the Mirabilia Urbis, which, over the course of centuries, informed generations of travelers—pilgrims, scholars or those who were simply curious—about the legacy of the Eternal City, this book pursues new and different pathways that lead to a discovery of Rome in the year 2000. Thus, while it is accurate and exhaustive in every fact that pertains to historical Jubilee events, it also plays a secular role by presenting a wealth of cultural and tourism information. The coexistence of sacred and profane, which makes Rome such an interesting sociological phenomenon, has long prevailed along the banks of the Tiber.

Rome is a profoundly hospitable city, and it offers a warm welcome to all. This welcome is part of the spirit of the Romans, who have been practicing it for centuries, turning it into a deeply rooted tradition. For us, the foreigner is a friend, to be welcomed with friendliness, interest, and in a spirit of fraternity.

Francesco Rutelli
Mayor of Rome

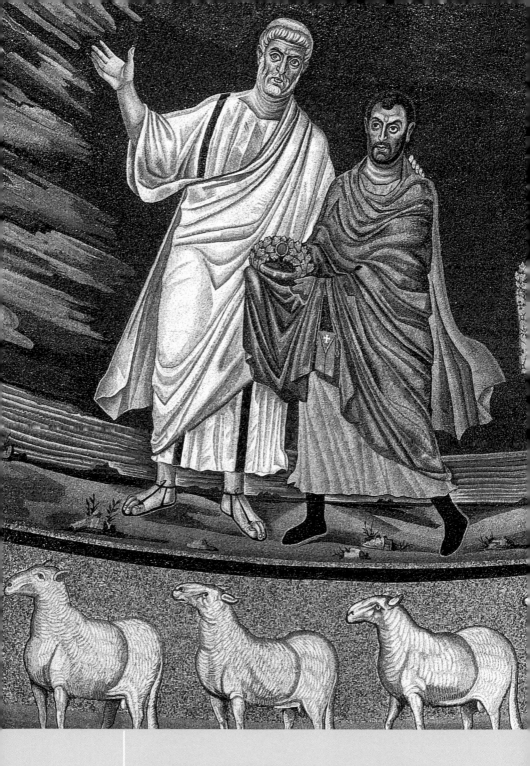

ROME OF SAINTS

AND MARTYRS

WHO DECIDES WHO IS A SAINT?

Today an individual achieves sainthood in the Catholic Church via canonization—that is, inclusion in a canon, a type of list. Canonization occurs only after a long inquiry by ecclesiastic authorities that involves the presentation of arguments for and against sainthood. One party provides proofs in favor of a candidate, while another party—the so-called devil's advocate—seeks to present counterproofs. If it is determined that the individual has accomplished at least two miracles after death, then he or she is beatified. Beatification, which confers the title of "Blessed," is the first step on the road to sainthood. Formal canonization, which may take decades, if not centuries, requires that other miracles be proved as well, and can be approved only by the pope. In the early centuries of Christianity becoming a saint was much simpler. A community could simply proclaim a person a saint by acclamation (*vindicatio* in Latin), as depicted in a scene in a panel on the wooden portal of S. Sabina (☞ 122).

The apostle Peter; detail of the mosaic in S. Maria Maggiore.

Rome's spiritual ties are deep, rooted in the early centuries of Christianity, and the city has always been known in Italian as "Roma Santa"—Holy Rome. This is in no small part because of the close ties it has had with its saints and martyrs and their relics through its entire history, up until the modern era.

Saints have been associated with Rome since St. Paul's letter to the Romans, which he addressed "to all God's beloved in Rome who are called to be saints" (Romans, 1:7, *Oxford Bible*). This use of the word "saint," applied to the Christian community's spiritual leaders at the time, had a much broader significance then than now. For the early Christians, "saint" ("devoted to worship," *sanctus* in Latin, *hagios* in Greek) was applied to those who played an important role in the community. According to another interpretation, which came to Christianity from the Jewish tradition, "saint" meant "separate" or "distinct." In the Christian religion all people could potentially become saints because Christ had sacrificed himself to redeem humanity from sin, but in the new Christian society, a category was created almost immediately for people who were "different," in that they were saints and officially recognized as such after death.

THE AGE OF PERSECUTIONS

When Paul arrived in Rome in AD 61, Christians were subject to no specific restrictions, nor did they endure threats from public institutions. But just three years later, during the summer of AD 64, when much of the city was devastated by fire, the emperor Nero, himself suspected of having caused the blaze, initiated the first persecution of the Christians. It was an isolated episode that took place only in Rome. Persecutions that involved all the empire's territories began in the 3rd century.

The idea of continuous persecutions sowed terror throughout the Roman world for 400 years after Jesus' death, but the systematic murder of hundreds of thousands of victims belongs more to the medieval imagination than to actual events. In the same way, the image of crowds of Christians hunted down

PETER AND PAUL IN ROME

Information about the martyrdom of these two saints is contradictory. Nevertheless, Rome is filled with sites that commemorate their presence and their suffering.

① Basilica di S. Pietro (☞ 52)
The largest sanctuary in Christendom is dedicated to the first apostle. The Crypt of St. Peter's contains the tomb of Peter, who suffered martyrdom a short distance away, in the Vatican circus.

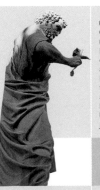

A statue of the apostle in Piazza S. Pietro.

② Carcere Mamertino (☞ 110)
In this ancient water cistern transformed into a prison (opposite the Forum, on the slopes of the Campidoglio), Peter and Paul were held. Legend has it that they both baptized their jailers.

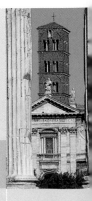

S. Francesca Romana's church and bell tower.

and hiding in the catacombs has it roots more in its portrayal in 19th-century paintings or novels such as *Quo Vadis?* and 1950s films such as *The Robe* and *Ben Hur*, than in historical sources. Although no one will never know how many early Christians were sent to their deaths for their beliefs, it is not impossible that, as historian K.T. Ware wrote in his *Orthodox Church*, more Christians died for their faith between 1918 and 1948 than in the 300 years following the crucifixion.

What inspired the persecutions is not clear. In the 1st century AD, far from looking upon Christians as a danger, Rome viewed them as a possible stabilizing political factor in the eastern Mediterranean, a means for pacifying a rebellious Judea. The messianic Christian "barbarians" could be more easily tamed, the reasoning went, than extremists such as the Zealots. After the death of Nero in AD 68, Christians enjoyed a period of tranquillity, and imperial authority seemed more concerned with protecting Christians than persecuting them; episodes of intolerance arose from the desire of certain provincial governors to display their power or to a specific emperor's politics and not from any deep-rooted policies held by the central government.

Nonetheless, Christians troubled the Roman world. Their belief in Jesus' sole authority set them apart from their fellow Romans and made them appear to be enemies of the state. Their belief in another God was disputed, although Rome had a policy of religious tolerance and even adopted the beliefs of conquered peoples on occasion. But the Christians' refusal to submit to imperial authority could not be supported, particularly in the provinces, which were perpetually under pressure to demonstrate their loyalty. In addition, Christians not only wanted to worship as they pleased, they also wanted to impose their new morality on the empire. To Romans, such proselytism was incomprehensible. Christians' ways were deemed subversive, but the line between lawful and unlawful behavior was blurred, and the decision to order a persecution often depended on a particular emperor's politics.

During this era, as emperors struggled to maintain the political balance or to distract impoverished classes from yet another social crisis, systematic persecutions alternated with restrictions

PLINY'S DOUBTS, TRAJAN'S RESPONSE

In AD 110 writer Pliny the Younger was governor of Bithynia and Pontica, and in his correspondence with Trajan about various political problems, he referred to the Christians. Pliny asked advice "about the great number of persons accused; in fact, without consideration of age, social class or sex, many are put on trial.... The contagion of this superstition now has become widespread, not only in the cities, but also in villages and in the countryside." Trajan responded in temperate fashion: "In general, one cannot establish a valid rule.... They should not be sought out; if they are denounced and are found guilty, they should be punished.... And as for anonymous denunciations, these mustn't be taken as valid in any trial, for they have the characteristics of the worst precedents and are not fitting for our times."

③
S. Francesca Romana
(☞ *113*)
The church contains two stones said to bear the knee prints of the apostles, who knelt and prayed for the sorcery of Simon Magus to be revealed. In an attempt at flight the latter did indeed fall to his death.

④
S. Pietro in Vincoli
(☞ *108*)
Housed in this church are the chains that bound Peter. For some time they were divided in two pieces, one in Rome, the other in Jerusalem. When they were placed next to each other, they miraculously fused.

⑤
S. Prassede (☞ *108*)
Tradition has it that this 5th-century church was built on the site of a house where Peter stayed. The house belonged to Praxedes, sister St. Pudentiana and daughter of Senator Pudente.

A bronze of the emperor Trajan in Via dei Fori Imperiali.

STRANGERS AMONG US

In Rome, the debut of a religion that arose from the Judaic world and that was expressed in Greek concepts and terms had more or less the same effect as the arrival of aliens in a spaceship. It is no wonder that great writers such as Svetonius or Tacitus described the Christians as a "race of men devoted to a new, strange and sorcerous cult" (*Vite dei Cesari*, Nero, XVI) and spoke of "ruinous superstitions" (*Annali*, XV, 44). To gain acceptance among the Roman cultural elite, the countercultural Christian community had to respond with traditional arts and letters. Such a task was left to intellectuals such as Minucius Felix, a lawyer who converted to Christianity. He used his oratorical talents in the *Octavius*, a three-way dialogue in which he lists and disproves, one by one, all the rumors about the Christians, including one about fried children.

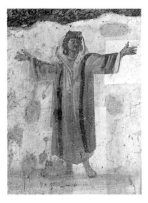

A figure praying; a 4th-century fresco in the spaces beneath the basilica of Ss. Giovanni e Paolo.

and periods of tolerance. The worst persecutions were under emperors Decius (250), Valerian (258), and Diocletian (303–313).

"THERE IS NO RAIN, THE CHRISTIANS ARE TO BLAME"

Romans of all social levels accused the Christians of ignorance, atheism, immoral conduct, incest, and cannibalism. Intellectuals and higher social classes depicted the followers of the new religion as a sect of gullible dupes, because they refused to sacrifice to the gods. This was not because the accusers believed in the efficacy of their pagan cults, but because they remained deeply wary of the wrath of gods whose honor had been wounded. They could not comprehend the moral rigidity of the early Christians, who would not make sacrifices to the spirit of the emperor. Christians' refusal to observe pagan rites was tantamount to a rejection of the essence of being Roman.

Roman rancor was also rooted in misunderstandings. Imagine what might have happened if a Christian and a pagan—both members of the middle class, working as artisans, small merchants, or the like—decided to discuss Christianity. It shouldn't have been hard for them to communicate, because they probably had many things in common, including the same cultural background and even the same tastes. But when the Christian tried to enlighten a pagan about the principles of Christianity or the mystery of the Eucharist, the pagan would simply not have understood. The pagan might have thought that members of the strange sect practiced incest, since they all called each other "brother" and "sister," and that, since they claimed to eat the body and blood of their god, they also practiced cannibalism.

Soon Romans blamed Christians for all sorts of things. Today's Italians joke, "If it rains, the government is to blame," but during the mid-4th century people would say, "There is no rain, the Christians are to blame."

"MARTYRS FOR GOD" AND OTHER SAINTS

Until the 5th century, the victims of persecutions in the Christian community were recognized in two categories of martyrs of God: confessors of the faith and martyrs. Threatened with torture, confessors survived for various reasons. Martyrs

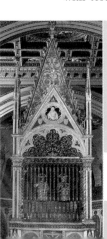

⑥
S. Giovanni in Laterano
(☞ *105*)
This ancient basilica, erected immediately following the edict of Constantine, is the cathedral of Rome; above the high altar (*at right*), two silver cases enclose the remains of the heads of Peter and Paul.

⑦
Chiesa del Domine Quo Vadis (☞ *129*)
This church was built on the Via Appia, on the site where Peter, fleeing Rome, saw Jesus. "Quo vadis Domine?" ("Where are you going, Lord?") Peter asked. Jesus' response led Peter to return to the city to face his death.

⑧
Abbazia delle Tre Fontane
(☞ *128*)
(Abbey of the Three Fountains)
This site on the Via Ostiense is where Paul was beheaded. Tradition has it that the saint's head fell and bounced on the ground three times, bringing forth three springs of water.

sacrificed their lives. ("Martyr," a word of Greek origin, means "witness," and these people are so-called because they gave witness to the truth of their beliefs with their death.) At first martyrs outnumbered confessors, but after the persecutions ceased the numbers switched. The term "saint" acquired widespread use only at the end of this period. To these two categories, the church soon added the worship of other saints, mainly those mentioned in the Bible: the Virgin Mary, John the Baptist, Joseph, the Magi, and Old Testament patriarchs, prophets, certain kings, and other figures. Angels, whose existence has been an article of faith since 325, were also venerated and considered saints in every respect. In 745, the Council of Rome sanctioned the worship of Michael, Raphael, and Gabriel, who served as messengers of God and defenders of men from evil.

A THOUSAND WAYS TO DIE

In the early centuries after Christ's death, martyrs automatically became saints in the eyes of the church. Their canonization was taken for granted, and the memory of their specific martyrdom was carefully preserved (and if the facts weren't well known, they were created). The attention the church paid to the sometimes macabre details, replayed in the accounts of the martyrs' sacrifices, arose partly out of a desire to present examples for the faithful, but was also a legacy of ancient Roman culture. Roman mythology assigned symbolic significance to different types of torture and execution.

The symbolism of a Christian's death often took second place to the Romans' desire to mount a spectacle, as seen in their circus games, and for this, the Greco-Latin literature offered a compendium of brutalities as sources of inspiration. During the games, mythological episodes of a tragic nature were staged, using Christians as stand-ins for the archetypal heroes: Hercules burning on the mountain, Marsyas flayed alive, Adonis torn to pieces by wild boars, Queen Dirce tied to the horns of a bull.

ICONOGRAPHY OF THE CRUCIFIXION

According to many historians, the oldest representation of the crucifixion, dating from the 2nd century and preserved in the Palatine Antiquarium, is a blasphemous graffito that depicts a crucified Christ with a donkey's head. A phrase, in Greek—"Alexamenos worshiping his God"—accompanies the pagan sneer. In this blasphemous graffito, as in the early Christian Eastern iconography, Christ's feet are apart. One of the oldest Christian representations of this kind of crucifixion is on S. Sabina's (☞ 122) carved wooden door, which dates from the first half of the 5th century. In the churches of S. Maria Antiqua (☞ 113) and Ss. Cosma e Damiano (☞ 116), Jesus still appears with his feet apart and dressed in a short-sleeved tunic known as a *colobium*. After the 9th century, this image becomes rare and is replaced by what has become the traditional iconography: the Christ figure with feet together, dressed only in a loincloth.

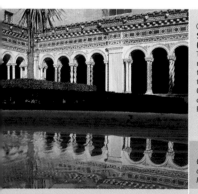

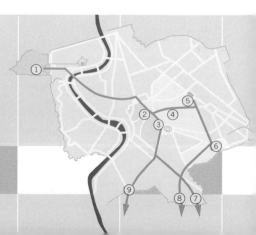

⑨
S. Paolo Fuori le Mura
(☞ *131*)
This large basilica marks the site of the tomb of Paul; inside the church, the Chapel of the Relics contains the chains of Paul's imprisonment.

Cloister of the basilica of S. Paolo Fuori le Mura.

SOLDIERS OF CHRIST

In the military, many refused to sacrifice to the gods and went from being defenders of the empire to defenders of Christ. St. Sebastian is one of the most eminent "soldiers of Christ." He served in the emperor Diocletian's personal guard, a prestigious position in the Roman army. After declaring himself a Christian, he was tied to a stake and pierced by arrows aimed by his fellow soldiers. His body rests in the basilica dedicated to him on the Appian Way (☞132); his head lies in church of the Ss. Quattro Coronati (☞117).

Crucifixion, the punishment for which the Romans were most famous, was traditionally inflicted on fugitive slaves and was a dishonorable way to die; it was used on a large scale during the slave revolts of the 1st century BC. Many Christians were crucified after Jesus, including the apostles Peter and Andrew.

The way martyrs died could also indicate legal status. Decapitation was reserved for Roman citizens, so many of the martyrs who were beheaded came from patrician Roman families. Pope Sixtus II, a patrician, was decapitated by order of the emperor Valerian in 258, and his Spanish deacon, Laurence, was crushed between two white-hot slabs and then roasted over a gridiron. Laurence is particularly venerated in Rome, and many churches are dedicated to him, in part because of his gestures toward the poor, to whom he donated the wealth of the church upon the orders of Sixtus II.

BREAKING DOWN THE SOCIAL BARRIERS

In martyrdom as in life, one of Christianity's disruptive effects, at least at the beginning, was the abolition of social barriers. Christian martyrs came from all walks of life: patricians, plebeians, soldiers, and even women and children, the "weak links" of Roman society. Many women—extremely young women, often little more than children—were raped and then martyred. Rape was a punishment in Rome because of the shame it entailed and because it forced the young girl to break the vow of chastity she had made with her God. Roman law, although more advanced than its Greek counterpart, failed to protect women and children, and the new religion wrought a cultural revolution. Women had a new central role that was founded in Christ's words. They were witnesses to his sacrifice and active participants in the new faith. Female saints greatly outnumber their male counterparts.

Christianity not only helped women embark on the long road to social liberation, but also encouraged its adherents to love children, a rare sentiment in a world

Guido Reni.
St. Sebastian (detail),
Musei Capitolini.

● ● ● VIA DELLA GRATICOLA

Gridiron Road is the name given to the tour of churches dedicated to Laurence, patron saint of Rome, with a direct connection to the episodes of his martyrdom.

① **S. Lorenzo in Lucina**
(☞99)
This church (*at rigtht*), which has interesting subterranean vaults, houses the gridiron and chains used to imprison the saint. These are exhibited on his feast day, August 10.

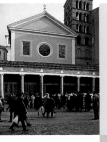

② **S. Lorenzo in Miranda**
(☞113)
The Temple of Antoninus and Faustina, in the Roman Forum, was transformed to create this 7th- to 8th-century church, supposedly on the site of the saint's trial (*at right*).

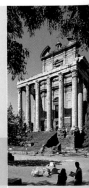

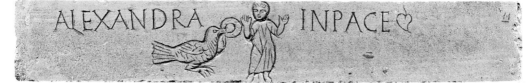

that viewed children as an economic burden. After Christ said, "Let the little children come to me," (Matthew 19:14, *Oxford Bible*), children became a symbol of purity and were treated with increasing respect, if only symbolically. In the catacombs, tombs of thousands of children (most of whom died of natural causes) are inscribed with epithets such as Unsullied Lamb, Dove Without Gall, Sweeter Than Honey, Sweetest Son. These signs of sincere and profound grief are mitigated by the conviction that the children's souls are making their way toward heaven.

THE SOURCES: PART HISTORY, PART FICTION

Everything that is widely known about the saints in the early centuries is based on the examination of two types of sources: archaeological evidence and texts, both liturgical and literary. In addition to the Bible, the writings of the church fathers, and imperial edicts, texts include the *Acta Martyrum* (Feats of the Martyrs), reports of the martyrs' trials; the *Vite* (Lives) of the confessors; and sermons, discourses, and brief biographies, including tales of their good deeds and miracles.

For devotional purposes, the church immediately collected its martyrs' names, death dates, and burial places, and recorded them in calendars. The Roman Calendar, one of these documents, dates from 313, and the *Depositio Martyrum* to 354. Martyrologies, in which saints' names appear with some biographical data, were compiled on the basis of these calendars; the oldest of these date from the 5th century. Martyrologies compiled between the 5th and 9th centuries were used to draw up the *Martyrologium Romanum* (1584), which was adopted by the Catholic Church.

Starting between the 3rd and 4th centuries, the *Acta* were read in churches on the anniversary of a saint's martyrdom, but the number of interpolations and apocryphal additions quickly expanded beyond the control of the church, so their liturgical use was eventually prohibited.

ABANDONED CHILDREN

In the Roman world, it was accepted practice to abandon newborns; Infants were left out in the open, in the Holitorium Forum, at the foot of the Lactaria Column (the column of milk), whose name derived from this custom. Most of these children died, a few were adopted and were thereafter known as "pupils," and the rest were enslaved. The great number of children's tombs in the catacombs seems to indicate that Christians took on the task of burying the abandoned children who died. In memory of their children, parents left inscriptions, many of which are now in the Vatican Museums or encased in cloister walls of basilicas outside the city. These are often embellished with simple designs such as a cross, the monogram of Christ, a dove (representing the soul), an anchor (symbolizing salvation), a tree (referring to Paradise), or a fish (because the Greek word for fish is an acronym for Christ's name.

Above: inscription of Alessandra (4th century) praying, next to a dove. Museo Pio Cristiano.

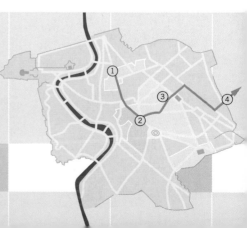

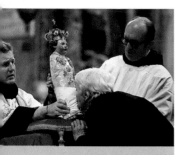

A VERY SPECIAL CHILD

The Christ child, widely worshiped in the Catholic world, is the cause and effect of the new emotional role children played among early Christians. The popularity of this figure has its origins in medieval times. St. Francis of Assisi constructed the first crèche with Jesus in a cradle. In 19th-century Rome, S. Maria d'Aracoeli's (☞ 115) image of the Christ child, which is thought to work miracles, was brought out to comfort the sick and dying. Now it is carried in a procession on January 6th (above).

Each angel on Ponte S. Angelo carries a symbol of Christ's Passion.

THE HISTORY OF A WORD

Both the *Acta* and the *Vite*, summarized and combined into various volumes, continued to be read, no longer as official texts but for instructional purposes, particularly in monasteries. These books, known as *comes* ("companions," because they were read during mealtime) or *legenda* ("things to read"), contained an incredible number of strange facts and popular elements that often borrowed from pre-Christian cults and symbology. The *legenda* enjoyed particular success beginning in the 13th century with the establishment of the Franciscans and Dominicans, monastic orders of preachers who used them in their homilies to illustrate the exemplary life. These collections were the source of the Middle Ages' major hagiographic texts, the most famous of which was the *Legenda Aurea* by the Dominican Jacopo da Varagine (ca. 1228–1298), who was also bishop of Genoa.

The transition from *legenda* to "legend" was anything but brief, and throughout the Middle Ages, the *legenda* were considered faithful accounts, to the extent that practically the entire iconography of saints is based on Jacopo da Varagine's work. If the word "legend" now implies an "altered, falsified account," it is because of Martin Luther, who rejected all the saints and all the literature about them, branding them as false. The Catholic Counter-Reformation (1545–1563), a movement of conservation and renewal that followed the Protestant Reformation, responded with a gigantic revision of its writings on the saints, culminating in the publication of the *Acta Sanctorum* (1643), edited by the Jesuit Jean de Bolland.

A NAME, A DESTINY

"*Nomen omen*" is a Latin saying that describes a belief still deeply rooted in the popular conscience: that a name has the capacity to indicate a person's destiny (in Latin, as in English, *omen* means "prediction"). This idea contributed in no small way to the development of many of the saints' legends. In the absence of other information, people looked to a saint's name for some clues about his or her life. Thus, St. Christopher (in Greek, "bearer of Christ") began to be depicted with the Christ child on his shoulders. St. Chistopher is patron saint of travelers, and his image is

●● GUARDIAN ANGELS

Deriving from Greek, *Anghelos* means messenger. Angels, in flight between man and God, are more spiritual than mortals, but are also endowed with free will. They are often pure voice, song, and idea. They listen and advise those who believe in them.

①
Cappella Sistina (☞ 55)
In his immense depiction of *The Last Judgment*, Michelangelo assigns the human body a central role and nudity a value of primordial significance. In an indeterminate sky, wingless angels, also nude, rise upward, futilely supporting souls held by demons.

②
Ponte S. Angelo (☞ 61)
The bridge, built by Hadrian during the imperial period, was embellished by Clement IX with the addition of 10 statues of angels bearing the symbols of the Passion. Bernini provided sketches and supervised students, who executed the sculptures.

③
S. Maria della Pace (☞ 71)
In the Chigi Chapel, created by Raphael, a bronze by Cosimo Fancelli depicts Christ transported by angels. To the right of the nave, at the sides of the arch, are prophets and angels by Vincenzo de Rossi.

extremely common along streets and in Alpine passes. Hippolytus's name derives from "divided by horses" (from the Greek *hippos*, "horse," and *lyo*, "undone, divided"), and hagiography has deduced that Hippolytus was quartered by horses. Other saints' characteristics can also likely be attributed to name interpretation. Agnes is represented with a lamb (*agnus* in Latin, symbol of purity); the distinctive features of Lucy of Syracuse are her eyes (in Latin *lux* means "light"), which are depicted resting on a plate. Legend has it that she was blinded during her martyrdom. She has become the patron saint of sight, and Rome's churches of S. Lucia del Gonfalone (☞ 72) and S. Lucia in Selci (☞ 106) are dedicated to her. Worshippers leave eyes made of wax as offerings in the former; in the latter, holy oil, considered soothing for the eyes, is distributed on her feast day, December 13.

ERRORS AND STEREOTYPES

Legends about the saints have also developed as a result of errors of interpretation. St. Caecilia, for instance, is the patron saint of music (her attribute is an organ) because of an error of translation of the word *organum,* which in Latin has several meanings, from the text about her martyrdom. In other cases, saints acquired unfounded military histories because the term "soldiers of Christ," occurring in eulogistic texts, was taken literally. Over the centuries, true soldier martyrs, such as Sergius and Bacchus, came to be depicted wearing a heavy chain because of erroneous interpretations of the gold collars they wore as members of the imperial guard.

Those who wanted to recount the lives of saints but had little or no information about them also resorted to stereotyping. If it was known that a certain martyr was brought to trial, then it could be supposed that more or less all martyrs must have stood before a judge. So trial scenes are inserted into practically every martyr's life story, especially for women. A well-known example is depicted in the iconography of St. Catherine of Alexandria, in particular in the frescoes of the chapel dedicated to her in S. Clemente (☞ 105).

A SAINT WHO COLLECTED BLOOD

St. Praxedes, sister of St. Pudentiana and daughter of Senator Pudens, was one of the few saints who did not suffer martyrdom during the centuries when Christianity was practiced in secrecy. Supposedly baptized by the apostle Peter himself, she is famous for having collected the blood of martyrs, after washing their remains and gathering them in a well. This is how she is depicted on the altar of the church dedicated to her (☞ 108). A porphyry circle on the floor of the main nave indicates the site of the sacred well.

Below, the saint and St. Paul are portrayed in a detail of the church's mosaics.

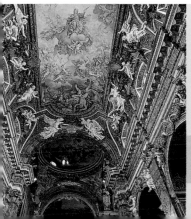

④
S. Maria della Vittoria
(☞ 126)
The frescoed vault of this church dedicated to St. Teresa, founder of the Carmelite order, is crowned by a circle of stuccowork angels that depict the *Assumption of the Virgin and the Fall of the Rebel Angels* by Giovanni Cerrini *(at left).*

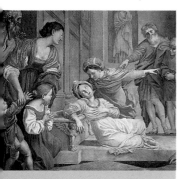

ST. CAECILIA

Often depicted with an organ
because of an error in the
translation of the text that
recounts her martyrdom,
Caecilia is the patron saint of
music. In 821, nearly six
centuries after her death in 230,
her remains were moved from
the catacombs of St. Calixtus
(☞ 129) on the Via Appia to the
church in Trastevere that is
dedicated to her. She is widely
venerated in Europe and is
associated with organs,
harpsichords, cellos, lutes, and
other images relating to music;
she often wears a crown of
roses or lilies, and her neck may
show the marks of her
beheading. Among the most
beautiful works of art in her
honor are the splendid sculpture
(1600) by Stefano Maderno in
the church of S. Cecilia (☞ 63),
which depicts her as she was
found when her tomb was
opened in 1595, and a fresco
cycle (1616–1617) by
Domenichino in S. Luigi dei
Francesi (☞ 84).

Stereotypes were also applied to hermits. Probably based on the
model of the temptations of Christ in the desert, hermits were
usually said to have been subjected to temptations by the devil.
They were also believed to have the power to tame ferocious
beasts, as did some martyrs: St. Thecla is modeled after Daniel in
the lion's den; St. Jerome is often depicted translating the Bible
with a tamed lion at his feet. Early bishops seized on these images
as part of their commitment to combating paganism and heresy.

CROSSES, SWORDS, AND STAFFS: HOW TO IDENTIFY THE SAINTS

Saints' faces were not very important in early Christian art.
Martyrs, particularly, were thought of as exemplary models
rather than as real people. Their physiognomic characteristics
were pronounced relatively unimportant in a polemic against
pagan art, which had reached great formal heights in Hellenistic
portraiture and continued to influence Roman art until the end
of the empire. This art must have appeared too individualistic in
the eyes of the church. Instead of identifying saints by portraying
physical features, a name sufficed to identify a saint, and names
often appear next to images in the mosaics in early Christian
churches. From the 4th century on, elements of the late ancient
tradition began to reappear, including facial features and halos,
which had once been an attribute of emperors. Images of the two
principal saints repeat the iconography of ancient philosophers;
Peter has white hair and a white beard, and Paul appears bald and
lean-faced, with a short, black beard.

All the other saints could be identified at first glance only by their
clothing, which indicated the category to which they belonged.
Apostles were depicted wearing royal mantles and pallia, hermits
and anchorites were shown in habits, soldiers in cuirasses, bishops with a shepherd's crook and miter, kings with a crown, and
so on. Intellectuals, including evangelists, prophets, church
fathers, and doctors, hold a book or scroll; knights a weapon; pilgrims and hermits a staff. It is only in Western Christianity, particularly with the flowering of the Gothic style, that personal
attributes became common. These referred to a salient event,
often martyrdom, in the saint's life: a gridiron for St. Laurence, a

FACES OF SAINTS

Many saints and
prophets appear in the
altarpiece of the
Adoration of the Trinity
(1592), by Francesco
Bassano, in the Chiesa
del Gesù, and they are
almost always depicted
with their attributes.
Here are some of them.

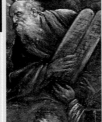

Moses with the tablets
of the Law.

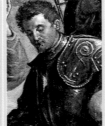

St. Martin with his cloak.

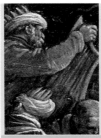

King David with his harp.

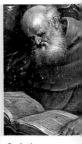

St. Anthony
Abbot with
a book.

wheel for St. Catherine, an organ for St. Caecilia, eyes for St. Lucy, the Christ child for St. Christopher, keys or a cross for St. Peter, a sword for St. Paul (who was beheaded), and the like.

PAINTINGS AND SCULPTURES: THE ICONOGRAPHY OF SAINTS

Dignity, heroism, devotion, and controversy describe the representational universe of the saints. Throughout the Middle Ages and until the late 15th century, saints were portrayed in dignified fashion. Images were almost never violent, not even the rare depictions of scenes of martyrdom. Violence appeared only in representations of the Last Judgment that were meant to admonish and frighten the viewer. Saints were presented as examples of how good Christians should live their mortal lives. During the Renaissance, with its humanistic attitudes, saints were shown as heroic, following newly rediscovered classical models.

The Counter-Reformation, which sought to return Christianity to the purity of its early days, inherited the image of the saint as hero but pushed for a more devotional, less titanic characterization.

Counter-Reformation doctrine dictated that images must be immediately recognizable, even by laypersons. In the struggle against the contempt of the Protestant world toward saints and images of saints, sacred art became charged with polemical significance. The more iconoclastic the Protestant countries became, the more the Roman Church urged the worship of images. Jean de Bolland brought attention to saints who were previously unknown, such as Praxedes, Pudentiana, and Agnes. Ironically, just as the representations of saints were taking on a universal, atemporal quality, historical studies uncovered new facts about saints, and the information found its way into works of art, to the point of esotericism (with the consequence that in certain altarpieces, there are saints whose names we still don't know). Martyr saints were depicted in increasingly bloody fashion as role models in the Catholic struggle against the Protestant Reformation, which did not recognize their cult. These representations served a

ST. CATHERINE OF ALEXANDRIA

Removed from the liturgical calendar after the Vatican II (1969), St. Catherine of Alexandria was one of the most venerated martyr saints. Martyred around 306, she was immensely popular from the 13th century until the end of the Middle Ages, and again during Baroque times, during which time she was honored and worshiped almost as much as the Virgin. Many legends exist about her life, and her protection is believed to extend to children, virgins, wives, and everyone working in any occupation that requires the use of wheels and knives. Before being beheaded, she was placed between two hooked wheels, which were meant to turn and lacerate her flesh. Lightening destroyed the infernal machine, and the iconography typically represents her with a fragment of hooked wheel or a sword. Two Roman churches— S. Caterina dei Funari (☞ 84) and S. Caterina della Rota— and two chapels—in S. Maria Maggiore (☞ 126) and in S. Clemente (☞ 105)— are dedicated to her.

Masolino's St. Catherine Freed by the Angels, detail of the fresco (1428–1431) in S. Clemente.

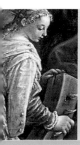
St. Catherine with the wheel.

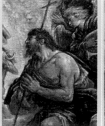
St. John the Baptist with his cross-shaped staff.

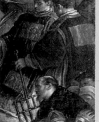
St. Laurence with a gridiron.

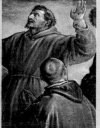
St. Francis with the stigmata.

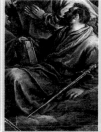
St. Paul with a sword.

SAINTS WORTHY OF DEVOTION

Almost all saints, particularly the oldest ones, are attributed to one or more patronages, whose origins, whether rooted in history or legend, have often been lost. The following are some of the patron saints widely venerated in Rome (and their feast days):

St. Sebastian (January 20): Martyred in 288 in Rome, he is the patron saint of the dying, merchants of hardware, potters, plumbers, gardeners, soldiers, and fountains. He also protects livestock from disease and plague.

St. Blaise (February 3): Martyred in 316 in Sebaste, Armenia (now Turkey), St. Blaise is the patron saint of doctors, cobblers, tailors, plasterers and bricklayers, bakers, milliners, musicians, and domestic animals. He is also patron saint for good weather and protector against sore throats, coughs, hemorrhages, toothache, and plague. On his feast day, candles, wine, and bread are consecrated and are still distributed in the church of S. Biagio della Pagnotta (☞76).

St. Vitus (June 15): A popular child saint who, according to tradition, was martyred in Rome in 304, at the age of 7, Vitus is patron saint of innkeepers, actors, blacksmiths and miners, domestic animals, springs, and people who are deaf or mute. He is also protector against epilepsy, hysteria, cramps, lightening, and bad weather.

dual purpose as devotional icons and as didactic mementos for novices destined for Protestant or non-Christian lands. Future missionaries filed past the *Martyrology* in S. Stefano Rotondo (☞*108*), to better know the fate that awaited them.

The Counter-Reformation was neither brief nor painless for religious art. Clement VII attempted to obliterate Michelangelo's *Last Judgment*, and hundreds of other works that did not follow the prescriptions laid down by the Council of Trent were renounced or destroyed. The church sometimes intervened directly, issuing directives about the postures and attributes that artists could depict and even the colors that they could use. Perhaps this was the beginning of the transformation of religious art, to which the West owes so much, into an art frozen in time, an art that with rare exceptions has seemed unable to absorb and reflect contemporary culture since the 19th century.

THE WORLD PROTECTED BY SAINTS

In addition to being models of behavior, saints almost immediately became intercessors with God and patrons (a term derived from the Latin for "protector" or "supporter"). The concept of protection by a saint is deeply rooted. Almost all Indo-European divinities presided over some activity and protected something or someone, and in this sense the saints performed a function of the old gods. In the frescoes of the Catacombs of Domitilla are the earliest examples of "personal" protection, where the patron saint places a hand on the shoulders of the person being protected. The idea of the saint as protector began to spread in the 11th century, when Europe experienced urban and economic rebirth, and continued to grow during the 14th century, when the Western world underwent one of its longest crises as a result of famine, the Black Death (1347–1348), and a sharp decline in population, which would not be restored to its original levels until the second half of the following century. During both these periods, everyone and everything—person, house, profession, confraternity, corporation, religious order, city, domain, or nation—had a patron saint; nothing in the world was without one. Particularly during the 14th century,

THE TRIUMPH OF GOLD

On the city's altars, light filtering through windows, or flickering from a multitude of candles, is reflected in warm colors by Rome's gilded treasures.

① **S. Pietro** (☞*52*) In front of Bernini's tribune, an immense gilded sunburst (detail at right) hangs over the monumental black and gold bronze throne, which encloses the so-called Chair of St. Peter.

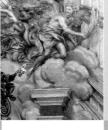

② **S. Eustachio** (☞*84*) This church was founded by Constantine on the site where St. Eustace suffered his martyrdom. In the church a high altar in bronze and polychrome marble, by Nicola Salvi, is surmounted by a beautiful baldacchin by Ferdinando Fuga.

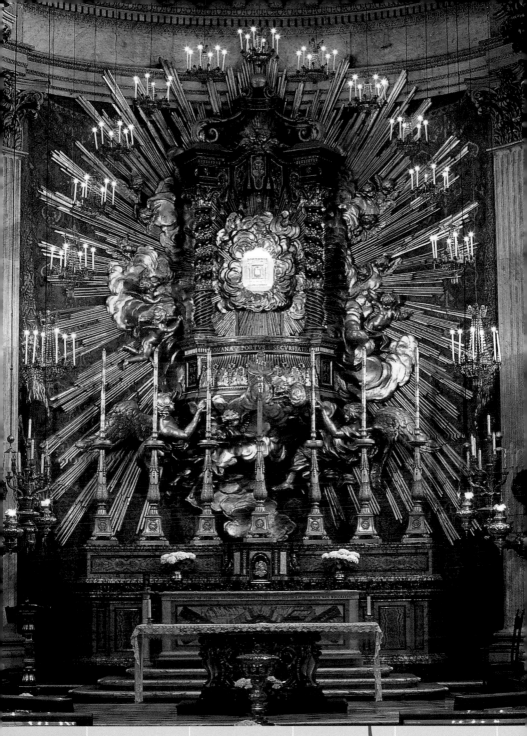

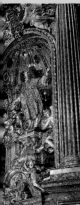

③ **Chiesa del Gesù**
(☞ 80)
The altar of St. Ignatius is emblematic of the splendor and decorative richness of Jesuit art. Four monumental lapis lazuli columns surround a statue of the saint, whose tomb lies beneath the altar (*left*).

④ **S. Maria in Campitelli**
(☞ 115)
This "glory" of gilded angels (*above*) is a splendid Baroque composition by Carlo Rainaldi, with a miraculous image of St. Maria in Portico Campitelli (11th century) at the center.

SAINTS WORTHY OF DEVOTION

St. Ignatius of Loyola (July 31): Patron saint of soldiers, children, spiritual exercises, and pregnant women, He is protector against guilty consciences, livestock diseases, and plague.
In Rome, the waters of St. Ignatius (holy water in which a relic of the saint or a small medal with his image has been immersed) are thought to have miracle-working properties.

St. Laurence (August 10): Patron saint of librarians, archivists, cooks, brewers, innkeepers, laundresses, ironers, firemen, vinedressers. He is also protector against eye and skin maladies, sciatica, fevers, and fires.

St. Bibiana (December 2): Martyred in Rome in 367, she protects against cramps, headaches, alcoholism, epilepsy, and accidents. Until the 18th century, the dust from the column to which she was bound during martyrdom (☞124), and the mint that grew around her tomb were used as a remedy for epilepsy.

Fra Angelico's St. Laurence distributing alms to the poor, detail, Cappella Niccolina, Palazzi Vaticani.

patron saints functioned as talismans against evil; they were protection against specific illnesses, storms, attacks from pirates, and so on. By invoking the right saint, it was believed that evil could be kept at bay.

PATRON SAINT OF ROME

Agnes, whose name means pure and innocent, is patron saint of Rome, along with Peter, Paul, Laurence, and Frances of Rome. Very little is known about Agnes; her martyrdom occurred during the persecution of Diocletian. The epigraph on her tomb, written by the poet-pope Damasus I (366–384), mentions her age: 12. She became a symbol of virginity because it was said that a mass of hair grew to cover her body, preventing her violation. As a result of this legend, hair became an attribute of virgins. The episode is depicted in a bas-relief in the vaults of the church dedicated to her in Piazza Navona (☞70). Tresses completely cover the body of the young girl, who is accompanied by two soldiers. The vault area is part of what remains of the stadium of Domitian, presumably the site where the girl's martyrdom took place. Agnes' head is kept in the same church, and her tomb is in the catacombs on Via Nomentana, where the basilica of S. Agnese Fuori le Mura stands (☞130).

THE WORSHIP OF RELICS

Before and after the era of Diocletian (284–305), when the last great persecutions took place, two dates are significant in the Christian world. The first is 260, when emperor Gallienus granted Christians the right to practice their religion freely and ordered the restoration of church property that had been confiscated. The second is 311, just two years before Costantine's edict that established freedom of worship to all religions, when co-emperor Galerius issued an edict that authorized the end of the great persecution. Although there were still innumerable obstacles in the late ancient world, these decrees allowed Christians to practice their religion openly. Homage began to be paid to the martyrs. The deification was accompanied by a phenomenon of relic-

---

● ● IN THE NAME OF MARY

"...You are blessed among women and blessed is the fruit of your womb...."
The populace has always exhibited great passion for the Mother of God and has always asked a great deal from her—healing, recovery from wounds, intercession...

① S. Maria in Trastevere (☞65)
This was the first church dedicated to the Madonna and probably the first in the city officially open to her worship. Domenichino painted the *Assumption of the Virgin* in the central section of the coffered ceiling (*below*).

② S. Maria in Aracoeli (☞115)
According to legend, Augustus, after seeing a vision of the Virgin, ordered that an "altar to the Son of God" be built. On the fourth column to the left, in the central nave, a fresco depicts the Madonna "Refugium peccatorum."

③ S. Agostino (☞82)
One of the earliest Renaissance churches in Rome, S. Agostino contains Jacopo Sansovino's *Madonna del Parto*, widely venerated as a protectress of women in childbirth. The church also houses the *Madonna of the Pilgrims* by Caravaggio (*right*).

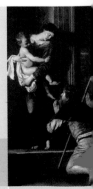

creation, and places and objects that came into contact with the diva or "divine one" (from the Latin *divus*, "divine") became relics. Temples were built on the sites of the martyrs' tombs or places of martyrdom, and parts of their bodies—known as relics (from the Latin *reliquus*, "that which remains")—were safeguarded and became objects of veneration. Relics were protected by specially commissioned containers, known as reliquaries, that were often masterpieces of goldsmithery. Everything connected to the saints became invested with a certain sanctity. During the Middle Ages, when saints' relics were venerated with particular fervor, European cities and monasteries vied and paid high prices for real and presumed bones of martyrs and fragments of clothing; one even acquired feathers from the archangel Gabriel. As the center of Christianity, a holy city, and the destination of a constant stream of pilgrims, Rome has always been rich in relics related to the best-known saints and to the life of Christ.

AN EXCEPTIONAL CASE: RELICS OF CHRIST

The remains of Christ's time on Earth are located in three of the four patriarchal basilicas, seat of the patriarchs, the highest ranking bishops in the Church of Rome. These relics are tied almost exclusively to two events: his Passion and his death. The so-called Column of the Flagellation was brought from Jerusalem to the church of S. Prassede (☞*108*) in 1223. S. Croce in Gerusalemme (☞*124*) houses the relics of the true cross—three pieces of wood, a nail, and part of the inscription (INRI), that hung at the top of the cross. S. Giovanni in Laterano (☞*105*) contains the table from the Last Supper, four columns that during the Middle Ages were thought to correspond to the height of the Savior, the stone slab on which the soldiers played dice for his tunic, and the so-called Well of the Samaritan. Near the Basilica of S. Giovanni is the Scala Santa (☞*109*), the largest relic in the Christian world. These so-called Holy Steps are said to be the staircase from the Praetorian Palace, where drops of Jesus' blood fell after he was flagellated in front of Pontius Pilate. The spots where the blood fell

ALEXIUS, THE BEGGAR SAINT

Several saints renounced all material possessions for a life of mendicancy on the fringes of society. One of the most famous of these so-called beggar saints, who lived almost semisecret lives in Rome, was St. Alexius, patron saint of beggars and vagabonds. He lived in the 4th or 5th century and was the son of a wealthy Roman family. According to some sources, he renounced his wealth on his wedding day and went to live in Edessa (Turkey); returning to Rome, he hid beneath the staircase of his paternal home, unknown to his family, and lived on charity. Baroque Rome celebrated his person—the Jesuits pointed to him as a model of chastity—and he became the subject of musical and theatrical portrayals. Bernini staged one of these, commissioned by the Barberini family, and traces of the sets, in the form of a monumental reliquary in stuccoed wood by Andrea Bergondi, can be seen in the church of S. Alessio (☞*119*).

④
S. Maria della Concezione in Campo Marzio (☞*90*)
The present-day church, probably buit on a preexisting 7th-century structure and rebuilt in the 17th century, houses on the high altar a 12th-century Byzantine icon of the *Madonna Advocata*, originally from Constantinople (*above*).

⑤
S. Maria Maggiore (☞*126*)
In the world's largest church dedicated to the Virgin Mary, a beautiful mosaic by Jacopo Torriti depicts one of the nine choirs of angels that take part in the coronation of the Virgin by the Redeemer, in the *Triumph of the Virgin*.

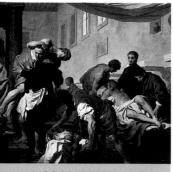

A GOOD DEATH

Given the high mortality rates until the modern era, the church calendar is full of patron saints of the so-called "Good Death" saints dedicated to the physical and spiritual assistance of people who are ill and dying. St. Camillus de Lellis (1550–1614), friend of St. Philip Neri and founder of the Camillini (1586), is one of the most beloved of these saints in Rome and was venerated for quite some time as the patron saint of the city. The Camillini, also known as the Ministers of the Sick, contributed significantly to health reform in Rome: they taught people to isolate those with contagious diseases, they considered diet as a function of illness, and they reorganized the hospital ward system.

St. Camillus is buried in the church of S. Maria Maddalena (☞99), whose walls are frescoed with scenes from his life.

St. Camillus de Lellis healing the sick during the 1598 flooding of the Tiber (1746) by Pierre Subleyras, Museo di Roma.

are now well protected, framed in metal and glass. In reality this is the stairway of honor from the Lateran Palace, installed here to provide access to the popes' private chapel. The steps were identified with the Praetorian Palace during the 15th century, and pilgrims today still climb them on their knees in profound devotion. The church makes pronouncements of authenticity only after very thorough examination, but as with the Scala Santa, veneration of a relic often persists, even when it may not be warranted.

The Basilica di S. Pietro (☞52) in the Vatican contains the veil of Veronica, who stopped to wipe Jesus' face when she met him on the road to Calvary. His image remained on the cloth, which was brought back from Jerusalem by the crusaders. The church also contains part of the wood from the cross and part of the lance with which Longinus pierced the Savior's side. All three relics are exhibited to the faithful during Holy Week.

"WE DESCEND LIVE INTO THE INFERNO"

"As a boy, when I was studying in Rome, my friends and I used to visit the tombs of the apostles and martyrs on Sundays. We would enter the tunnels carved out of tufa stone and entirely covered with tombs, so that the prophetic saying, 'We descend live into the inferno,' seemed to be fulfilled. Occasional rays of life from the surface lessened the shadows a bit.… We proceeded slowly, one step at a time, completely enveloped in darkness" (Commentary to Ezekial, 40:5).

When you visit the catacombs today, you may well have the kind of experience recounted above by St. Jerome (347–420), the church father who translated the Bible into Latin. For centuries an aura of legend—related to the worship of saints' relics, places of martyrdom, and tombs—has surrounded the catacombs. These intricate networks of underground tufa passages were never hiding places or places of worship. They were immense cities of the dead, the bodies buried in niches carved into the walls. The names of Rome's catacombs are those of the saints, martyrs, and popes who were entombed there, including

●● UNDERGROUND ROME

This hidden city is rich in itineraries to its ancient core: tombs of early Christians, forgotten and buried churches, sites of esoteric sects and cults.

The Good Shepherd, 2nd- to 3rd-century, Catacombs of St. Calixtus.

① **Catacombe di S. Callisto** (☞129)
The official burial ground of the Roman church lay along the Via Appia Antica. Fifty martyrs and some 16 popes from the early centuries of Christianity are buried here.

② **S. Sebastiano** (☞132)
Built at the behest of Cardinal Borghese, this church occupies the site of a Constantinian basilica and stands above the catacombs. The *triclinium*, a porticoed space with graffiti-painted walls, is where early Christians used to worshipped Sts. Peter and Paul.

③ **Catacombe di Priscilla** (☞129)
This catacomb complex stands along the ancient Via Salaria, where Romans buried their dead. In one of the burial chambers is a Madonna and child fresco (*rigth*), the oldest representation of the Madonna (mid-2nd century).

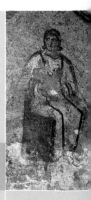

Sebastian, Callistus, Agnes, and others; or of the people who gave the land where they were established, such as Priscilla and Flavia Domitilla. Many catacombs contain significant pictorial decorations that document the transition of art from Roman to early Christian styles. Even after the catacombs' funerary function ended in the 5th century, pilgrims continued to come—to worship and to look at and touch the tombs and even the bodies of the saints. Here and there *fenestellae*, or small slits, were opened, through which pilgrims would reach in and touch the remains with small pieces of fabric. Others were content to leave with a bit of oil that burned in the lamps near the tombs. It is not difficult to understand how, in the pilgrim's tales of their visits, those bits of fabric that had touched the body of a saint became parts of the saint's clothing. These, too, became relics, precious memories of the long and dangerous voyage to Rome.

ROME OF THE DEAD

At the foundation of Roman culture was the peoccupation, even obsession, with boundaries. In ancient times a boundary—the walls—separated the city of the living from the city of the dead, who reposed in necropolises along the consular roads. In the 5th century, the dead began to be buried inside the city walls, in orchards, churches, crypts, vaults, and monasteries. Those who could afford it were buried near the tomb of a martyr or next to a high altar. One way or another, people tried to be close to one who had been closer to God. Thus the dead entered the city.

As barbarian incursions and earthquakes made life appear increasingly precarious, and the distance between the world of the living and that of the dead began to shrink, Christians stood fast in their belief that life and death were stages on the path toward eternal life. Faith in the Resurrection and the new concept of a hereafter, where the just were rewarded and the wicked punished, made death seem less traumatic.

Throughout the Middle Ages and for much of the modern and contemporary era in the West, death was a familiar presence. Famines, wars, epidemics, and poor hygiene took lives indiscriminately. In his *Cantico di Frate Sole*

FRANCIS IN ROME

St. Francis of Assisi, patron saint of Italy since 1939, lived in Rome between 1181 and 1226. During the period he worked to have his new order approved, first by Pope Innocent III in 1210, then by Pope Honorius III in 1223 (who granted definitive approval). In 1224, the saint received the stigmata—bodily marks resembling the wounds of the crucified Christ that miraculously appeared on him— and some of the bandages that covered his wounds are housed in S. Francesco alle Stigmata, next to the Pantheon. In the church of S. Francesco a Ripa (☞ 64), a monk accompanies visitors to a small room where the saint resided, the only remaining portion of the ancient Hospice of S. Biagio; there, a stone that St. Francis used as a pillow is preserved (protected by a grate), along with a spectacular reliquary dating from 1696

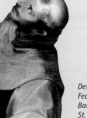

Detail of Federico Barocci's St. Francis receiving the stigmata, Vatican Pinacoteca.

④
S. Prisca
(☞ 121)
Beneath this church, built prior to the 5th century on the remains of a Roman structure, is a 2nd- to 3rd-century Mithraeum. Preceded by a vestibule where victims were sacrificed, the room has frescoed walls.

⑤
Basilica di Porta Maggiore
(☞ 124)
Hidden beneath the roadbed of the Rome—Naples railway, this church is believed to have been the site of a neo-Pythagorean worship. Perfectly preserved, it is divided into three naves, its walls and vaults covered with beautiful stuccowork.

THE COMPANY OF IGNATIUS

St. Francis Xavier (1506–1552), co-founder of the Jesuits, proselytized throughout Japan, China, and India, and the church proclaimed him the patron saint of the Indies, of missionaries, and of missions in the East. His body remains in Goa, but his arm is housed in the chapel dedicated to him in the right transept of the Chiesa del Gesù (☞ 80) opposite the chapel dedicated to his confrère, Ignatius of Loyola, with whom he was canonized in 1622. In 1679, Carlo Maratta painted the altarpiece illustrating his death (below).

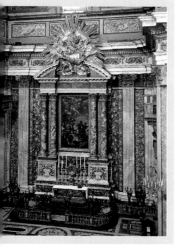

(1224), St. Francis of Assisi praised God for "Bodily death our sister." The everyday relationship with death gave meaning to burial; it was one of the acts of mercy. Joseph the carpenter, one of the world's most venerated saints and the protector of grave diggers and the dying, was one of the saints to whom people prayed for a good death. Confraternities and religious orders, the first of which were the Franciscans, were founded to bury the dead and assist the dying or those condemned to the gallows.

Baroque Rome dramatized death through spectacular and in some cases macabre representations of the passage from life. With advances in anatomical knowledge, decorations imitating tibias, femurs, and skulls were used on tombstones or monuments inside churches. The Franciscans decorated crypts and chapels with real bones; in the church of S. Maria della Concezione dei Cappucccini(☞ 126) the remains of 4,000 cadavers create a complex of chapels decorated with friars' bones and mummies. An hourglass and scythe motif emphasizes the precariousness of life, and an inscription reminds the visitor: "I am what you will become. I was what you are."

ROME OF THE LIVING

The image of Rome as a city of God has been shaped by more than the worship of the dead and their relics. A great many saints, some of whom are inextricably bound to the Eternal City, lived, studied, and worked here. St. Frances of Rome (1384–1440), forced by her parents to marry, was an exemplary wife and mother. Upon her husband's death in 1436, she became the Mother Superior of the Benedictine Oblates of Tor de' Specchi, a community dedicated to charitable work. One of the 15th century's great mystics, she was in constant contact with her own guardian angel, in whose company she is often depicted, and many prayed to her for help and counsel. Her body rests in the church dedicated to her (☞ 113).

Rome owes a great deal to the Spaniard Ignatius of Loyola (1491–1556), founder of the Society of Jesus and author of the *Spiritual Exercises* (1548), which was in the vanguard of the Counter-Reformation. This militant order, which would become one of the most powerful in the church, was dedicated to mis-

● ● THE TOUR OF THE SEVEN CHURCHES

The first great Roman basilica dedicated to St. Peter and the six other basilicas have always been pilgrimage destinations. In 1577 St. Philip Neri introduced the Tour of the Seven Churches, a route necessary to obtain plenary indulgence.

① **S. Pietro** (☞ 52)
This is the largest church in the world. In 326 Pope Sylvester consecrated the first basilica, which had been established by Constantine on the site of the apostle's martyrdom and burial. A symbol of Christianity, it houses priceless treasures

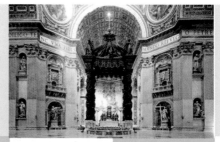

Above S. Pietro's central nave and baldachin.

sionary work and, from the beginning, active in every sector of public life. To combat heresy and convert non-Christians, Ignatius expected his followers to undergo rigorous cultural and educational preparation. Jesuit colleges became famous throughout the world and provided instruction for the ruling classes of Europe. The Chiesa del Gesù (☞80), one of Rome's most beautiful churches, was erected on the occasion of Ignatius's canonization (1622). Beneath the ornate altar in the left transept, the saint's remains rest in an urn; next to the church are the rooms where Ignatius lived.

"BE GOOD, IF YOU CAN"

St. Philip Neri (1515–1595) was extremely popular among Romans, who nicknamed him Pippo Bono (Good Phil). An itinerant preacher in the city, he was known as the Apostle of Rome, and the entire city wept at his funeral. He took in poor children for instruction, removing them from squalor. Immensely patient, he told the children to "be good, if you can," a phrase that became almost a refrain in Rome. The saint was a friend and counselor to popes and cardinals, including St. Charles Borromeo, archbishop of Milan. He is also the patron saint of humorists, and there are many anecdotes about his cheerfulness and ready wit. When an aristocrat slapped him, tired of Neri's continual requests for money for orphans, Neri responded, "This is for me; and for my children?" The rooms where he worked and an altar dedicated to him are in S. Maria in Vallicella (also know as the Chiesa Nuova ☞68). In this church he taught the faithful to sing religious hymns and invented the musical form of the oratory; the order he founded in 1575 goes by the name Oratorians.

A MILANESE IN ROME: CHARLES BORROMEO

One of the most beautiful domes in Rome belongs to Ss. Ambrogio e Carlo al Corso, a church dedicated to two Milanese bishops that lived 12 centuries apart. St. Ambrose, who died in 397, is one of the distinguished Doctors of the Church; St. Charles Borromeo (1538–1584), patron saint of pastoral workers and seminarians, left an indelible mark on church his-

ST. BENEDICT, FATHER OF WESTERN MONASTICISM

Benedict of Norcia (c. 480–547) spent little time in Rome: he studied here and immediately fled, horrified by the dissoluteness of his schoolmates. But his influence on church history was profound, and in 590, Gregory I, a member of the order St. Benedict founded and that bears his name, was elected pope. The remains of Benedict's room are in the church of S. Benedetto in Piscinula (☞63), which was built around them; the saint is depicted in a 15th-century panel with a gold background on the high altar and a fresco at the church entrance. One of the most beautiful images of St. Benedict, Pierre Subleyras's *The Miracle of St. Benedict* (1744), depicts Benedict raising a gardener's son from the dead; it is in the sacristy of the church of S. Francesca Romana (☞113).

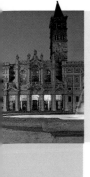

② S. Maria Maggiore
(☞126)
Legend has it that the basilica stands on the site of a miraculous snowfall, which is why it is also known as S. Maria della Neve (of the Snow). Built by Sixtus III, it is held up by 40 monolithic columns and has a beautiful mosaic pavement.

S. Maria Maggiore at night (left)

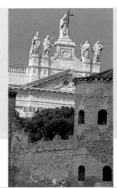

③ S. Giovanni in Laterano
(☞105)
Pope Miltiades established this basilica in the 4th century, on property owned by the Laterani family. Damaged and pillaged numerous times, it was renovated by Borromini for the 1650 Jubilee.

The facade emerges from behind the Roman walls of Porta S. Giovanni (left).

④ S. Croce in Gerusalemme
(☞124)
This church was founded by Constantine in 320 to house the relics of Christ's Passion, brought back from the Holy Land by his mother, St. Helena. In addition to these important relics, soil from Calvary is said to lie beneath the floor of the church.

ST. ANDREW

Among the many churches in Rome dedicated to Andrew, at least three are well known: S. Andrea delle Fratte (☞ 97), S. Andrea al Quirinale (☞ 104), and S. Andrea della Valle (☞ 70). This apostle's popularity dates from 1462, when his remains were brought to Rome at the request of Pope Pius II. Churches, paintings, and sculptures were dedicated to the saint from that time on, especially during the first half of the 17th century. Outside Italy in the late 15th century, iconography of St. Andrew began to include an X-shape cross, as seen in in the paintings by Domenichino in S. Gregorio Magno (☞ 113) and those by Mattia Preti in S. Andrea della Valle (*below*), and it is with this cross that the saint has almost always been depicted since then.

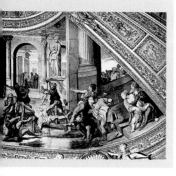

tory. Charles Borromeo spent a few years in Rome, as special secretary to his uncle, Pope Pius IV. He became archbishop of Milan in 1564, but his work had a broader resonance in the Italian church, as did his reputation as a model pastor. He was an important figure during the Council of Trent and a promoter of the immediate application of its provisions. He is one of the exemplary saints of the Counter-Reformation, along with Ignatius of Loyola and Philip Neri. His activity during the plague of 1576 in Milan made him so popular in Rome that he displaced as a protector from plague medieval saints such as St. Roch. Fine portrayals of St. Charles in prayer, in procession, and among those afflicted by plague may be seen in the church of Ss. Ambrogio e Carlo al Corso (☞ 92) and in the churches of S. Carlo ai Catinari (☞ 82) and S. Carlo alle Quattro Fontane (☞ 104).

ROME WITHOUT SAINTS

The last 300 years of the millennium seem like one long conspiracy against the saints. The Eternal City was secularized first by the Enlightenment; then by the Risorgimento (the "Resurgence," a nationalist struggle angainst the Austrian-Hungarian Empire), which culminated in the unification of Italy and taking of Rome (1870); and finally by the modern era. During these times saints appeared to wane from the capital of Christianity. But 2,000 years of faith—and an almost equal period of secular power for the papacy—are not easily erased. In this holy city, saints have left a tangible legacy, as present as the churches and the monuments of Rome. The many religious orders established by them are strongly rooted in the city and throughout Italy: Jesuits, Oratorians, Piarists, Trinitarians, Camilliani. The dozens of religious orders, whether strictly cloistered or fully involved in charitable works, were and continue to be the tool through which the church remains in continuous touch with the world of men

Facing page:
Detail of the opulent decoration of the church of S. Andrea al Quirinale.

⑤
S. Lorenzo Fuori le Mura (☞ 131)
The present-day basilica was formed by merging two ancient churches: S. Lorenzo (4th century) and the Chiesa della Vergine Maria (8th century). The current 13th-century appearance is the result of restoration work following World War II bombings in 1943.

⑥
S. Sebastiano (☞ 132)
This basilica was built in the 4th century on the site of a Christian necropolis. Initially dedicated to Sts. Peter and Paul, it was later named for St. Sebastian, the Roman soldier martyred during the persecutions of Diocletian.

⑦
S. Paolo Fuori le Mura (☞ 131)
After S. Pietro, this is the largest basilica in Rome. It was built by Constantine on the site of a small existing chapel and was dedicated to St. Paul.

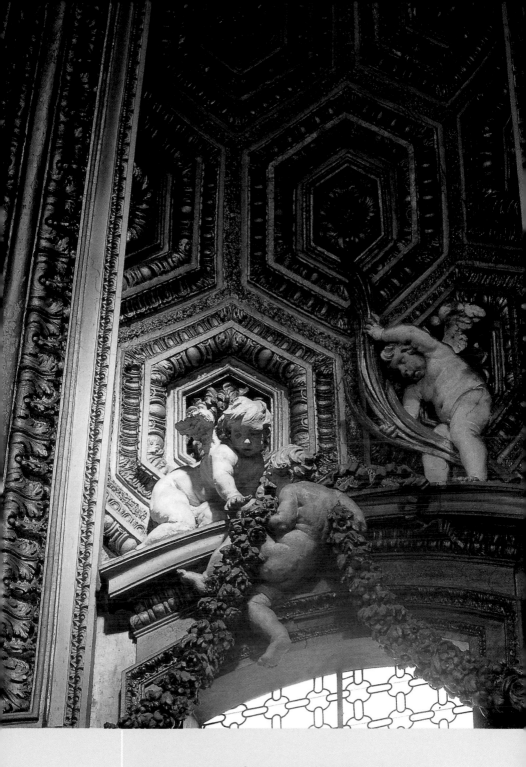

ROME'S JUBILEES
Origins and Chronology

In the Beginning

I n the Old Testament (Leviticus, 25), one of the dictates God communicated to Moses on Mount Sinai was that of the Jubilee, a sabbatical celebration of a year of remission, to be held every 50 years. During this year, normal work activities were to cease, slaves were to be freed, and debts and punishments forgiven. It is difficult to say if this tradition came from Egypt or if it was imported there. A hieroglyphic describes Ramses II, the ruling pharaoh at the time of Moses, as "rich in jubilee celebrations." The festive trumpeting of the ram's horn that announced the year of remission was called a *yôbêl*, the derivation of the Latin term *iubilaeum* and the English word jubilee.

When Christianity adopted the concept of a great periodic indulgence, the idea of the forgiveness of accumulated material debts was replaced by the remission of spiritual and moral debts—that is, sins. Medieval man was much more concerned with these debts than with material ones, because of his vivid conception of hell and purgatory, places where eternal and interim punishments were carried out.

During the Middle Ages, a pilgrimage was the best means of obtaining forgiveness for sins and redemption from guilt. Although the tradition of making pilgrimages to holy sites dates from the early centuries of Christianity, starting in the 8th century pilgrimages could earn sinners expiation from even the gravest sins, including murder and adultery. Special manuals indicated the number of pilgrimages and penances required to atone for each sin, a tariff calculated to correspond with the severity of the crime. In a liturgical ceremony, the worldly clothing of the guilty was removed and replaced with the garments of pilgrims: a staff with a metal point, a long dress of rough texture, sandals, a short cape, and a leather bag to carry food and money. In their quest for rehabilitation, pilgrims could travel as far as their pilgrimage destination under church protection, but they remained excluded from society until they had redeemed their sins.

With the advent of Benedictine monasticism in the 9th and 10th centuries, this practice was more strictly regulated, in part because of the social disorder that the presence of criminals in

RELICS AND RELIQUARIES

Mortal remains of saints, martyrs, and heroes of the church are relics, treasures of faith, and objects of intense devotion.

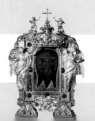

Reliquary of the image of Christ of Edessa. Papal Sacrist (left).

① **S. Pietro** (☞ 52)
The basilica, which rises above the tomb of the apostle Peter, houses the veil of Veronica, a portion of the wood of the cross, and part of the lance that pierced Christ's side. The Treasury of S. Pietro contains an extensive collection of reliquaries.

② **S. Clemente** (☞ 105)
The apse mosaic of the Triumph of the Cross (*detail, above left*) contains fragments from the holy cross of Golgotha. The crypt beneath the ciborium contains the saint's body.

③ **Scala Santa** (☞ 109)
Sixtus V had this building constructed to preserve the ancient private chapel of the popes (the chapel of S. Lorenzo, known as the Sancta Sanctorum). The stairway has been falsely identified as the one traversed by Jesus during his trial (*right*).

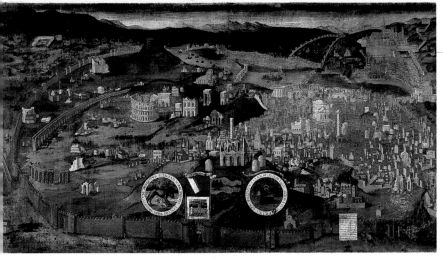

View of Rome
at the time of
Pope Sixtus IV
(oil on canvas,
c. 1550)
Mantua,
Palazzo Ducale.

free circulation inevitably might provoke.

Principal pilgrimage destinations at that time were Jerusalem, considered the center, not only of Christianity, but also of the universe; Rome; and Santiago de Compostela, in Galicia, a region of northwest Spain, where the tomb the apostle James, evangelizer of Spain, is located. During this period, although Rome housed the tombs of Sts. Peter and Paul, the city was just a stop along the route to the Holy Land. Italy served as a natural and cultural bridge between West and East.

The Crusades for the liberation of Jerusalem from the "infidels," —as Muslims were called by medieval Christians—marked the apex of the armed pilgrimage movement. By participating in the Crusades, even financially, Christians were able to obtain plenary indulgence, or the remission of all temporal penance inflicted on the sinner in expiation for his or her sins.

FROM JERUSALEM TO ROME

With the passage of time, Arab incursions throughout the Mediterranean made pilgrimages to the Holy Land increasingly difficult. For centuries Arab forays constituted a threat to the Christian West, particularly to Spain. From the late 11th century to the mid-13th century, Crusades ensured European access to Biblical sites. But by the late 13th century, Christian Europe had lost control of the Holy Land. In 1270, the Seventh (and final) Crusade, against Tunisia, ended in defeat for the Christians, whose forces were decimated by plague; France's Louis IX, later St. Louis, was among the dead. Then, in 1291, the Crusades lost

ROME'S APPEARANCE

Throughout the Middle Ages and almost until the dawn of the Renaissance, pilgrims coming from the most distant locales, from as far away as northern Europe, arrived in Rome after a long and tiring trek. Looking down on the city for the first time from the surrounding heights, they saw hundreds of fortified and crenellated towers rising up amid the classical ruins. Each of these towers corresponded to one of the families that were vying for control of the city. Writer Piero Bargellini described the city, which stood amid vast areas of countryside:

"[Rome] still looked Medieval, with its enclosing walls, crenellated towers and campaniles pierced with windows: a city without domes, other than the flattened one of the Pantheon. The four major basilicas, with sloping roofs, formed arch-vaulted islands, spread out in four locations, distant from one another: S. Pietro, near the Tiber, S. Paolo Fuori le Mura, S. Giovanni in Laterano and S. Maria Maggiore."

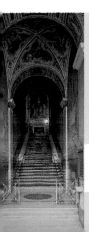

④
S. Croce in Gerusalemme
(☞124)
Also called the Basilica Sessoriana (*Sessorium* was the term for the imperial residence in the late empire), the church was erected by Constantine to house and honor relics of Christ's Passion, brought back from the Holy Land.

⑤
S. Susanna(☞100)
During the Middle Ages, this church was a pilgrimage destination because of its numerous relics of martyrs and saints (including St. Susanna), and well as relics of the cross, the tomb of Christ, and the Virgin's garments and hair.

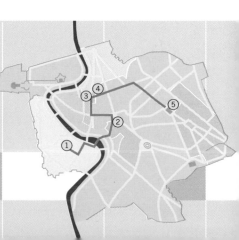

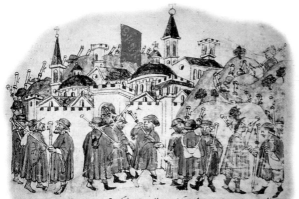

Pilgrims arriving in Rome, from Giovanni Sercambi's Chronicles, early 15th century. Lucca, State Archives.

"DISCOUNTS" FOR VISITING THE BASILICAS

At the end of the 14th century, the city's four patriarchal churches were S. Giovanni in Laterano, S. Pietro, San Paolo Fuori le Mura, and S. Maria Maggiore. Pilgrims who visited each basilica were granted an indulgence "bonus": a deduction of one year plus 40 days from the length of the punishment to be suffered in the afterlife. Those who visited other less "important" churches in Rome received a partial indulgence of only 40 days.

the last Christian bulwark in the Near East, St. John of Acri (now Akko, in Israel).

The likelihood of a reconquest of the Holy Sepulcher became increasingly remote, and the center of the Christian world almost naturally shifted to Rome, site of the papacy and a holy place because of the presence of the tombs of Sts. Peter and Paul.

Many evangelical sites were difficult to reach, so sanctuaries where relics were kept and venerated, even relics of dubious authenticity, became pilgrimage destinations in the West. These relics arrived in Europe by two routes: some came from the Holy Land, having been donated by crusaders or bought by monasteries, and others were plundered from the imperial treasury in Costantinople, the capital of the Eastern Empire and, in a major turn of events, the site to which the Venitians had diverted the Fourth Crusade (1202–1204) from its original intended destination, Egypt. In this way the West, lacking in sacred objects, was able to satiate its hunger for relics. News spread through the Christian world of miracles wrought by the relics, and the relics' new homes—churches, monasteries, sanctuaries—became centers of Christianity and destinations of popular devotion.

HOLY ROUTES

As the major monastic and mendicant orders were established, numerous abbeys and routes were constructed to connect them, which made it less difficult and dangerous to reach holy sites. The routes to Santiago de Compostela and Rome were dotted with sanctuaries that housed miraculous relics, which in turn transformed the sanctuaries into cultural centers and ultimately commercial hubs. New settlements developed because of the presence of pilgrims, and they vied with one another for the presence of worshippers, who came searching for parts of saints' bodies and

● ● ● A REFUGE FOR PILGRIMS

Foreign communities had *scholae*, recognized institutions equipped with churches, hospitals, cemeteries, and hospices for the benefit of pilgrims from specific countries.

①
S. Maria dell'Anima (☞71)
Approved by Boniface IX, this was a hospice for Germans, who were guaranteed food and lodging for 10 days.

②
Nostra Signora del Sacro Cuore (☞68)
Next to the church of S. Giacomo degli Spagnoli (the original name) was a Spanish hospice, which offered food and lodging for three days.

③
S. Luigi dei Francesi (☞84)
Since the late 15th century, this institution welcomed French pilgrims, who could stay up to three days and received a cash subsidy upon leaving (*right:* the church's ceiling).

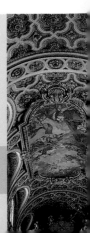

objects connected to their memories.

As stories of miracles multiplied, and as the number of new cults surrounding martyrs and saints mushroomed, restoration projects were undertaken to create glorious settings worthy of the sacred mementos. The acquisition of precious objects of worship took on economic as well as spiritual importance, and a speculative market in relics soon developed.

INDULGENCES

Visiting sacred sights yielded indulgences of various types, either partial or plenary. Bishops were soon granting indulgences in exchange for money and subcontracting their distribution, and the privilege was abused to the point where the practice was compromised irremediably.

The 13th century brought a canonic examination of the practice of indulgences, and the bishops' assembly convoked for the Lateran Council IV (1215) reestablished full papal authority, the *plenitudo potestatis*, over this matter. St. Thomas Aquinas (1225–1274), the great philosopher and theologian of the time, addressed the issue in definitive terms: "The power to grant indulgences resides exclusively with the pope."

Doctrine legitimized the principle of indulgence when it affirmed that the church is not only the fiduciary custodian of the Communion of Saints—that is, the saints' community—but also the guardian of the treasury of merits acquired by them. The church may distribute part of this limitless "moral capital" to the faithful. When Boniface VIII proclaimed plenary indulgence for the Jubilee of 1300, he simultaneously seized for himself, as representative of Peter on Earth, the right to distribute this immense reserve of salvation.

In 1295, just five years before that first Jubilee, plenary indulgence was granted to pilgrims who had gone to the church of S. Maria in Collemaggio in Aquila and to Assisi, while those who had visited the patriarchal basilicas in Rome received only a partial indulgence. At the same time, the prized remissions of sins were also granted, for a variety of different reasons, to believers who had not made pilgrimages. Among the beneficiaries were

KEEP TO THE RIGHT

The first Jubilee brought about innovations in transportation and traffic. In 1300, one-way traffic was introduced on the two sides of the Ponte S. Angelo. Dante Alighieri may have participated in this Jubilee, of which he wrote:

"thus the Romans, because of the great throng, in the year of the Jubilee, have taken measures for the people to pass over the bridge, so that on one side all face toward the castle and go to S. Pietro, and on the other they go toward the Mount."

—Dante's *Inferno*, translation by Charles S. Singleton, 1970, Princeton University Press (Bollingen Series)

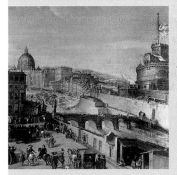

Papal procession over the Ponte S. Angelo. 17th century.

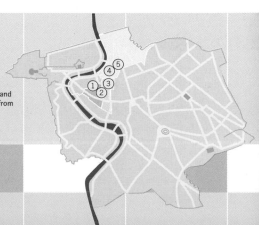

In Medieval Latin, a *bulla* was a seal of authentication on official documents; it was affixed to the parchment with a silk or hemp thread. The word later came to mean the documents promulgated by papal or imperial authority. Thus a papal bull is a letter from the pope that can address various issues (subjects of faith, but also affairs of state), and which is proclaimed or delivered to recipients. Papal bulls are still written in Latin, the official language of the church, and in the historiography they are identified by the first words of the text. The first Jubilee (1300), for example, was declared with the papal bull *Antiquorum habet fida relatio* ("The elderly are circulating a trust-worthy account").

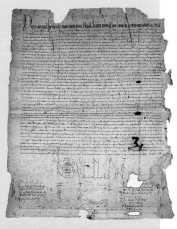

Papal bull by Honorius III, dated March 15, 1218.

Franciscans, missionaries to the Tartars; the pope's allies in the war against the Sicilians; and all those who fought against the Colonna, Rome's powerful patrician family and mortal enemies of Pope Boniface VIII, who was a member of the rival Caetani family.

ROME, THE NEW JERUSALEM

For centuries, Jerusalem was the center of the world of the faithful, but now this role fell to Rome. Calling itself the Cradle of Christianity and site of the throne of Peter, the city designated itself the direct heir to Jerusalem. Where it was once necessary to join the Crusades to obtain an indulgence, the establishment of the Jubilee put indulgences within the reach of anyone who completed a penitential journey, *ad limina apostolorum*, to the tombs of the apostles. Important relics—such as the veil of Veronica (the sudarium of Christ, with the impression of his face) and fragments of the true cross and the holy lance, all preserved in Rome—attracted multitudes of pilgrims.

Legend has it that the pilgrims who went to Rome for Christmas 1299, when Christmas coincided with New Year's, spread the word that the pope was about to proclaim a grand indulgence on the occasion of the century's close. An account of the events, written by Cardinal Jacopo Stefaneschi, relates that Boniface VIII, looking for a precedent, consulted the archives to see if there was any mention of such a custom, but he found no doctrinal justification that might endorse such an initiative. It was at that point that an elderly pilgrim came forward with a story in support of a precedent. He told the pope that he had participated, along with his own father, in the plenary indulgence granted at the close of the preceding century. His father had then requested that the son, if still alive a century later, return to Rome to complete a similar pilgrimage.

> *"The elderly are circulating a trust-worthy account that those who go to the honored Basilica of the Prince of Apostles in Rome are granted great remissions and indulgences of sins."*

FAITH ENROUTE

Beautiful shrines, with painted Madonnas, signs of widespread and popular devotion, decorate corners of Rome's pilgrimage roads. Like beacons at the sea's edge they capture the traveler's eye.

① Via della Lungara (☞67) Designed by Bramante, this street, along with the parallel Via Giulia, is considered a sacred route because of the flow of pilgrims that traveled it, en route to S. Pietro. The street is a continuum of 16th-century villas and palaces.

② Via del Pellegrino (☞79) Opened in 1497, this was part of the ancient Via Peregrinorum that lead toward the Vatican; at the corner of the Arco di S. Margherita is a beautiful stucco shrine with a Madonna and child.

③ Via dei Coronari (☞73) Many pilgrims traveled this street to cross Ponte S. Angelo and arrive at the basilica of S. Pietro. *Coronari*, or rosary-makers, gave the street its name; they were merchants who sold rosaries to the faithful along this route.

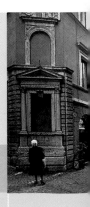

The oldest shrine in Rome, on Via dei Coronari.

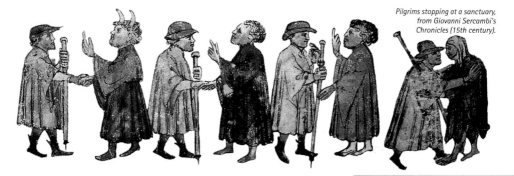

Pilgrims stopping at a sanctuary, from Giovanni Sercambi's Chronicles (15th century).

Thus begins the papal bull *Antiquorum habet fida relatio*, in which Pope Boniface VIII proclaimed the first Jubilee year in 1300. The first Jubilee marked the beginning of a custom that has endured many ups and downs ever since. In the papal bull *Antiquorum habet*, the pope decreed that the Jubilee would take place in every centennial year. But one of Boniface VIII's successors, the French pope Clement VI (1342–1352), proclaimed a second Jubilee as early as 1350 and decreed that the Jubilee should be celebrated every 50 years. This schedule would be changed numerous times, and extraordinary Jubilees were added to ordinary ones. As a result, Jubilees have long been held every 25 years. Over the centuries, Jubilee celebrations have reflected the political, social, and cultural situations of their times, but the principal players remained the pilgrims, who faced the long, difficult journey to Rome, full of hope and faith that their path would lead to salvation.

A DANGER-FILLED JOURNEY

During the Middle Ages, only soldiers, merchants, and pilgrims habitually traveled the perilous roads that linked different cities and countries. Merchants and pilgrims, particularly, ran numerous risks along the way. Merchants traveled to acquire material riches; pilgrims hoped to acquire gifts and wealth of another nature: indulgences and grace. Both abandoned familiar, safe places to face the unknown and danger, with no certain guarantee of ever returning home.

THE SPECTACLE OF FAITH

Michel de Montaigne, a 16th-century philosopher and traveler, wrote in his *Italian Travel Journal* (1580–1581):

"The splendor of Rome and its principal grandiosity consist in the conspicuousness of devotion; it is quite wonderful, these days, to observe the religious zeal of so vast a multitude. . . . The most notable and amazing thing I have ever seen, here or elsewhere, was the incredible quantity of people scattered throughout the city that day for devotions, and above all the quantity of confraternity members. For in addition to the great number of those who were seen by day, gathering in S. Pietro, as soon as the city grew dark, a fire appeared for each of those monks, who set out in a line, toward S. Pietro, each holding a torch, in most cases a white candle. I believe that at least 12,000 torches passed before me, since this procession filled the street from eight in the evening until midnight, during which time I saw neither space nor interruption."

④ **Piazza di Tor Sanguigna (Piazza Navona) (☞70)**
A theatrical shrine, depicting the Assumption of the Virgin, dominates the piazza in front of the facade of Palazzo Grossi. A painting inserted within an exuberant frame is surrounded by putti (*above right*).

⑤ **Via del Plebiscito (Galleria Doria Pamphilj) (☞80)**
On Palazzo Pamphilj's facade, an opulent shrine with a sunburst design, with an image of the Madonna at the center.

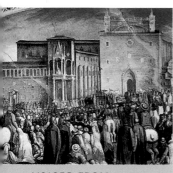

VOICES FROM THE PAST

In his description of the millennial Jubilee celebrations of 1300, German historian Ferdinand Gregorovius quoted Giovanni Villani, a Florentine merchant and banker, eyewitness of the event, and author of the *Nuova Cronica*:

"Rome offered the spectacle of throngs of pilgrims coming and going ... such a mob of people ... Men from their own countries were ready to welcome them at the gates ... and urban officials ... who pointed out to them places where they could find lodgings

... For an entire year, Rome was a seething field of pilgrims, a true Babel in its confusion of languages. They say that every day, 30,000 pilgrims came and went and every day there were 200,000 foreigners in the city..."

It is difficult for the modern traveler to imagine the significance of the sacrifices that a pilgrimage implied in the Middle Ages. The pilgrim left his land and loved ones, and they, in turn, were deprived of his labor for as long as he traveled. The journey also entailed additional expenses for the family, which had to supply their pilgrim with a sum sufficient to live on for a period of time that was difficult to estimate.

Once a pilgrim made the decision to go, the bishop blessed him in a solemn ceremony and presented him with the pilgrim's staff of penitence, a curved staff that symbolized his new condition. The pilgrim was then accompanied in a procession beyond the city gates. A few privileged pilgrims departed on horseback or astride mules, but most went on foot. Before leaving, many made their wills.

All roads led to Rome, it was said, because it was from there that, in ancient times, pilgrims had departed. In antiquity, the efficiency of communication routes contributed to the expansion of the empire, but since its collapse in AD 476, the Roman system of well-constructed roads, which had led from the capital of the ancient world through Europe to the East and to Africa, had slowly and inexorably deteriorated. Time had damaged the paving, bridges had collapsed, and major routes often changed because of interruptions and detours. Along the principal routes, pilgrims found a dense network of inns and places of shelter, as well as numerous minor sanctuaries and abbeys where they could rest and take refreshment. At dusk, a bell, called the *smarrita* (for "those gone astray") rang out from places of shelter, to indicate the way to those who were still on the road. The *smarrita* was renamed the Ave Maria (Hail Mary) when St. Bonaventure ordered his monks to recite a prayer three times for those who might be lost during the night.

During medieval times, those who could took advantage of water routes, which were quicker and more direct, although made dangerous by Saracen pirates, who all too frequently intercepted pilgrims' ships and sold the travelers as slaves in distant lands. The difficulties, dangers, and sufferings of a pilgrimage—including the tolls, duties, and taxes along the road; the perpetual danger of bandits; and the threats of illness and inclement weather—served

●● CHRISTMAS IN ROME

Christmas crèches of all sizes and styles are scattered throughout the city, in the piazzas and in almost every church in Rome. They can be visited in a citywide itinerary from mid-December mid-January.

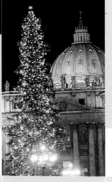

① S. Pietro (☞ 52)
During the festivities, city residents and tourists gather in the embrace of Bernini's colonnade to admire the tall fir tree decorated for the holiday, and the traditional crèche at the foot of the obelisk. The recent custom of a Christmas tree in Piazza S. Pietro was introduced by Pope John Paul II. (*left*).

② Piazza Navona (☞ 70)
Both before and after its Baroque transformation, the piazza was a theater for famous festivals and processions. Today, during the Christmas season and until Epiphany, the piazza is filled with stalls selling small figures for crèches and toys.

③ Ss. Ambrogio e Carlo al Corso (☞ 92)
The church contains an elaborate 18th-century crèche that reflects, in its details, the period of its creation (*below*).

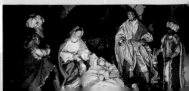

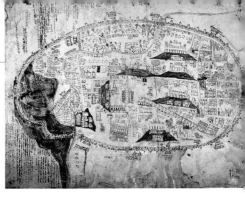

to increase the value of the venture as an atonement for misdeeds and a source of indulgences.

HELP ALONG THE WAY

Since antiquity, guidebooks have described the itinerary to Rome from the most remote parts of Europe. Some, such as the *Itinerary of Einsiedeln* and the *Notitia ecclesiarum urbis Romae*, both dating from the Carolingian era, limited themselves to written descriptions of the route and stopping places. Others were embellished with images or maps and included information about distances, in days on foot, and suggestions about which direction to take. Two of the most well-known were the *Chronica Maiora* by Matthew Paris, written in the 13th century, and the *Tabula Peutingeriana*, a 23-foot scroll taken from an original source dating from late antiquity.

These precious aids were accessible to very few pilgrims, both because of their value and because most people were illiterate or did not know Latin. The majority of wayfarers trusted oral descriptions and information, and they reached the principle communication routes and joined forces with other pilgrims who had the same destination. From throughout Europe, they gathered en route to Rome along Via Francigena (the road from France) also called Via Romea (the road to Rome), which, depending on the era, coincided with stretches of Via Aurelia, Via Cassia, and Via Flaminia. The route arrived at Rome over the Ponte Milvio (Milvian bridge) and passed through the Porta del Popolo, or from the present Via Trionfale, descending from the Monte Mario hill.

Once in Rome, the *Mirabilia Urbis Romae*, an illustrated, handwritten guidebook, described for voyagers the legends, between history and myth, about the ruined monuments of antiquity. The vestiges of ancient Rome were scattered among the urban outgrowths that crowded around the major churches, separated from one another by vast areas of countryside and vineyards.

In subsequent centuries, the institution of Jubilees in Rome contributed significantly to the renewal of the city and to its return to a splendor that, even today, attracts millions of visitors—pilgrims and non-pilgrims alike.

Plan of Rome in 1345.

Opposite: Pilgrims at S. Giovanni in Laterano; detail from a fresco in the Biblioteca Apostolica Vaticana.

VOICES FROM THE PAST

"A chronicler who was among the pilgrims in 1300 described it thus: 'Bread, wine, meat, fish and oats were traded in abundance and at reasonable prices; but hay was rather expensive and inns extremely so.

... The Romans claim to number 2 million men and women in all. And in that crowd, I often saw someone fall and be crushed beneath the feet of the multitudes and it was only with great effort that I myself, more than once, escaped such misfortune.'

... We can imagine the quantity of ancient artifacts, coins, gems, rings, sculptures, marble fragments and manuscripts—which pilgrims took back to their countries."

—Storia della Città di Roma nel Medioevo (1859–1873)

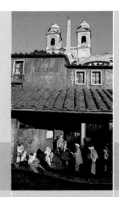

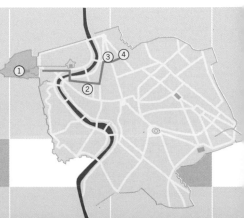

④
Piazza di Spagna
(☞ 89)
As in many Italian cities, life-size crèches are installed in the piazzas of Rome. On January 6, on the Spanish Steps, the Three Kings arrive, bearing gifts for the infant Jesus (*left*).

The Tumultuous Middle Ages in Rome

1300 THE FIRST JUBILEE

Pope Boniface VIII (1294–1303) issues the papal bull *Antiquórum habet fidu relutio*, proclaiming the first Jubilee. It is written to address popular expectations at the century's end and is promulgated two months after the New Year. Approximately 200,000 pilgrims are in Rome. Giotto is commissioned to execute a fresco in S. Giovanni in Laterano, depicting Boniface VIII proclaiming the Jubilee, and a mosaic of the Navity in S. Pietro.

1302 With the papal bull *Unum Sanctam*, Boniface VIII proclaims the supremacy of the papacy over secular authority. This is the first sign of a rupture between the church and the French monarchy, the most powerful of the time.

1303 Boniface VIII establishes the Rome's university, now the Università della Sapienza (from the name of the Palazzo della Sapienza, where it was located from the 15th century until 1935). Philip IV, king of France, reacts to the publication of *Unam Sanctam* by having Boniface VIII captured while at his residence in Anagni (south of Rome). Freed by popular insurrection, the pope returns to Rome, where he dies in October of that year.

1309 Pope Clement V (1305–1315) transfers the papal see to Avignon, France, marking the beginning of the so-called Avignon captivity, which lasts until 1377, during which time the papacy is subject to the French crown.

1341 The River Tiber floods the city.

1343 Motivated by the success of the Holy Year, particularly for the city's economy, a Roman delegation appears before Pope Clement VI (1342–1352) in Avignon, to convince him to proclaim a new Jubilee before the end of the century

1347 For a few months, Cola di Rienzo, a common man, assumes power in a popular revolt as tribune of the people, with the initial support of the papacy. His political model, based on republican and imperial Rome, contributes to reawakening interest in the monuments of antiquity. He is killed on the Campidoglio in

1354, during an uprising.

1348 The stairway of S. Maria in Aracoeli (☞115) is opened. In September, the most terrible earthquake since the founding of Rome destroys both recent structures and ancient monuments. The facade of S. Giovanni in Laterano collapses and the basilica of S. Pietro is damaged. The Black Death strikes the city.

1350 THE JUBILEE WITHOUT A POPE

Clement VI remains in Avignon and sends two cardinals to celebrate the Holy Year. A visit to S. Giovanni in Laterano (☞105) is added to the visits to the basilicas of S. Paolo Fuori le Mura (☞131) and S. Pietro (☞52) recommended by Boniface VIII for the first Jubilee. To gain indulgence, Romans must visit the three basilicas once a day for 30 days; pilgrims coming from outside the city must make the daily visit for 15 days.

1377 The end of the Avignon captivity is confirmed by Gregory XI's reentry into Rome. The pope's residence is moved from the Lateran to its new headquarters at S. Pietro. This move reflects the shift of Rome's city center, which now lies in the area within the bend of the Tiber, between the Campidoglio and the Vatican. Because of the plague and the continuing economic crisis, the population, which stood at approximately 35,000 inhabitants in 1300, declined to approximately 25,000.

1383-1388 The plague further decimates the population of Rome.

1389 With the papal bull *Salvator Noster Unigenitus*, Pope Urban VI (1378–1389) proclaims a new Jubilee year for 1390 and changes the interval between one Jubilee and another from 50 to 33 years (the number of years in the life of Jesus). The change is meant to accommodate the average human life span, which at the time was less than 50 years, but the unexpected proclamation also has several political motives, such as addressing the

A crusader; 14th-century fresco. Naples, Cathedral.

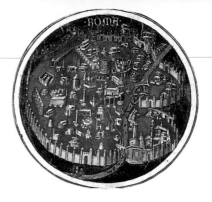

Taddeo di Bartolo's plan of Rome (early 15th century). Siena, Palazzo Pubblico.

antischismatic struggle against the antipope in Avignon and papal control over the city of Rome, which is torn by clan rivalries.

1390 | THE UNEXPECTED JUBILEE

Pope Boniface IX (1389–1404) has only a few months to organize and manage an unforeseen Jubilee in a devastated city. Within the city's walls, vast uninhabited areas alternate with small settlements; the layout of the road network has almost disappeared; churches are crumbling, and the baronial families have taken possession of the ancient ruins, transforming them into fortresses from which they control urban points of access and transit. The church is without funds, and to face its grave economic problems, it is forced to seek loans and take out mortgages from Tuscan bankers. S. Maria Maggiore (☞ 126) is added to the list of three basilicas to be visited. To prevent an outbreak of plague, a decree is issued on May 31, specifying that pilgrims need only visit the basilicas for a single week, but the plague returns nonetheless. The pope retreats to nearby Rieti. The church reaps considerable income from the Jubilee, in part because of a new practice of granting of indulgences outside Rome. For the first time, penitents' economic situations are taken into account in determining the amount that they must pay to obtain indulgences without making a pilgrimage to the city.

1399

In the spring, the Flagellanti Bianchi (White Flagellants), members of a popular religious movement, traverse Italy to the cry of *pace e misericordia* (peace and mercy). They flagellate themselves as a sign of penitence, dress in white (hence their name), and wear hoods. They enter Rome, where the pope receives them on September 7.

1400 | THE UNOFFICIAL JUBILEE

This Jubilee is not officially proclaimed by the usual papal bull, but rather is commanded by throngs of the faithful flocking to the city

(120,000 according to some sources) in September 1399. With the arrival of hot weather, the plague returns, claiming up to 800 victims a day. On the outskirts of the city, roads are littered with corpses. The Hospice of S. Maria dell'Anima (☞ 71) is established to accommodate German pilgrims. The pope institutes a building commission for the restoration of S. Paolo Fuori le Mura.

1415 | A flood strikes Rome.
1422 | An outbreak of the plague and a flood devastate the city.

1423 | AN UNKNOWN JUBILEE
1425

Scant documentation provides differing accounts of the precise date of this Jubilee. As soon as he is elected by the Council of Constance to remedy the Western Schism, Pope Martin V (1417–1431) initiates the difficult task of restoring the social, economic, and cultural life of the city. He begins reconstruction projects to improve the image of the papacy and the church, and basilicas, churches, and palaces are renovated. During this period, various painters work under the patronage of the pope and cardinals: Gentile da Fabriano (the frescoes in S. Giovanni in Laterano that depict scenes from the life of John the Baptist), Pisanello, Masaccio, and Masolino (*Triptych of the Snow* in S. Maria Maggiore). For the first time, papal documents mention the opening of the Porta Santa (Holy Door) in S. Giovanni in Laterano.

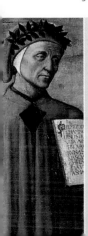

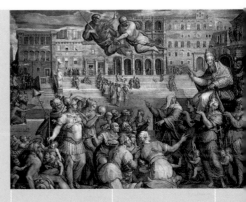

1271
Marco Polo (1254–1324) begins his voyage to the East.

1290–1375
Dante Alighieri (*left*, in a fresco by Domenico di Michelino in the Florence Cathedral), Francesco Petrarch, and Giovanni Boccaccio lay the groundwork for modern Italian literature.

1377
The Avignon captivity ends. Pope Gregory XI reestablishes the seat of papal power in Rome (*right*: the event in a fresco by Giorgio Vasari, in the Sala Regia of the Vatican). The election of this French anti-pope leads to the Western Schism (1378–1417).

The Splendors of Rome's Renaissance

1450

THE NEW FACE OF ROME

Nicholas V (1447–1455), the humanist pope, continues restoration work in the city. He establishes the basis for the Vatican Library's first collection of books, acquiring codices and manuscripts; he is also establishes the Vatican Botanical Garden. A period characterized by patronage and advances in the arts begins. The contract for the Holy Year treasury is granted to Cosimo de' Medici, who strikes a medal called a Giubileo, which pilgrims take home as souvenirs, along with copies of Veronica's veil. The areas traversed by pilgrims traveling from one basilica to another are sparsely inhabited and unsafe. On the occasion of the Jubilee, to encourage development of these areas, the pope resorts to incentives, exonerating inhabitants from payment of taxes and lining streets with new elm trees. A new outbreak of plague forces pilgrims to spend only five days in the city. The pope blesses the pilgrims every Sunday at S. Pietro, and the Veronica's veil is exhibited to the public every Saturday. Parts of the old Constantinian basilica of S. Pietro are demolished, others expanded. Architect Leon Battista Alberti begins construction of the Vatican Palaces (☞54–58).

1452

Two important projects took place during this year: the improvement of three roads (Via dei Pellegrini, which leads into the present-day Ghetto; Via Papale, which leads to the Campidoglio; and Via Recta, the present Via dei Coronari) and the rebuilding of the Leonine City that lies between Castel S. Angelo and S. Pietro. The latter calls for the demolition of the old medieval Borgo district and the creation a new small city layed out on three rectilinear streets.

1455

The construction of Palazzo di Venezia (☞81) begins.

1458

Enea Silvio Piccolomini, humanist, patron, one of the leading figures in the cultural renewal of Rome, is elected pope. He takes the name Pius II (1458–1464).

1462

With the papal bull *Cum Almam Nostram Urbem*, Pius II promotes the protection of ancient monuments.

1473-1475

In preparation for the Jubilee of 1475, Sixtus IV (1471–1484) begins an urban renewal plan that addresses problems with roads, sanitation, the restoration of monuments, and the construction of new buildings, with attention paid to the aesthetic and commemorative aspect of the new architecture. Some of the many projects include the construction of the Ponte Sisto (☞76), the only bridge built over the Tiber between antiquity and the 19th century; the straightening of many medieval streets; the demolition of exterior stairways, overhangs, and balconies from residential buildings; and the enclosing of porticoes and passageways. These measures were also meant to reduce crime in a city where pilgrims were frequently assaulted in the dark recesses of porticoed streets. Renaissance Rome begins to take shape.

1475

THE SISTINE JUBILEE

Plague affects this Holy Year, which is extended until Easter 1476. The pope sanctions the 25-year Jubilee period and the cancellation of all indulgences outside Rome during the Jubilee year. The city becomes the definitive center of the Catholic world. Pilgrims included many crowned heads: King Ferrante of Naples; Queen Dorothy of

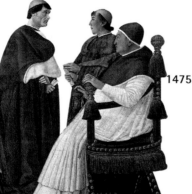

Above: Sixtus IV nominates Platina prefect of the Vatican Library (1477), in a painting by Melozzo da Forlì. Pinacoteca Vaticana.

1402
The Visconti of Milan repelled Robert of Bavaria's attempted invasion.

1407
The Banco of S. Giorgio, Europe's first public bank, is established in Genoa.

1427
Masaccio paints the fresco of the Trinity in S. Maria Novella in Florence. He dies a year later in Rome at age 27.

1443
Brunelleschi's (1377–1446) cupola is completed on Florence's Duomo.

1451
Christopher Columbus (*below*) is born in Genoa

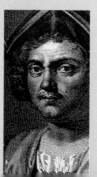

1455
Beato Angelico dies in Rome

1469–1492
Florence is ruled by Lorenzo de' Medici (1449–1492), known as "the Magnificent," one of history's greatest patrons of the arts.

1498
Dominican friar Girolamo Savonarola (1452–1498), right in a painting by Fra' Bartolomeo della Porta, was hanged and burned in Florence as a heretic. After the expulsion of the Medici family (1494), he had established a democratic republic based on a moralistic philosophy.

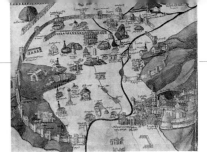

Denmark; Mattia Corvino, king of Hungary; Federico da Montefeltro, duke of Urbino; and Charlotte of Lusignano, former queen of Cyprus. With the papal bull *Ad decorem militantis Ecclesiae*, Sixtus IV establishes the Biblioteca Apostolica Vaticana (☞55). Reconstruction projects continue under Sixtus IV, including S. Maria del Popolo (☞92) from 1475 to 1477; S. Agostino (☞82) from 1479 to 1483; S. Maria della Pace (☞71) in 1482; the Sistine Chapel (☞55) from 1475 to 1481; the Ospedale di S. Spirito in Sassia (☞61) from 1473 to 1478; and the Palazzo della Cancelleria (☞69) in 1485.

Domenico del Massaio's plan of Rome, 1472. Biblioteca Apostolica Vaticana.

1500	**THE JUBILEE OF THE GREAT MASTERS** Pope Alexander VI (1492–1503) establishes the ritual of the opening and closing of the Porta Santa in each of the four major basilicas. The passage through the door becomes a condition for obtaining indulgence. Resuming a project of Pope Nicholas V, the Via Alessandrina is constructed, corresponding to the new Porta Santa of S. Pietro (inaugurated December 24, 1499, with the beginning of the Holy Year). Bramante designs the cloister of S. Maria della Pace and the tempietto of S. Pietro in Montorio (☞71), his first two projects in Rome. Michelangelo creates the *Pietà*, his first work in Rome.
1503	Julius II (Giuliano Della Rovere), one of Rome's greatest patron of the arts, is elected pope. He is pope until 1513.
1508–1512	Michelangelo paints the frescoes for the Sistine Chapel.
1509	Raphael (1483–1520) begins work on his Stanze in the Vatican (☞52).
1510	Martin Luther visits Rome and is scandalized by the dissolute habits of the popes and by the sale of indulgences.
1517	Lateran Council V concludes in Rome, during which Pope Leo X declares that the church's work of self-reformation is completed.
1523	Another devastating plague strikes the city.

1525 THE TRIUMPH OF MONEY

The sale of indulgences flourishes; believers are no longer required to complete a pilgrimage and can simply pay to receive absolution. The plague and the possibility of obtaining indulgence without going to Rome result in a very small number of pilgrims during the Jubilee. Pope Clement VII (1523–1534) opens the Via del Babuino (formerly the Via Clementia, then the Via Paolina, completed in 1543, under Paul III). Thus the so-called trident of the Campo Marzio district takes shape, with its vertex at Piazza del Popolo (☞88), the principal northern point of entry for pilgrims. In subsequent centuries, numerous inns and hotels open here to houses artists and travelers. Antonio da Sangallo and Baldassarre Peruzzi continue working on S. Pietro in the Vatican. Raphael designs the Hall of Constantine.

1526	The first historically reliable census in the modern era counts 55,000 inhabitants.
1527	Charles V's imperial troops pillage the city in what will be known as the Sack of Rome.
1542	Paul III establishes the congregation of the Santo Uffizio as a custodian of Catholic orthodoxy.
1546	Antonio da Sangallo, who is overseeing the construction of the new basilica of S. Pietro and the Palazzo Farnese, dies. Michelangelo Buonarroti takes over these projects.

Above: a gold ducat coined by Clement VII for the Jubilee of 1525. Museo Nazionale Romano.
Below: S. Pietro and the Vatican. Vatican, Barracks of the Noble Guards.

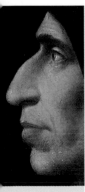

1499 Leonardo da Vinci (1452–1519) completed the *Last Supper* for the refectory of S. Maria delle Grazie in Milan. **1513** *The Prince* by Machiavelli (1469–1527) was the strongest expression of Renaissance political thought.	**1521** Pope Leo X (Giovanni de' Medici, 1513–1521) excommunicates Martin Luther (1483–1546), precipitating the Protestant Reformation. **1545–1563** The Council of Trent formulates the Catholic response to the Reformation.

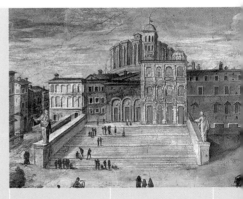

Counter-Reformation and the Baroque Era

1550 | ### THE JUBILEE OF THE "NEW" ROME
The death of Paul III in 1549 delays the opening of the Holy Year, which is inaugurated by Julius III (1550–1555) during Carnival of 1550. To avoid speculation and unjustified price increases, rents are frozen for pilgrims' lodgings. Ignatius Loyola and Philip Neri actively participate in the Jubilee. Julius III allows Michelangelo, now elderly, to visit the seven churches on horseback. The appreciation and restoration of ancient monuments continues, intended to spur an ideological revival of classical Rome's pomp and splendor, and to sanction the continuity between the Roman empire and the papacy.

1551–1555 | Julius III builds a suburban villa, the Villa Giulia (☞*134*), a compendium of Mannerist culture.

1555 | Pope Paul IV (1555–1559) issues a papal bull that establishes the Ghetto (☞*81*) in the area of the ancient Circus Flaminius; it will be the compulsory residence of the Jewish community until 1870.

1561 | Pius V (Antonio Ghislieri), persecutor of the heretics, is elected pope. He will later become saint.

1568 | Construction of the Chiesa del Gesù (☞*80*), designed by Vignola, begins.

1575 | ### THE JUBILEE OF THE COUNTER-REFORMATION
At the height of the Counter-Reformation, the Holy Year becomes an ideological celebration of the church in defense of the Catholic religion and a call for unity among believers. The law *Quae Publice Utilia*, written at the behest of Gregory XIII (1572–1585), introduces the concept of building for the public good. The pope grants a permanent headquarters to the Archconfraternity of the

Portrait of Pope Julius III, in the Galleria Spada.

Santissima Trinità, which will play an important role in welcoming pilgrims during this and future Jubilees. Carlo Borromeo, archbishop of Milan, participates in a pilgrimage and travels barefoot over the prescribed itineraries. With the establishment of the Itinerary of the Seven Churches, an initiative by Philip Neri, work on the roads connecting the major basilicas becomes necessary; the Via Merulana and Via Gregoriana are opened (1576).

1584 | The Vertuosa Compagnia de' Musici (Company of Virtuous Musicians), also known as the Academy of S. Cecilia, is established; it will remain the most important musical institution in Rome.

1585–1590 | These years mark Sixtus V's papacy, during which the advent of the use of carriages mandates the broadening or redesign of numerous streets, including Via Felice, Via Panisperna, Via dei Serpenti, and Via Maggiore.

1586 | Under the direction of Domenico Fontana, the Vatican obelisk is placed in the center of Piazza S. Pietro (☞*54*); the "memorable undertaking," as contemporary accounts call it, takes six months to complete.

1592 | A malaria epidemic strikes the city.

1598–1599 | Once more, the Tiber overflows its banks and floods the city.

1599–1602 | Caravaggio paints three canvases dedicated to St. Matthew for the church of S. Luigi dei Francesi (☞*84*).

1600 | Philosopher Giordano Bruno is burned as a heretic in Campo de' Fiori (☞*74*).

1600 | ### THE JUBILEE OF THE GREAT PROCESSIONS
In preparation for the Jubilee, Clement VIII (1592–1605) creates two commissions to oversee the organization of the spiritual and material aspects of the event. New piazzas are created in front of various churches, including S. Prisca

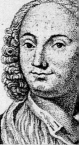

1571
A multinational fleet defeated the Turks in the Battle of Lepanto.

1633
Galileo Galilei (1564–1642) faces the Inquisition.

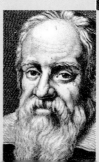

1678
Composer Antonio Vivaldi (*above*) was born in Venice. He died in 1741 in Vienna, totally forgotten.

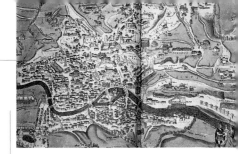

Plan of Rome, 1588.

(☞*121*), S. Gregorio Magno (☞*113*), S. Nicola in Carcere (☞*85*), and S. Giovanni in Laterano; the titular basilicas are restored; and new churches are consecrated, among them Chiesa Nuova (☞*68*).

Approximately 500,000 pilgrims converge on the city. Confraternities, many of which are founded during this period, organize retinues and processions. Members and participants wear cloaks and mantles of different colors. The spectacle of processions, with standards, banners, and the sound of liturgical songs against the backdrop of ancient and modern monuments, gives this Jubilee an air that is more theatrical than pious.

1614	Rome's first public library, the Biblioteca Angelica, is founded.
1622	Carlo Maderno creates the dome of S. Andrea della Valle (☞*70*), the second tallest in Rome after that of S. Pietro; the church is consecrated in 1650.
1623–1624	Gian Lorenzo Bernini begins work on the bronze baldachin for S. Pietro, using bronzes from the Pantheon portico; this project is completed in 1633.

1625 THE WARTIME JUBILEE

The city suffers a new plague and another flood. Fearing contagion, visits to the basilicas outside the city walls are replaced with visits to S. Maria in Trastevere (☞*65*), S. Lorenzo in Lucina (☞*99*), and S. Maria del Popolo. With the papal bull *Pontificia Sollicitudo*, Pope Urban VIII (1623–1644) grants indulgence to hermits, monks, prisoners, the ill, and all those who are unable to make to journey to Rome, as well as to those who pray for peace in a Europe suffering the torment of the Thirty Years' War.

1626	The new basilica of S. Pietro is consecrated.
1638	Francesco Borromini begins construction of the church of S. Carlo alle Quattro Fontane (☞*104*).

1650 THE HEIGHT OF BAROQUE ROME

For the Jubilee of Innocent X (1644–1655) there is a great flow of pilgrims (approximately 700,000), and once again the confraternities, particularly the Filippini and the Gonfalone, distinguish themselves in welcoming the multitudes. The tone of this Jubilee is worldly, with retinues, receptions, and gaudy processions organized by rival confraternities. On Easter, the Spanish confraternity sponsors spectacular fireworks in Piazza Navona. Bernini conceives the Fontana dei Quattro Fiumi (Fountain of the Four Rivers) for the piazza; the project is completed the following year. Borromini designs the church of S. Ivo alla Sapienza (☞*84*).

1667	The colonnade of Piazza S. Pietro, designed by Bernini, is completed; the project was begun in 1656.

1675 THE QUEEN'S JUBILEE

The elderly and tired Clement X (1670–1676) inaugurates the 15th Jubilee in the presence of Queen Christina of Sweden, who converted to Catholicism. For the papacy, her conversion is a symbol of the victory of the church over the Lutheran religion. Bernini creates a statue of the *Blessed Ludovica Albertoni*, housed in the church of S. Francesco a Ripa (☞*64*).

1694	Carlo Fontana completes the Palazzo di Montecitorio (☞*97*), begun in 1653 by Bernini.

Ponte Sisto in a series of views of Rome by Gaspare Vanvitelli, housed in the Musei Capitolini.

1707	Austrian domination over Italy replaces the French.
1714	With the Peace of Rastadt, France recognizes the new Italian possessions: Lombardy, Sardinia, and the kingdom of Naples.
1720–1790	The Great Age of the Grand Tour: northern Europeans visit Italy and start the vogue for classical studies. Among the famous visitors are Edward Gibbon (1758), Jacques-Louis David (1775), and Johann Wolfgang von Goethe (1786).

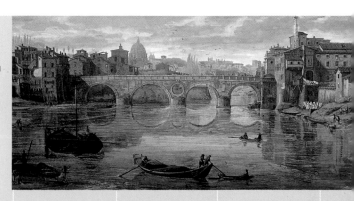

From the Enlightenment to the Present Day

1700 | **THE JUBILEE OF THE TWO POPES**
The Jubilee proclaimed by Innocent XII (1691–1700) is brought to conclusion by Clement XI (1700–1721). The tone of this Holy Year is sober, with less of the pomp and frivolity that had distinguished previous Jubilees. The city administration issues edicts for street cleaning and for the maintenance of churches. Indulgences are granted to pilgrims who visit S. Giovanni in Laterano on St. Thomas's feast day and to those who follow the pope on his visit to the four basilicas.

1704 | Reconstruction of the Porto di Ripetta, Tiber's ancient port "della Posterula," used for small river traffic from Tuscany and Umbria, begins. This is Rome's largest urban renewal project in 18th century.

1725 | **THE JUBILEE OF THE NEEDY**
Pope Benedict XIII (1724–1730), a Dominican, emphasizes providing pilgrims with hospitality and assistance during their journey. He visits the ill and the imprisoned, devotes himself to assisting the needy, and shows little interest in the political vicissitudes of the time.

1726 | Piazza di Spagna is linked to the Pincio by the steps of Trinità dei Monti (☞ 88,90).
1729 | The Hospital of Ss. Maria e Gallicano (☞ 62), designed by Filippo Raguzzini, is completed; it is a model for 18th-century hospital architecture.
1743 | The names of the various rioni are placed on plaques and nailed to the walls of houses at street intersections.

1750 | **THE JUBILEE OF ENLIGHTENMENT**
Religious fervor and participation in the celebration of the Holy Year (as well as the flow of pilgrims) decreases. Benedict XIV (1740–1758) entrusts Frà Leonardo da Porto Maurizio with the spiritual preparations for the Jubilee; he preaches in Piazza Navona,

S. Maria in Trastevere, and S. Maria sopra Minerva. The Stations of the Via Crucis are moved into to Coliseum, reinterpreting this ancient monument in Christian terms as a place of martyrdom. Luigi Vanvitelli reorganizes the interior of the Basilica of S. Maria degli Angeli (☞ 125) and is involved in the building of S. Pietro.

1762 | Pope Clement XIII (1758–1769) inaugurates the Trevi Fountain (☞ 94).
1763 | German archaeologist Johann Joachim Winckelmann (1710–1768), spiritual father of neoclassicism, is put in charge of Rome's antiquities.
1771 | Clement XIV (1769–1774) establishes the Museo Pio-Clementino (☞ 57); the transformation of the Vatican Palaces into museums begins.
1773 | Clement XIV disbands the Jesuits. The order will be reinstated in 1814.

1775 | **THE LAST JUBILEE OF THE ANCIEN RÉGIME**
The Jubilee is celebrated by Pius VI (1775–1799), who welcomes Maximilian of Austria and Tanucci, minister of the Kingdom of Naples, to Rome; both these men harbor Enlightenment and anticlerical ideas, a sign of the church's opening to modernity.

1789 | Antonio Canova creates the funerary monument of Clement XIV, housed in the basilica of SS. Apostoli (☞ 101). It is his first work in Rome.
1798 | Napoléon's French troops occupy Rome; the Republic of Rome is proclaimed, and Pope Pius VI is exiled and dies in France.
1799 | A conclave is held in Venice, and Pius VII (1800–1823) is elected pope. He arrives in Rome on July 3, after traversing an Italy occupied by the French. The Jubilee of 1800 is not celebrated.
1816–24 | Architect and urbanist Giuseppe Valadier redesigns Piazza del Popolo.
1823 | Fire destroys the basilica of S. Paolo Fuori le Mura.

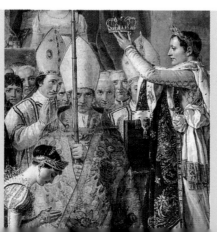

1778
Teatro alla Scala is completed in Milan.

1796
Napoléon begins his Italian campaigns, annexing Rome and imprisoning Pope Pius VI four years later.

1804
Napoléon crowns himself emperor (*right:* a detail of a painting by J.-L. David) in the presence of Pope Pius VII.

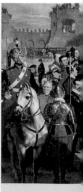

1815
Austria controls much of northern Italy after Napoléon's downfall.

1820–1831
Insurrections and revolutionary movements strike many Italian States and cities.

1848–1849
New popular revolts for national independence from Austria.

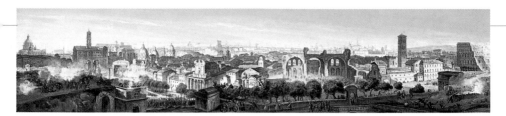

1825	**THE JUBILEE OF THE RESTORATION**

After the riots of 1820–1821, Leo XII (1823–1829) proclaims the Jubilee amid a tense climate, full of suspicion and fears that the crowd of pilgrims will be infiltrated by revolutionary elements. The confraternities of SS. Stimmate di S. Francesco, Orazione e Morte, and SS. Trinità dei Pellegrini oversee hospitality; special new laws prohibit improper behavior and regulate women's clothing.

1848 Riots, inspired by Giuseppe Mazzini's republican ideals, result in the creation of the short-lived Roman Republic, defended militarily by Giuseppe Garibaldi's volunteers. Pope Pius IX (1846–1878) retreats to Gaeta, near Naples, and doesn't return to Rome until April 1850, after the French troops of Napoléon III retake the city.

1850 The Jubilee of 1850 is not declared.

1863 Poet Giuseppe Gioachino Belli (1791–1863) dies; his work in Roman dialect, published posthumously, reveals him to be one of the greatest writers of italy's dialect literature.

1868 Cholera claims 8,500 victims in Rome.

1870 Vatican Council I pronounces the dogma of papal infallibility in matters of faith. The Tiber floods the city. After a short siege, Italian troops occupy Rome, the last city to fold in this 10-year-old kingdom. This event completes the Italian territorial unity and constitutes the end of the church's secular power.

1871 Rome becomes the new capital of Italy.

Above: View of Rome after the breaching of Porta Pia (1870). Museo del Risorgimento.
Below: Carlo De Paris's Presentation of the keys of the city to Pius IX, who returned to Rome on April 12, 1850. Museo Storico Vaticano.

1875	**THE JUBILEE OF POLEMICS**

After the proclamation of the unification of Italy, and in open polemics with the Italian State, the Holy Year, proclaimed with the papal bull *Gravibus Ecclesiae et huius Saeculi Calamitatibus*, is celebrated stealthily, without public ceremonies and without the opening of the Porta Santa.

1876 After the disastrous 1870 flood of the Tiber, construction begins on river embankments, a project that is completed in 1900.

1881 With more than 270,000 inhabitants, Rome is now the third largest city in Italy, after Naples and Milan.

1891 Pope Leo XIII (1878–1903) publishes the encyclical *Rerum Novarum*, which signals an attempt to seek a political balance between the Italian State and the church, and a new social role for the church within the new state.

1900	**THE JUBILEE OF THE NEW CENTURY**

Contributions to the Jubile by welfare and charitable organizations, which played such a large role in assisting pilgrims, is sharply reduced by political transformations. The pope appoints a permanent pontifical commission to assist pilgrims.

1922 The fascist march on Rome concludes with Benito Mussolini assuming the task of forming a new government.

1924 Socialist House Representative Giacomo Matteotti is assassinated by the fascists.

1925 The governorship of Rome is established; the city administration depends directly on the Ministry of the Interior, and the capital assumes unique administrative status.

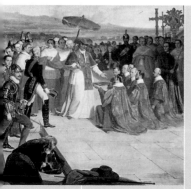

1860
Garibaldi (*right*) defeats the Bourbon rulers in Sicily and Naples. The Kingdom of Italy is established a year later.

1870
Rome is captured by Italian troops and is declared capital of Italy.

1900
King Umberto I is assassinated by an anarchist; he is succeeded by King Victor Emmanuel III.

1915
Italy enters World War I on the side of the Allies.

1925 | **THE JUBILEE UNDER FASCISM**
During the Jubilee, pilgrims can obtain indulgences by praying for the unity of Christians, peace among people, and a solution to the Palestinian problem. Different commissions organize the reception of pilgrims, and a large Missionary Exposition spreads the word about the activities of Catholic missions in the world and celebrates the church's evangelical work. Pope Pius XI reopens the exterior loggia of S. Pietro and gives the blessing *Urbi et Orbi* ("to the city and the world").

1929 | The Lateran Treaty is signed. The treaty defines the relationship between church and state and declares the independence of the Vatican City; the Italian State grants payment to the church for expropriation of its property.

1933 | The Via dell'Impero, the present-day Via dei Fori Imperiali, opens.

1943 | On July 19, U.S. planes bomb the S. Lorenzo quarter; on September 10, Italian and German soldiers clash at Porta S. Paolo; on October 16, the Jewish community of Rome is rounded up and deported.

1948 | Pope Pius XII (1939–1958) establishes the Holy Year Central Committee, which will oversee Jubilee preparations.

1950 | **THE JUBILEE OF RECONSTRUCTION**
Pilgrims flow into the city, and the Casa del Pellegrino is established, on the new Via della Conciliazione, to accommodate them; the Hospice of SS. Trinità dei Pellegrini is restored. The pope proclaims this Holy Year a "year of great return, a year of great forgiveness."

1957 | The Treaty of Rome is signed, and Italy becomes a founding member of the European Economic Community.

1975 | **THE JUBILEE ON TELEVISION**
This Jubilee, proclaimed by Paul VI (1963–1978), is the first to be broadcast on worldwide television. The world has changed a great deal, and the pope expresses his opinion about the church with regard to social and moral changes through numerous encyclicals, which address issues of birth control, celibacy of priests, and the relationship between the church and the world. Paul VI undertakes numerous pastoral trips worldwide.

1991 | Rome's population numbers more than 2,700,000 inhabitants.

1996 | The Italian State votes into law its commitment to the Jubilee. The law sets aside money for development of accommodations, transportation, and infrastructures for the health and safety of pilgrims in the new millennium. A large number of sites undergo restoration and improvement, following what has become a centuries-long tradition of preparing the city for the event.

2000 | **THE JUBILEE OF THE THIRD MILLENNIUM**
With the papal bull *Tertio millennio adveniente*, Pope John Paul II (1978) proclaims the Jubilee for the year 2000. It acquires special significance because of its dual role of celebrating the Holy Year and marking mankind's path toward a new millennium.

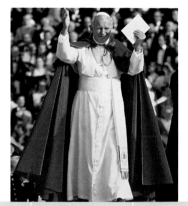

1925
Mussolini, prime minister since 1922, establish a fascist dictatorship.

1940–1944
During World War II, fascist Italy fights with Axis powers until it is forced to capitulate (1943), and Mussolini flees Rome. Italian partisans and Allied troops compel the eventual withdrawal of German troops from Italy.

1968–1979
Years of violence, when terrorists from both the extreme left and the extreme right resorted to bombs, destruction, and attacks, culminate in the kidnapping and murder of former prime minister Aldo Moro (1916–1978).

1991
Waves of refugees from neighboring Albania flood southern ports on the Adriatic.

1993
Italians vote for sweeping reforms after scandal exposes widespread political corruption.

1999
NATO alliance planes bomb Yugoslavia in an effort to resolve a situation of ethnic strife in Kosovo.

Above:
Pope John Paul II.

Facing page:
One of two 17th-century fountains at the focal point of the ellipse of Piazza S. Pietro.

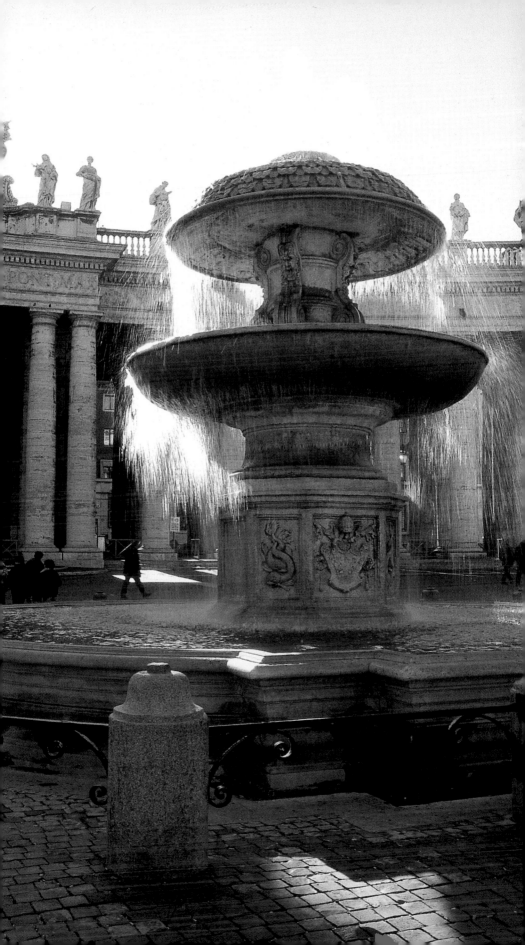

Holy
Rome

Area by area, churches, ancient temples, palaces of the powerful and pilgrims' routes, catacombs and relics. These sites have been part of the history of the Church and have transformed the Eternal City into the Holy City.

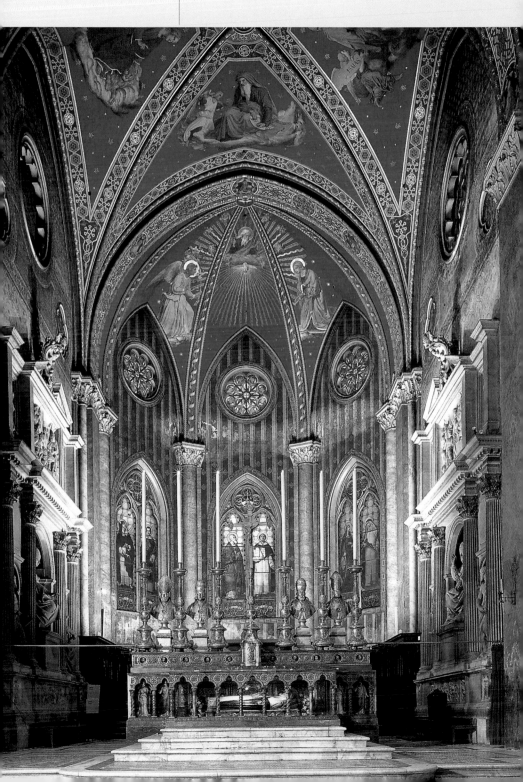

1

Vatican, Borgo, and Prati

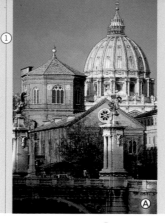

①

(A) The majestic dome of the basilica of S. Pietro, seen from the Ponte Vittorio Emanuele II.

(B) The baldacchino and the throne of St. Peter, created by Bernini for the basilica of S. Pietro.

VATICAN CITY

Much of the history and development of this tiny state was determined by the presence of St. Peter's tomb, located a short distance from the Circus of Caligula, where the apostle was martyred between AD 64 and AD 67. In 800, Charlemagne was crowned emperor in the basilica founded by Constantine, and the district acquired worldwide political significance. In the Middle Ages, after the construction of the city walls by Pope Leo IV, the area became a fortified citadel and, after the Avignon exile, the definitive seat of the pontiffs. The Renaissance and Counter-Reformation patron-popes were responsible for majestic projects that remodeled the city as the capital of a modern state, while later interventions organized the immense art collections into museums. After the Lateran Treaty of 1929, the Vatican City became independent from Italy, with the pontiff granted full legal, political, and administrative sovereignty. In addition to the area contained within the walls, the Vatican also has sovereignty over the Lateran, Cancelleria, and Propaganda Fide palaces; the Hospital of the Bambino Gesù; Castel Gandolfo; and the Cybo and Barberini villas. The Vatican has its own armed forces, police, and mint; maintains its own communications network; and publishes L'Osservatore Romano, *the official newspaper of the Holy See.*

Basilica di S. Pietro ①
(St. Peter's Basilica)

⊞**2 D3.** In approximately AD 320, in honor of the first apostle and commemorating his divine investiture ("You are Peter…"), the emperor Constantine had an impressive basilica constructed on the site of the hallowed tomb of St. Peter. Ancient documents marvel at the magnificence of this church, resplendent with mosaics, art treasures, and gold, a sight that rewarded the arduous travels of pilgrims who arrived from every corner of the world. When the popes returned from exile in Avignon (1377), the more than 1,000-year-old basilica was in disrepair. After some ineffective restorations, Julius II decided to demolish it to make space for a new, even grander edifice to symbolize the supremacy of the Church of Rome. Famous architects succeeded one another in directing the works, but the turning point came with Michelangelo, who designed the monumental dome. In 1626 (before the construction of Bernini's colonnade), the basilica was opened, following innumerable polemics. The enormous facade by Carlo Maderno, too wide in proportion to the height, seems more suitable to a palace than to a religious edifice. Five doors lead to the sanctuary, which is symbolically guarded by the equestrian statues of Constantine and Charlemagne. The last door to the right is the **Porta Santa**, or Holy Door, that is opened and closed by the pope only during Jubilee years. At the center of the facade is the grand loggia, set aside for the traditional blessing, *Urbi et Orbi* (to the city and to the world). The basilica was conceived as a symbol of the church's eternity, and most of its fragile decorations have been removed over the years. Pieces that do remain include the beloved statue of St. Peter and Michelangelo's *Pietà*. Tradition has

it that the former, attributed to Arnolfo di Cambio (13th century), was created by melting down a statue of Jupiter; the right foot has been worn away from being rubbed by the hands and lips of the faithful. The *Pietà* is the only statue signed by Michelangelo, supposedly because he became furious at hearing it attributed to another sculptor. The basilica's interior bears the dominant and sumptuous imprint of Baroque art, particularly that of Bernini, who is responsible for the dramatic *cattedra* (throne) of St. Peter and the majestic *baldacchino* (canopy) above the apostle's tomb. The loggias inserted between the piers of the dome safeguard the basilica's most precious relics, including Veronica's veil, which has an imprint of a male face that, since the early Middle Ages, has been believed to belong to Jesus. The pontiffs' many funerary monuments, created over the centuries by illustrious artists, make this vast Christian sanctuary a "triumphal" space.

Beneath the central nave of St. Peter's Basilica is the **Sacre Grotte Vaticane** (Crypt of St. Peter's), which occupies the space between the current basilica and the old basilica of Constantine. In addition to the tombs of numerous popes, the grottoes also hold early Christian sarcophagi, architectural fragments, and monuments from the old basilica. Excavations have determined the location of the Circus of Caligula (beneath the left nave) and, just next to it, a pre-Constantinian necropolis. This cemetery area, with pagan and Christian tombs, was in use from the 1st to the 4th centuries AD and includes well-preserved mausoleums belonging to the families of wealthy freedmen, with interiors decorated with stuccowork, frescoes, mosaics, and sarcophagi. The presence of Christians can be ascertained from the inscriptions and

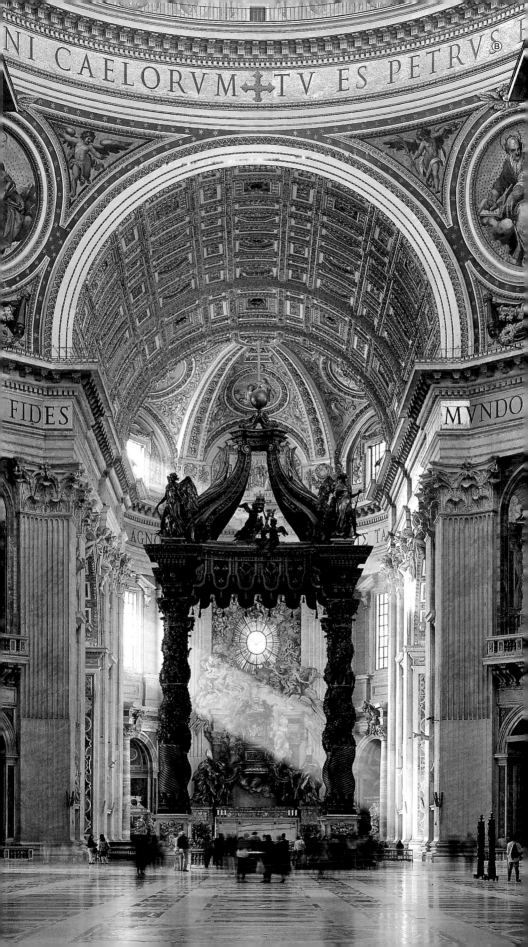

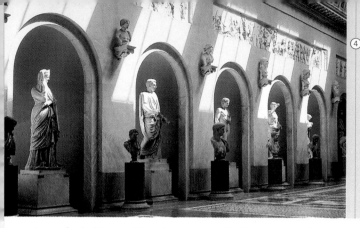

personal tribulations of the artist take shape in a terrible image that brings to mind the gloomy verses of the *Dies Irae* rather than the words of the Bible, with an almost unbearable emphasis on the tragedy of man, shattered by divine turmoil. Michelangelo spent five years working alone, and the immense fresco, which is organized in superimposed bands, revolutionized the traditional iconography of the subject. All partitions are filled with the swirling motion of the resurrected and the damned. Even the Madonna seems to draw back in fright at the explosive power of Christ. Among the saints, the solemn figures of Peter and Paul can be identified, and Michelangelo left an anguished self-portrait in the flayed skin of St. Bartholomew. Below, angels sound the trumpets of judgment, and all around a battle rages between angels and devils vying for souls. The work is one of the milestones of European culture. When it is time to elect a new pope, the College of Cardinals meets in conclave here, surrounded by these images.

Cortile della Pigna
(Courtyard of the Pinecone)
⊞2 C3. The vast Belvedere Courtyard, designed by Bramante and famous during the Renaissance for its tournaments, was subsequently divided into three sections, one of which is this courtyard. In the Middle Ages a colossal bronze pinecone was discovered on an ancient public building in the Campo Marzio, which is the derivation of the Pigna district's name. For centuries the pinecone adorned the atrium of the ancient basilica of St. Peter before being moved to its current location.

Galleria delle Carte Geografiche
(Map Gallery)
⊞2 B3–C3. The gallery's name comes from the 40 geographical maps of Italian regions and church possessions that Pope Gregory XIII had painted between 1580 and 1583, based on cartoons by Egnazio Danti, an eminent mathematician and cosmographer of the time. To distribute the maps clearly on the walls, Danti adopted the Appenines as a dividing element. On the walls facing the Belvedere Courtyard he represented the regions bounded by the Ligurian and Tyrrhenian seas, and on the wall facing the gardens, the regions bounded by the Alps and the Adriatic. Many of the maps show panoramic views and city plans, and some indicate sites of famous battles. As a group, they constitute an important document of 16th-century geography and cartography.

Museo Chiaramonti ④
(Chiaramonti Museum)
⊞2 C3. The Museo Chiaramonti, which takes its name from its founder, Pope Pius VII (1800–1823), was laid out and organized by Antonio Canova. It displays almost 1,000 ancient sculptures and a rich collection of epigraphs. The Museo Chiaramonti proper occupies part of a gallery designed by Bramante and contains Roman copies of Greek statues, portraits, reliefs, urns, and sarcophagi from the Roman era. The **Galleria Lapidaria** (Gallery of Stone Tablets), located in the remaining part of the gallery, displays pagan and Christian epigraphs that were first collected by Pope Clement XIV. The **Braccio Nuovo** (New Wing) is a Neoclassical gallery created after the return of sculptures removed by Napoléon. It contains some famous and important works: a statue of Augustus, found in Livia's villa in Prima Porta, is the most famous portrait of the first Roman emperor. Other Roman copies of Greek sculpture include the *Wounded Amazon*, restored by Thorvaldsen; the *Satyr in Repose*; the *Spear-bearer*; and the *Athena Giustiniani*. A colossal statue of the Nile, flanked by sphinxes, crocodiles, and 16 putti, which symbolize the fertility guaranteed by the river's flood, is based on a Hellenistic original.

Museo Gregoriano Egizio
(Egyptian Museum)
⊞2 B3. Established by Pope Gregory XVI in 1839, the museum was first organized by Luigi Ungarelli, one of the first Italian scholars of Egyptology. It was reorganized in 1989 by Jean-Luc Grenier, who regrouped the exhibits according to dynasty. The museum houses a significant collection of epigraphs ranging from the 3rd century BC to the 6th century AD, numerous statues, sarcophagi, mummies, steles, and other remains from funerary rites. The works from the Roman era, inspired by Egyptian art, are of particular interest and bear witness to Roman society's enthusiasm for Egyptian culture. Many of the pieces came from Hadrian's villa in Tivoli, others from the important sanctuary of Isis in Campo Marzio in Rome.

Museo Gregoriano Etrusco
(Etruscan Museum)
⊞2 B3. Created by Pope Gregory XVI in 1837, this museum contains materials that, for the most part, were obtained from excavations carried out by the church in southern Etruria during the 19th century. The princely Regolini-Galassi tomb (named for the men who discovered it) from Cerveteri yielded splendid jewels and furnishings from the 7th century BC. The famous *Mars of Todi*, one of the masterpieces of Italian bronze work, from the 5th century BC, depicts a young warrior pouring an offering before leaving for battle. According to the epigraph engraved on the breastplate, the donor was

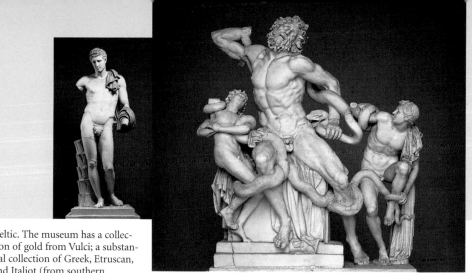

Celtic. The museum has a collection of gold from Vulci; a substantial collection of Greek, Etruscan, and Italiot (from southern Hellenized Italy) ceramics; and a small collection of antiquities from Rome and Lazio.

Museo Gregoriano Profano
⊞2 B2–B3. This collection of antiquities was established by Pope Gregory XVI in 1844 in the Lateran Palace and moved to its current location by Pope John XXIII in 1970. It includes materials from excavations within the papal state. A significant section is devoted to original Greek works, including some sculpture fragments from the Parthenon, an Attic funerary relief (5th century BC), and a head of Athena. Roman copies of Greek sculptures include a statue of Marsyas, copies of a famous bronze group by Myron (460 BC) that once stood at the entrance to the Acropolis in Athens, and the *Niobid Chiaramonti*, probably after a work by Skopas or Praxiteles. There are numerous significant examples of Roman sculpture, including the monumental funerary edifice of Vicovaro, the imperial statues from Cerveteri, fragments from the tomb of the Haterii, and an impressive series of sarcophagi.

Museo Missionario Etnologico
(Ethnological Missionary Museum)
⊞2 B3–C3. Established by Pope Pius XI in the Lateran Palace, the museum was transferred here by Pope John XXIII. It displays materials from the 1925 Jubilee missionary exhibition and various gifts from individuals and missionary congregations, presenting extensive documentation of cultures and traditions outside Europe. On exhibit are objects, reconstructions, and texts related to local religions, death rituals, the introduction of Christianity, social organization, artistic production, and daily life (with a vast array of garments, furniture, household goods, arms, and furnishings).

Museo Pio Clementino ⑤
⊞2 B3. This first major component of the Vatican Museums was a result of the efforts of popes Clement XIV and Pius VI. Its founding went beyond the mere organization of a papal collection, and occurred within the framework of a broader plan to safeguard works of art that were well known in the late 16th century. Clement XIV wanted to design a location for the substantial collection that had been accumulating in the Belvedere Palace since the times of Julius II. Pius VI completed the new installation, which was begun in 1771 and financed with proceeds from a lottery. For centuries, many of the sculptures exhibited here influenced art throughout the world: the *Apoxiomenos* (a Roman copy of a work by Lysippus, 4th century BC); the *Apollo di Belvedere*, *Laocoön*, and *Hermes* statues in the Octagonal Courtyard (all Roman copies of Greek masterpieces), and the *Perseus Triumphant* by Canova. The collection also includes the *Apollo Killing a Lizard* (from a bronze by Praxiteles, 4th century BC), the much-admired *Sleeping Ariadne* (from a 2nd-century BC Hellenistic original), and the *Torso del Belvedere* (1st century BC), which inspired Michelangelo for his Sistine Chapel nudes.

Museo Pio Cristiano
⊞2 B2–B3. Founded by Pope Pius IX in 1854, the museum contains artifacts from the catacombs and from the early Christian basilica. Housed here is an impressive series of early Christian sarcophagi, mosaics, architectural fragments, and sculpture. Also displayed is a comprehensive collection of Christian epigraphs of a funerary, public, commemorative, and religious nature dating from the 1st to 7th centuries AD. These objects provide a a glimpse into the religious ideas, social composition, everyday life, and spoken language of the early Christian communities. The most precious monument is the funeral pillar of Abercius, bishop of Hierapolis of Phrygia, who lived during the time of emperor Marcus Aurelius (AD 161–AD 180). An inscription in Greek bears the epitaph dictated by him: "Wherever my faith pushes me, and prepares for my meal, fish from streams . . . untainted, which the pure Virgin takes and each day places before her friends so that they might eat, with excellent wine that she offers, mixed with bread." If the Christian interpretation of the text is correct, this is the most ancient Christian epigraph about the Eucharist.

Museo Profano
⊞2 C3. This single exhibition room preserves the rich original furnishings designed by Luigi Valadier. Founded by Clement XII, the museum displays artifacts from the Etruscan, Roman, and medieval eras. Artifacts were culled from 18th-century collections such as those of Carpegna and Albani and from early 19th-century excavations.

Museo Sacro
⊞2 C3. Created by Pope Benedict XIV, this museum displays early Christian and Byzantine antiquities from various sources, including some from Roman catacombs. The

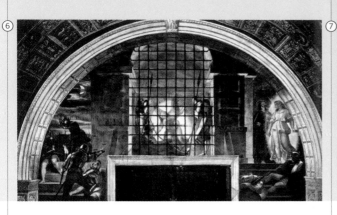

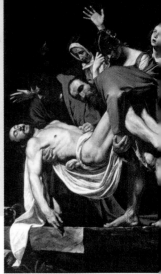

The night scene of the *Deliverance of St. Peter* in the Stanza d'Eliodoro, painted by Raphael in 1512–1514.

holdings of the museum include a Byzantine mosaic depicting St. Theodore (14th century); a case for the head of St. Sebastian (9th century), formerly in the church of the Ss. Quattro Coronati; early Christian and Coptic textiles; a rich collection of lamps and ceramics with Christian, pagan, and Jewish symbols; and an Eastern-style water vessel used for washing the hands after meals (8th–9th century), which, according to legend, was used by St. Laurence.

Museo Storico Vaticano
(Vatican Historical Museum)
▦**2 C3.** Located in the Lateran Palace, this is a department of the institution of the same name. Created by Pope Paul VI in 1973, it contains a collection of means of transport used by various popes and cardinals: black landaus, the daily means of transportation for popes until the early years of the papacy of Pius XI; coaches, designed to endure long trips over rambling roads; formal carriages, including one built for Leo XII by the celebrated Roman carriage builder Gaetano Peroni; and numerous sedans, such as the extremely elegant, red damask one used by Leo XIII.

Pinacoteca Vaticana ⑦
▦**2 C3.** This extraordinary collection of paintings was established by Pope Pius VII (1816), who welcomed the Congress of Vienna's decision that works plundered by Napoléon's troops should be returned from France and kept in public collections. Other works of art were added from various sources, creating a vast and multifaceted group of paintings, with emphasis on Italian works, ranging

from pre-Renaissance to 17th-century works. The museum also contains 10 tapestries made in Brussels from cartoons by Raphael, depicting scenes from the Acts of the Apostles; Pope Leo X commissioned these to decorate the walls of the Sistine Chapel. Giotto's *Stefaneschi polyptych,* originally painted for the high altar of the old St. Peter's, is the best preserved work by this 14th-century artist in Rome. The museum's Renaissance sections include other masterpieces, such as *Sixtus IV Nominating Platina Prefect of the Vatican Library* (1477) by Melozzo da Forlì; Raphael's *Coronation of the Virgin* (1503), *Madonna of Foligno* (1512), and *Transfiguration* (1517); and Leonardo da Vinci's *St. Jerome.* There is an extensive collection of works from the 17th century, the apogee of religious painting in Rome, including Caravaggio's dramatic *Deposition* (1604), Pietro da Cortona's *Pietà,* Domenichino's *Communion of St. Jerome* (1614), and Guido Reni's *Crucifixion of St. Peter.*

Stanze di Raffaello
(Raphael Rooms) ⑥
▦**2 D3.** These rooms constituted the official portion of the apartment of Julius II; the decorative scheme was entrusted to Raphael, who worked here between 1508 and 1525. The first room, the **Stanza della Segnatura,** illustrates the highest attributes of the human spirit: Divine Truth, investigated by Theology (*Disputation of the Sacrament,* depicting the debate about the mystery of the Eucharist), and Rational Truth, investigated by Philosophy (*School of Athens*); Beauty, represented by *Parnassus;* Goodness, expressed by the *Theological and Cardinal Virtues;* and Law, both civil (*Justinian, the Emperor, Handling the Pandects*) and ecclesiastic (*Gregory IX Handling the*

Decretals). Many of the figures in the two major scenes resemble men of Raphael's time: Julius II is portrayed dressed as Gregory IX, Leonardo as Plato, Bramante as Euclid. Frescoes in the second room, the **Stanza d'Eliodoro,** illustrate a series of divine interventions to protect the church: faith threatened (*Mass at Bolsena,* representing an episode when blood issued from the communion wafer held by a doubting priest); the person of the pontiff (*The Deliverance of St. Peter from Prison*); in its see (*Meeting of Attila with Leo the Great*); and the church's legacy (*Expulsion of Heliodorus,* portraying the thief trampled by the horse of the divine envoy). The **Stanza dell'Incendio** extolls the new pope, Leo X, in four episodes from the lives of popes with the same name (Leo III and IV). In the scene from which the room takes its name, the blessing given by Leo IV miraculously stops the fire that is destroying the Borgo district; in the *Battle of Ostia,* the same pope thanks God for a storm that dispersed the Arab fleet. Leo III is the protagonist of the *Coronation of Charlemagne* and the *Oath,* where he refutes the false charges of the nephews of Hadrian I. The **Stanza di Costantino** was decorated by pupils of Raphael from his drawings. The theme is the victory over paganism and the establishment of the church in Rome (*Baptism of Constantine, Battle of Ponte Milvio, Apparition of the Cross,* and the *Donation of Rome*).

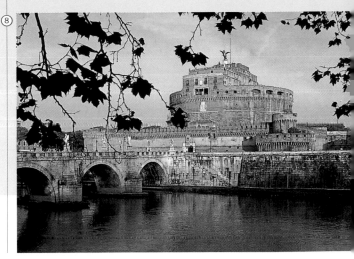

The Deposition ⑦, a work of rare dramatic power, painted by Caravaggio in 1604.

View of Castel S. Angelo ⑧, built in the 2nd century as a tomb for the emperor Hadrian.

BORGO AND PRATI

Beginning in late antiquity, Christian Rome emerged in the vast area defined by the right bank of the Tiber River, Castel S. Angelo, and the Vatican, almost in opposition to the pagan city on the opposite bank. As the numbers of pilgrims to the tomb of St. Peter increased, the communities of Christianized northern Europe urged that a permanent facility be established. The result was the Borgo district (the word "borgo" derives from the Gothic word "burg," or town). The sack of Rome by the Saracens (AD 846) pushed Pope Leo IV to build a wall, defining an area known as Città Leonina, which included St. Peter's, Borgo, and Castel S. Angelo. The development of the district, which did not become an official rione (region) until 1586, took place during the urban development of the Vatican. Its building fabric remained intact until the defacements of the 20th century, the most serious of which was the opening of the Via della Conciliazione. The Prati district, the last of the modern rioni, is also on the right bank. Prior to the postunification building explosion, the area was filled with meadows (prati), vineyards, orchards, and marshes that were scattered with huts and inns for hunters.

Castel S. Angelo ⑧

⊞2 C6–D6. Over the course of its long existence, Castel S. Angelo has played various roles, from mausoleum to fortress, from notorious prison to sumptuous papal residence, and it has been the setting for some of the most dramatic events in Rome's history. It was built as the monumental tomb of the emperor Hadrian (2nd century AD), who wanted to create a work that would convey the power and wealth of the Roman Empire, heir to the splendor of the Eastern monarchies. Its inclusion within the Aurelian Wall (AD 275) inaugurated its new purpose as a citadel, capable of resisting the assaults of the Visigoths (410) and the Ostrogoths (537). In addition to being a mighty fortress, it was located at a meeting point between ancient and medieval Rome and the new Vatican, which had grown up around the tomb of St. Peter. Its Christianization, including its name, dates from the year 590 and is linked to an apparition by the Archangel Michael, who announced to Pope Gregory the Great the end of the plague. The event is evoked in the large bronze statue atop the structure. Between the 10th and 15th centuries, the fortress passed into the hands of various patrician families and became the property of various popes. Each strengthened the building's military function and opulently decorated its interior spaces, turning it into an emblem of power and renewed authority after the exile to Avignon and the Great Schism. Today it is the site of the **Museo Nazionale di Castel S. Angelo,** which includes, in addition to a collection of ancient arms, the luxurious papal apartments, decorated stucco, friezes, frescoes, tapestries, and ceramics. Its terrace, made famous by Puccini's *Tosca,* provides one of the most beautiful views of the city's historic center. ⊠*Lungotevere Castello 50,* ☎*06/687–5036.*

Chiesa and Facoltà Valdese di Teologia
(Waldensian Church and Theological Institute)

⊞3 C2. The unique style of the facade, which brings together Romanesque, German, and Byzantine forms, was chosen to differentiate the building from Catholic churches and, through the cylindrical side towers, to resolve the problem of linking it to the structures that lie behind. The interior, which has a basilican plane and a women's gallery, has no sacred images, in accordance with Waldensian dictates; the stained-glass windows are embellished with Christian symbols and floral motifs. The church was erected between 1911 and 1914, a few years after the establishment of the adjacent theological institute, which has a vast library. ⊠*Via Dionigi 57.*

Museo delle Anime del Purgatorio
(Museum of the Souls of Purgatory)

⊞3 C3. In 1897 the priest Victor Janet began to collect textiles, skullcaps, breviaries, Bibles, wood panels, nightshirts, and other objects that, in his opinion, showed the traces of fire left by the souls of the departed. The small museum displays this disconcerting evidence of celestial life, submitted from various regions of Europe, although the Catholic Church has made no pronouncements as to the significance of the materials. The museum is contained within space belonging to

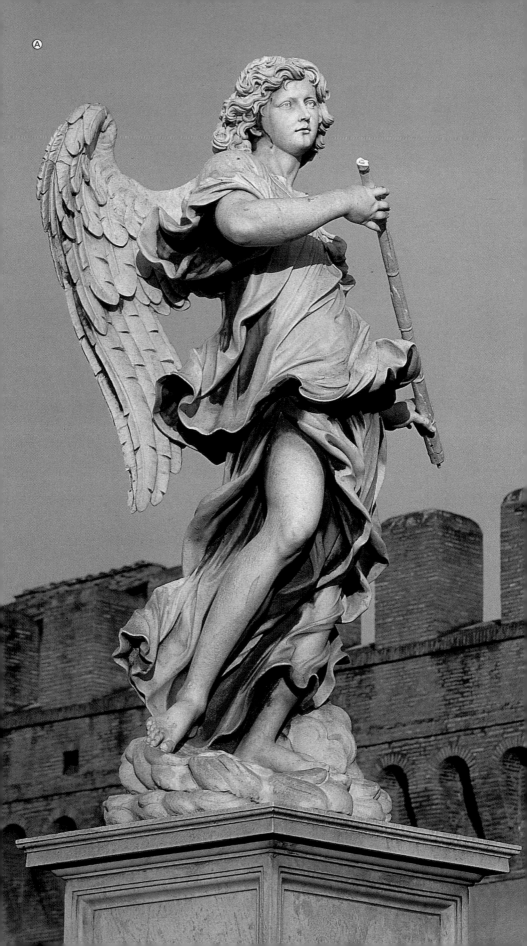

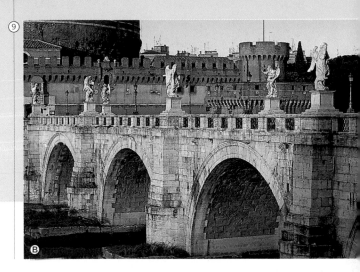

Ten statues of angels, bearing symbols of Christ's Passion, rise along the parapet of the Roman Ponte S. Angelo. They were created from drawings by Gian Lorenzo Bernini (the two sculpted by Bernini himself are now in S. Lorenzo alle Fratte).

the church of the Sacro Cuore del Suffragio (1894–1917), a rare example of neogothic architecture in Rome, apparently inspired by Milan's cathedral. ⊠*Lungotevere Prati 12*, ☎*06/688–06517.*

Ospedale di S. Spirito in Sassia
(Hospital of St. Spirito in Sassia)
⊞2 D5–E5. Created by Pope Innocent III in 1201 on the site of the Schola Saxonum (the hospice for Saxon pilgrims, from which the appellation "in Sassia" is derived), the Hospital of S. Spirito in Sassia was established to assist the sick, the poor, and orphans. It achieved considerable economic power, which was further consolidated in 1605 with the establishment of the Banco di S. Spirito. A religious order of the same name spread throughout Europe, with institutions similar to the Roman model. Sixtus IV completely rebuilt the edifice (1473–1478), and his successors added various wings. The hospital's long history as an important teaching and research institution is amply documented in the **Museo Storico Nazionale di Arte Sanitaria** (National Historical Museum of Health Services), which exhibits anatomical charts, gynecological and surgical instruments, and a collection of pharmacy vessels. The impressive and unfinished door of S. Spirito, designed by Antonio Giamberti da Sangallo the Younger at the time of Paul III, is clearly inspired by ancient triumphal arches. ⊠*Lungotevere in Sassia.*

Palazzo dei Penitenzieri
⊞2 D5. For many years this building was the center of operations for the Jesuits, who functioned as confessors (with particular powers for granting absolution) in St. Peter's Basilica. Erected between 1480 and 1490 for Cardinal Domenico della Rovere, it has an stately facade inspired by the

Palazzo Venezia, an unusual two-story courtyard, and refined frescoes attributed to Pinturicchio, who, at the time, was working on the Borgia Apartment. Today the building is used as a hotel and as offices for the Equestrian Order of S. Sepolcro di Gerusalemme. ⊠*Via della Conciliazione 33.*

Ponte S. Angelo ⑨
⊞2 D6. Built by the emperor Hadrian to link his mausoleum with the Campo Marzio, this bridge became the principal crossing point for pilgrims going to St. Peter's. Pope Clement VII (1534) had two statues, depicting St. Peter and St. Paul, placed on the end opposite the mausoleum. Pope Clement IX (1668) later transformed the bridge into one of the most theatrical monuments of the Roman Baroque, embellishing it with 10 statues of angels holding the symbols of the Passion. These were executed by various sculptors from drawings by Gian Lorenzo Bernini. These raging youthful figures, their faces misshapen by grief, their garments in disarray, summarize 17th-century devotion with a wedding of physicality and spirituality. The two angels created by Bernini himself (one with a scroll, another with a crown of thorns) were considered too fine to remain exposed to the elements and were moved to S. Andrea delle Fratte.

S. Maria in Traspontina
⊞2 D5. The name of the church comes from its location, beyond the S. Angelo Bridge ("Trans pontem," or "across the bridge"). Its monumental construction was part of a plan to renew the Borgo, which had been largely abandoned

by its most prosperous residents after the 1527 sack of Rome. Begun in 1566 and completed in 1668, the church has a Latin cross plan surmounted by a dome without a drum, so the artillery stationed at Castel S. Angelo could have an unencumbered range of fire. On the high altar, designed by Carlo Fontana with a crown-shaped baldachin surmounted by angels, is an icon of the Virgin brought to Rome from the Holy Land, perhaps in 1216 by the Carmelites. ⊠*Borgo S. Angelo 15.*

S. Spirito in Sassia
⊞2 D5. Currently part of the vast hospital complex of the same name, the church replaced the ancient S. Maria in Sassia, which was annexed to the hospice for Saxon pilgrims during the 8th century. It was rebuilt at the behest of Pope Paul III by Antonio Giamberti da Sangallo the Younger, who employed sober Renaissance forms, and completed by Sixtus V (1585–1590). The medieval church of S. Maria was the site of a solemn procession, instituted by Pope Innocent III in 1208, which brought Veronica's veil from the Vatican basilica. Pilgrims who were present were asked, in exchange for a year of indulgences, to make donations to the hospital, which had just been established. ⊠*Via dei Penitenzieri 12.*

2
Trastevere

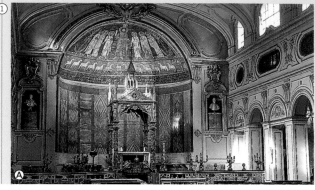

Trastevere's centuries-long separation from the rest of the city and its history have resulted in distinctive customs, traditions, and even a dialect, all of which contributed to the legendary pride of its population and the frequent disputes with the inhabitants of the opposite bank. The district's working-class character has origins in antiquity: in Roman times it was inhabited by foreign merchants who traded at the port of Rome and by the city's Jewish community (which later moved across the river). During subsequent eras Trastevere continued to be occupied by people devoted to trade and by settlements of foreigners, including Venetians, Corsicans, and Genoese. Until modern times very few buildings in the district had been restored, although there are a number of architectural treasures, particularly from the Renaissance and Baroque periods. During the second half of the 19th century, various initiatives transformed the structure of the neighborhood. The most drastic changes involved the construction of an embankment and the opening of the Viale Trastevere, which destroyed numerous historic buildings and much of the ancient street fabric. Today, large areas of the district retain the old mysterious, noisy, genuine flavor that constitutes Trastevere's unique charm.

Fontana dell'Acqua Paola
⊞5 D2. Buit in 1612 for Pope Paul V (from whom it takes its name), the fountain celebrates the restoration of the aqueduct of Trajan. Marble from the Forum of Nerva and columns from the first basilica of St. Peter were used. In 1690, Pope Alexander VIII commissioned Carlo Fontana to design the broad piazza, which offers an excellent view of the fountain, and the semicircular basin. The compact volumes of the structure, inspired by Roman triumphal arches, are extended by three arcades and surmounted by a multilinear coping, and the theatrical effect fits perfectly within the landscape of the Janiculum. ⊠ Via Garibaldi.

Gianicolo (Janiculum)
⊞5 A1–D2. The Janiculum was indispensable to the city's defense from ancient times until the arduous battles between Garibaldi and the French troops in 1849. But the hill, well known for its silhouette of pine and cypress trees highlighted at sunset and its splendid views, is one of Rome's most gentle and suggestive locations. Solitary and contemplative types such as Tasso, Leopardi, and Chateaubriand favored the site, as have legions of artists, who, since Renaissance times, have come here to capture some of the most beautiful images of the city. According to one legend, this is the site where St. Peter, crucified upside down, gathered the entire city in an unencumbered visual embrace. After 1870 the celebrated *passeggiata* (promenade) dominated the crest of the hill, which was thus preserved in its natural beauty and consecrated to patriotic memories.

Ospedale dei Ss. Maria e Gallicano
⊞5 D4. The hospital, built between 1724 and 1729, was founded by Benedict XIII to aid those suffering from skin afflictions (a tradition that has been maintained in today's dermatological hospital). These people were often rejected by other hospitals, with the exception of the Hospital of S. Lazzaro, on the Via Trionfale. Architect Filippo Raguzzini created a model for hospital architecture of the time, and the anatomy theater, a source of pride for this institution in the 19th century, still has a stuccowork frieze depicting the legend of Aesculapius and the Tiber Island and portraits of famous physicians. ⊠ Via S. Gallicano 25/A.

Ospizio Apostolico di S. Michele a Ripa Grande
⊞5 E5–F5. Established in the late 17th century as a boys' reformatory, the hospice later became the city's principal institution for education and welfare, named after the Archangel Michael, long the subject of special devotion in Rome. In the mid-18th century it opened its doors to orphans of both sexes, single women, the elderly, the disabled, and the destitute, and also served as a women's prison. The building, designed by Carlo Fontana and Ferdinando Fuga, incorporates the churches of S. Michele and the Madonna del Buon Viaggio. In addition to its function as an institution of public assistance, the hospice played an important role in Rome's artisanal history. It was the site of a wool mill, a famous tapestry factory, and a foundry (one of its last creations was the equestrian group for the Victor Emmanuel Monument). Today it houses the Ministry of Cultural Affairs. ⊠ Via S. Michele 22.

Palazzo Corsini
⊞5 B3. Built in the 16th century, the palace became famous during the 17th century, when it was inhabited by Queen Christina of Sweden, who made it the center of Rome's cultural life. In the 18th

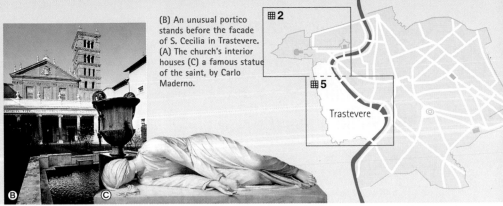

(B) An unusual portico stands before the facade of S. Cecilia in Trastevere. (A) The church's interior houses (C) a famous statue of the saint, by Carlo Maderno.

century it was purchased and expanded by the Corsini family to accommodate their gallery of paintings and their family library, which included a rich collection of early books and manuscripts. Since 1883 it has been the property of the state and the location of the Accademia Nazionale dei Lincei, the most authoritative cultural and academic institution in Italy, founded in 1605. The **Galleria Corsini** (which, together with the gallery in the Palazzo Barberini, constitutes the Galleria Nazionale di Arte Antica) was founded by Cardinal Neri Corsini, nephew of Pope Clement XII, and is the only 18th-century Roman collection to survive intact. It displays Italian and foreign painting from the 17th and 18th centuries. In 1883, the palace garden became the Botanical Garden of the University of Rome and now contains environments that simulate various climatic conditions. The 19th-century greenhouses shelter various species of citrus fruits, orchids, and succulents. ⊠ *Via della Lungara 10,* ☎*06/688–02323.*

S. Agata
⊞**5 D5.** The simple Baroque church of S. Agata is linked to the religious traditions of Trastevere because of its wooden sculpture of the Madonna del Carmine. Every year in July, the Festa de' Noantri is celebrated with a series of outdoor spectacles, illuminations, fireworks, and a tremendous consumption of watermelons and wine. It is an example of the secular festival, dating from the 1920s, superimposed on a traditional religious festival. The celebrations begin with a procession that transfers the statue (dressed each year in new embroidered garments) from the church of S. Agata to the nearby church of S. Crisogono. ⊠*Largo S. Giovanni de Matha 9.*

S. Benedetto in Piscinula
⊞**5 D5.** Erected between the 11th and 12th centuries, this church preserves the cell of St. Benedict, part of the saint's house according to tradition. It has a small Romanesque bell tower with two rows of mullioned windows and a Neoclassical facade. The Cappella della Madonna holds a 14th-century fresco of a *Madonna and Child.* The principal nave, flanked by columns with ancient and medieval capitals—plundered from other locations—has traces of a mosaic floor and, on the high altar, a gold-topped table with a 15th-century image of St. Benedict. ⊠*Piazza in Piscinula 40.*

S. Callisto
⊞**5 D4.** After being a slave to a Christian and leading a less than impeccable life, Callistus became papal secretary and then, in AD 217, pope. He was one of the most active and important of the early popes, and he was a protagonist in the first schisms in the church's history. About a century after his death he began to be venerated as a martyr. According to legend, he was thrown into a well, his neck tied to a stone (the well has been identified as the one in the garden of the former monastery annexed to the church). During the 8th century this small building was erected on the site of his presumed martyrdom, and it was rebuilt in the 17th century. Callistus was buried in the Calepodio Cemetery, on the Via Aurelia, not in the cemetery that bears his name. ⊠*Piazza S. Calisto.*

S. Cecilia in Trastevere ①
⊞**5 D5.** In addition to being one of the most interesting churches in the city, this is one of the very few oases of solitude in the turbulent Trastevere district. The Passion of the young martyr, who lived during the first half of the 3rd century and has been venerated in Rome since early Christian times, is in large part legendary. According to tradition, the first place of worship was the house of Caecilia's family or of her husband, Valerian, who was also a saint and martyr. The church encompasses the remains of a calidarium, the room with hot baths, where she was confined for three days, exposed to the steam in an attempt to suffocate her, before she was finally beheaded. Pope Paschal I rebuilt the edifice as a basilica in 821 to safeguard the saint's body, which was recovered intact in the catacombs of S. Callisto. In 1595, the sarcophagus was opened and the body was found exactly as it had been buried, turned on one side, the face turned down, and three of her fingers extended, which was taken to allude to the mystery of the Trinity. Stefano Maderno immortalized the miraculous event in his famous statue, which is located beneath the high altar (1600). The sarcophagus of this saint and other martyrs is kept in the crypt, where many tombs have been recovered (Christians aspired to be buried as close as possible to the martyrs), along with frescoes, including a 5th-century image of St. Caecilia at prayer. A magnificent 9th-century mosaic in the apse depicts Christ offering a benediction, flanked by saints and by Pope Paschal I, who commissioned the work. The pope is portrayed with a square halo, because he was still alive at the time the work was executed. The basilica contains two pivotal works by two late 13th-century masters of the figurative revival, both of whom attempted to restore the plastic values of the ancient world. At the center of the presbytery is a ciborium, or altar canopy (1293), by Arnolfo di Cambio, a masterpiece of Gothic sculpture, executed at the same time that Pietro Cavallini was completing his magnificent *Last*

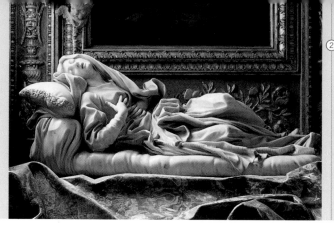

Judgment on the opposite wall. Today St. Caecilia is considered the patron saint of music and the makers of musical instruments, although without any precise historical reference. The Accademia Nazionale di S. Cecilia is one of the most famous conservatories in the world. ⊠*Piazza S. Cecilia 22.*

S. Crisogono

⊞**5 D5.** The current church is the result of a radical 17th-century restoration of a Romanesque (12th century) structure, which in its turn had been built above the remains of a 5th-century basilica (one of the most ancient in Rome) dedicated to St. Chrysogonus, who was martyred at the time of the Diocletian persecutions. There are some interesting fresco remains (8th–11th centuries) from the early Christian building, with figures of saints and hagiographic episodes: *Pope Sylvester Capturing the Dragon, St. Pantaleone Healing the Blind Man, St. Benedict Healing the Leper,* and the *Rescue of St. Placid.* The later building, with three naves and a beautiful mosaic floor, has seven altars, each with its own relics (as in great basilicas), and on St. Chrysogonus's feast day (November 24) pilgrims and worshipers receive plenary indulgence. The painted coffered ceiling from the Baroque era is one of the most beautiful in Rome. ⊠*Piazza Sonnino 44.*

S. Dorotea

⊞**5 C3.** The church appearance is a result of the 18th-century reconstruction of the original Romanesque building, first called S. Silvestro and later named after Dorothy, a 3rd-century Eastern martyr. At the beginning of the 16th century the church was the assembly place for a religious confraternity, the Oratorio di Divino Amore, established by St. Cajetan (1480–1547), co-founder (with

Peter Caraffa, later Pope Paul IV) of the Theatines religious order, which, along with the Jesuits, became one of the forces of the Counter-Reformation. In the adjacent house, St. Joseph Calasanctius opened the first free public school in Europe, in 1592. ⊠*Via S. Dorotea 23.*

S. Francesco a Ripa ②

⊞**5 E4–E5.** The church was built on the site of the former S. Biagio (10th century), where, according to a deeply rooted tradition, St. Francis of Assisi stayed during his sojourns in Rome. The current appearance dates from the partial renovation in the late 7th century. The side chapels, rich in works of art, bear witness to the particular devotion of certain Roman noble families to the saint of Assisi. In the Paluzzi-Albertoni Chapel is Gian Lorenzo Bernini's statue of the *Blessed Ludovica Albertoni* (1674), a masterful blend of mysticism and theatricality, along the lines of his *Ecstasy of St. Teresa* in the church of St. Maria della Vittoria. The architectural cornice and the skillful use of light focus attention on the vibrant figure of this Roman mystic (1474–1533), who had a gift for making miracles and prophecies. The only surviving space from the ancient Hospice of S. Biagio is the Chapel of S. Francesco, whose theatrical wooden reliquary (1696), inspired by Bernini, has a copy of a panel attributed to Margaritone d'Arezzo, considered an actual portrait of St. Francis. (The original is in the Pinacoteca Vaticana.) ⊠*Piazza S. Francesco d'Assisi 88.*

S. Giovanni Battista dei Genovesi

⊞**5 D5.** The Genoese community in Rome had its residences and mercantile warehouses near the port of Ripa Grande. In 1481, Meliaduce Cicala, a Genoese

nobleman, left a bequest for the construction of a church dedicated to the patron saint of Genoa and a hospital for sailors. The hospice building, completely renovated outside, has an evocative late 15th-century cloister with a portico with arches and octagonal columns and an architraved loggia. The church, which has been renovated many times (most recently in 1864), contains a beautiful funerary monument to its donor. The spaces above the cloister contain the Archive of the Confraternity of St. Giovanni, which includes hospital documents. ⊠*Via Anicia 12.*

S. Maria dei Sette Dolori

⊞**5 C3.** Beginning in 1643, Borromini built this church and convent for the Order of Augustinian Oblates. The master designed a facade (unfinished) almost completely without openings, animated solely by a double order of pilasters and niches, as if to express visually the strict cloistered life of the monastic order by turning the wall into an element of isolation and defense. As in the Oratory of St. Philip Neri, the church is developed along an axis parallel to the facade. Inside, a high cornice twists uninterruptedly around the arches of the side chapels and the presbytery; above the entrance, the cornice breaks into two curved volutes, the building's most significant element, unifying and strengthening the space. The atrium alternates curved and rectilinear segments, most likely inspired by a space in Hadrian's Villa in Tivoli. ⊠*Via Garibaldi 27.*

S. Maria dell'Orto

⊞**5 E5.** The current 16th-century church has its origins in a chapel erected during the 15th century to celebrate an image of the Virgin with child, which had been removed from a garden wall. The facade has two rows of columns

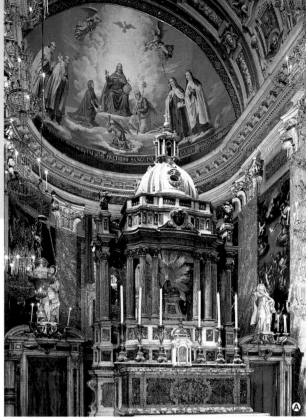

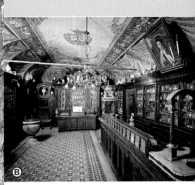

added to the 11th-century church, and the entire complex was completely renovated in the 19th century by the Doria Pamphili family to become Rome's first home for the aged. ⊠ *Vicolo S. Maria in Cappella 6.*

S. Maria in Trastevere ④

5 D4. The basilica of St. Maria in Trastevere is one of the most important churches in Rome, overshadowed only by the four patriarchal basilicas. Founded by Pope Julius I in the mid-4th century, it was the first place of worship dedicated to the Madonna. During Jubilee years afflicted by calamities or pestilence, this church was often preferred by pilgrims to the distant S. Paolo. Tradition links the dedication to Mary to the miraculous source of a fountain of mineral oil that was later interpreted by Christians as a sign auguring the birth of Christ. An inscription near the apse marks the spot where the miracle is said to have occurred. In the 9th century, Pope Gregory IV constructed a crypt to hold the remains of certain martyrs that had been moved from catacombs threatened by the Saracens' sack of Rome. The current church (12th century) was built by Innocent II and decorated with celebrated mosaics in the apse depicting Christ and Mary enthroned with saints. In 1291, another mosaic by Pietro Cavallini, illustrating *Scenes from the Life of the Virgin,* was added at the height of the windows. This mosaic's refined and delicate colors and the plastic strength of the figures were an innovative departure from Byzantine canons and can be compared with developments in the work of Cimabue and Arnolfo di Cambio. Bertoldo Stefaneschi, a member of one of the most important families in Trastevere, commissioned the frescoes. He is portrayed in prayer, in a lower

punctuated by pilasters, arched portals, and a crowning element of small obelisks. Inside, the exuberant 18th-century stucco and gilded decoration radically transform the spatial equilibrium of the Renaissance layout. The building was the site of numerous "universities" (corporations) of arts and crafts, the names of which are recorded in the dedication of the chapels. The Luigi Huetter Study Center on Roman Confraternities and Universities of Arts and Crafts, which has a library and a small museum, is annexed to the church. ⊠ *Via Anicia.*

S. Maria della Luce

5 D5. The name of the original church (3rd or 4th century) was S. Salvatore in Corte, perhaps refering to an ancient public edifice. It was rebuilt in the 12th century on a basilica plan, with an elegant bell tower with triforium and a transept with an apse (visible from the Vicolo del Buco). After the miraculous image of a Madonna, who restored the sight of a blind man, was transferred here, the name and structure of the church were changed. In 1730, the interior space was rebuilt in its current form, with luminous, late Baroque elements embellished by stuccowork. ⊠ *Via della Luce.*

S. Maria della Scala ③

5 C3. Like many churches in Trastevere, this was built (1593–1610) to house an image of the Madonna, painted above a stairway and considered miraculous. Inside the church are works by 17th-century artists, such as Carlo Rainaldi, Cavaliere d'Arpino (Giuseppe Cesari), and Pomarancio. Important works of art include the *Beheading of the Baptist* by Gerrit van Honthorst, a Dutch painter who was profoundly influenced by Caravaggio. Carlo Saraceni's *Death of the Virgin* replaced a painting of the same subject by Caravaggio, now in the Louvre, because the latter work was rejected by the monks as lacking in "decorum" and because they suspected that the model was a prostitute who had drowned in the Tiber. The adjoining monastery administers a famous pharmacy that dates from the 17th century, that supplied the papal court, and that still has the original furnishings and equipment. ⊠ *Piazza della Scala 23.*

S. Maria in Cappella

5 E6. The name is derived from the makers of *cupelle,* or barrels, who were given the church as the site for their confraternity in the 15th century. A hospital was later

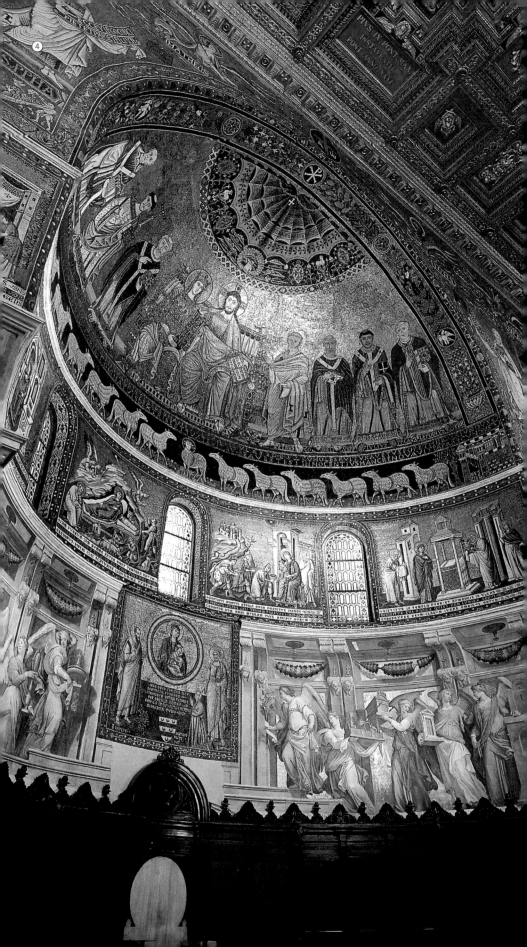

The apse mosaics (left), created in two phases (those in the spherical vault date from the 12th century, those in the lower band from the 13th), are among the treasures within S. Maria in Trastevere ④.

The tempietto of S. Pietro in Montorio ⑤, designed in the early 16th century by Bramante, is a milestone of Renaissance architecture .

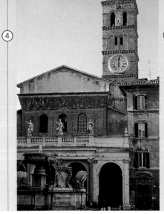
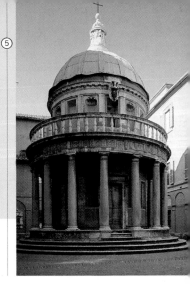

panel, with the Madonna and St. Peter and St. Paul. The most venerated image in the church is the monumental icon of the *Madonna of Mercy,* in the Altemps Chapel; this 6th- to 7th-century encaustic panel depicts the Virgin and child enthroned between two angels. Considered a miraculous sacred image, created by a direct emanation of divinity, it was the object of great care and devotion by certain Roman pontiffs. Gregory III (731–741) covered it in silver leaf, and Leo III (795–816) donated a large purple veil to hang in front of the sacred image. ⊠ *Piazza S. Maria in Trastevere.*

S. Onofrio al Gianicolo
⊞2 F5. Dedicated to the venerated 4th-century hermit, this monastery complex was built during the 15th and 16th centuries on the site of an ancient hermitage. It is linked to the poet Torquato Tasso, who stayed here, dying in 1595. He was posthumously granted a crown of laurel on the Campidoglio. Beneath the Renaissance portico of the church courtyard, three lunettes (1605) by Domenichino depict scenes from the life of St. Jerome (in memory of the hermits who resided here in the 15th century). The interior has an opulent decorative scheme by, among others, Domenichino, B.B. Ricci, students of Annibale Carracci, and, perhaps, Baldassare Peruzzi (*Scenes from the Life of Mary*). A cloister with frescoed scenes from the life of St. Onuphrius is attached to the church. The monastery houses the **Museo Tassiano,** which has manuscripts and editions of his works. ⊠ *Piazza S. Onofrio 2.*

S. Pietro in Montorio ⑤
⊞5 D3. Ferdinand and Isabella of Spain built this church (1481–1500) and dedicated it to St. Peter, who, according to an unfounded tradition, was crucified

here. The name "in Montorio" is derived from the ancient Latin name for the Janiculum, *Mons Aureus* (Mount of Gold), so-called because of the yellow sand that is visible at twilight. Numerous works of art decorate the church, including the *Flagellation of Jesus* (1518) by Sebastiano del Piombo, perhaps based on a drawing by Michelangelo. The site's main attraction is Bramante's **Tempietto,** commissioned in 1502 as a commemorative chapel to the martyrdom of Peter. This minuscule edifice holds a place of primary importance in 16th-century architecture, with its perfect elaboration of the central plan and its obvious reference (including its name) to Greco-Roman architecture. Bramante's rigorous treatment of the geometric elements of the circle and cylinder define an architectural model of universal value and symbolize the synthesis between Christian and Renaissance Rome and the ancient city. ⊠ *Piazza S. Pietro in Montorio 2.*

Via della Lungara
⊞2 E5–E6; 5 A2–B3. One of the roadways most frequently traveled by pilgrims on their way to S. Pietro, the Via della Lungara ("street along a river") was also called the Via Santa, or Holy Way. It was built between 1508 and 1512 by Pope Julius II, at the same time the Via Giulia was laid out, along the other bank of the Tiber. The task was entrusted to Bramante, who, in addition to being a talented architect, had a profound interest in designing urban spaces. The stately character of the street, which is flanked by villas, palaces, and churches built between the 16th and 18th centuries, is now diminished by the Tiber embankment that partially demolished and lowered what had been one of most spectacular streets in Rome.

Villa Farnesina
⊞5 B3. Agostino Chigi built this sumptuous residence (1507–1509) in the midst of suburban gardens along the Tiber. It was the principal backdrop for Roman society and cultural life at the culmination of the Renaissance, until the dramatic sack of Rome in 1527. Chigi welcomed as guests numerous cardinals, ambassadors, and princes, and the host of artists and intellectuals who gravitated around the court of Pope Leo X. Baldassare Peruzzi designed this "villa of delights," which was later acquired by the Farnese family, hence the building's name. Peruzzi combined a typical 15th-century city palace structure with a loggia and projecting side wings, emphasizing the relationship between building and nature. The best painters in Rome contributed to the opulent interior decorations, which are dominated by mythological and astrological subjects. In addition to Sebastiano del Piombo, Il Sodoma, and Domenico Beccafumi, Chigi engaged the painter Raphael, whose *Triumph of Galatea* (1513–1514) is a showpiece of classicism, both in its subject and in the figures and colors. The artist also conceived the decorative scheme for the loggia overlooking the garden, transforming the vault into a luxuriant pergola that frames scenes from the adventures of Psyche. ⊠ *Via della Lungara 230.*

3

Ponte and Parione

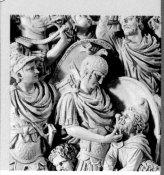

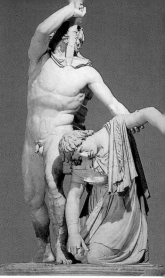

Detail of the Ludovisi sarcophagus (showing a battle between the Romans and the Barbarians) and a statue of a Galatian committing suicide, in the Museo Nazionale Romano in the Palazzo Altemps.

During the early Middle Ages, much of Rome's population was concentrated in the area within the bend of the Tiber that is closest to the Vatican. People were drawn here by the proximity to the Holy See and by the presence of the Ponte S. Angelo, one of the few ancient Roman bridges still standing and considered important enough to have lent its name to the entire district. The surrounding area was scattered with ruins of ancient monuments, and the name Parione may derive from the Latin paries ("wall"). Along today's Via dei Banchi Nuovi, Via Governo Vecchio, Via di S. Pantaleo, Via dei Banchi Vecchi, Via del Pellegrino, Campo de' Fiori, and Via dei Giubbonari, which closely follow the outlines of the ancient city, a dense urban fabric developed, full of small churches, inns, warehouses, and exchange banks. The urban renewal promoted by Renaissance and Baroque popes transformed the two districts, which were enriched with churches, palaces, and elegant houses. There was tremendous commercial activity, and the transfer of the market from the Campidoglio to Piazza Navona further contributed to the quarter's liveliness. The opening of the Corso Vittorio Emanuele II and other postunification projects altered the earlier urban plan and accelerated the deterioration of many structures.

Chiesa Nuova ②

⊞3 E2–F2. In 1575, the pope gave the little church of S. Maria in Vallicella to the Congregation of the Oratory, which was founded by St. Philip Neri, and they immediately began its reconstruction. The building's design recalls that of the Chiesa del Gesù, and the 10 side chapels, personally requested by St. Philip Neri, celebrate episodes from the life of the Madonna. The interior decoration expresses not only the ascetic orientation of the Oratorians, but also the ideals of the "triumphant" church of the Counter-Reformation and the diversity of tastes of the chapels' private patrons. These range from Federico Barocci's delicate *Visitation*, commissioned by St. Philip Neri, to typical Counter-Reformation devotional painting. There are also works by Caravaggio (*The Deposition*, 1604, now in the Vatican Pinacoteca); by Rubens, who was commissioned to paint the three presbytery paintings in 1608; by Guido Reni, who painted a famous altarpiece with the portrait of the saint; by Il Guercino; by Alessandro Algardi; and a by host of stuccoworkers, who, according to a writer at the time, bathed the church in a "shower of gold." Pietro da Cortona's frescoes cover the dome, apse, and nave and depict the apparition of the Virgin to St. Philip during the demolition of the ancient little church. The frescoes are the artist's most ambitious rendering of a sacred subject. Next to the magnificent church the Oratorians built a vast monastery complex, the **Palazzo dei Filippini,** characterized by an austere design.

Because of his esthetic and moral convictions and love of simple materials, architect and sculptor Borromini was perfectly suited to the order's spirit of charity and good works, and he carried out the assignment brilliantly, creating the oratory, the **Torre dell'Orologio,** and the extraordinary concave facade, a metaphor for the embrace of the faithful that was echoed by Bernini in St. Peter's. The palace houses many cultural institutions, including the Roman Newspaper Archive, which contains nearly all Roman newspapers from the 18th century to the present; the Capitoline Historical Archive; and the Vallicelliana Library, established by St. Philip Neri in 1581, also designed by Borromini, and one of the oldest libraries in Rome open to the public. ⊠*Piazza della Chiesa Nuova.*

Nostra Signora del Sacro Cuore

⊞3 F3. This is the real name of the church of S. Giacomo degli Spagnoli, built on the occasion of the 1450 Jubilee. The church was long the site of the Spanish court's celebrations and rituals of mourning. The solemn Easter celebrations in Piazza Navona organized by the Confraternity of the Resurrection, headquartered in the church, were particularly famous. After the focus of Spanish court life shifted to **S. Maria in Monserrato,** these activities declined, but the church continued to be used as a loggia for viewing spectacles in the piazza. The works of art and funerary monuments were transferred to the new Spanish church. Some Renaissance works remain, such as a chancel in polychrome marble, the marble backdrop behind the high altar,

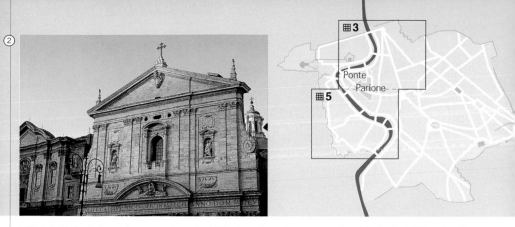

S. Maria in Vallicella, better known as Chiesa Nuova, was rebuilt at the request of St. Philip Neri, beginning in 1575.

and the S. Giacomo Chapel. ☒ *Piazza Navona.*

Palazzo Altemps, Museo Nazionale Romano ①

3 E3. Built at the end of the 15th century, the Palazzo Altemps is crowned by a beautiful covered roof terrace with arcades and four obelisks, the work of Martino Longhi the Elder, who also finished the extraordinary courtyard in travertine and stucco. The palazzo was restored so it is possible to appreciate fully the impressive pictorial scheme and the wooden ceilings inlaid with mother-of-pearl. But the contents are even more precious than the container: the palazzo is one of the locations of the **Museo Nazionale Romano** and contains more than 200 antiquities from collections of some of the city's aristocratic families. The most noteworthy group of works is from the Ludovisi collection, which was created by Cardinal Ludovico (1595–1632), nephew of Gregory XV, to embellish his immense villa. The cardinal's villa was demolished as a result of postunification building speculation and to make space for the neighborhood that now exists off the Via Veneto. The cardinal's collection, which was originally much richer, is a testament to the Roman aristocracy's passion for antiquities and classical art. ☒ *Piazza S. Apollinare 44,* ☎ *06/683–3566.*

Palazzo Braschi

3 F3. This Neoclassical edifice (1791–1811) is the last palazzo built in Rome for the family of a pope (Pius VI). The building's grand staircase was designed by Giuseppe Valadier and embellished with statues and stucco decora-

tions. In 1871, the palazzo became the property of the state, and it now houses offices for various cultural institutions. One of these is the **Museo di Roma,** which contains paintings, sculptures, drawings, and other art objects that illustrate various aspects of the city's life and culture, from the Middle Ages to the present. Some of the most interesting works are paintings inspired by Roman costumes and festivals and the collection of men and women's costumes from the 18th and 19th centuries. The palazzo also houses the **Gabinetto Comunale delle Stampe,** the municipal photo archive and print room, which contains precious documentation of transformations in the city and its territory between the 16th and 20th centuries. ☒ *Piazza S. Pantaleo 10,* ☎ *06/687–5880.*

Palazzo della Cancelleria

5 A4. Construction of the palazzo began in 1485, at the request of Cardinal Raffaele Riario, nephew of Sixtus IV, with contributions by the pope's other nephew, Julius II (both pontiffs' coats of arms appear on the facade). In 1517, Leo X confiscated the building from the cardinal, who was guilty of organizing a plot against the pontiff, and shortly thereafter it became (and still is) the location of the Apostolic Chancellery, the office that publishes papal decrees. Today it houses various cultural institutions and the Tribunale della Sacra Rota, the Vatican's highest court. The building's authorship is uncertain, although Bramante was certainly involved, most obviously in the courtyard. Other noteworthy elements are the extremely long facade, the elegant balcony overlooking the Campo de' Fiori and Via del Pellegrino, the Salone dei Cento Giorni (which Vasari claimed to have frescoed in 100 days), and the Study, with a vault

painted by Perin del Vaga. During the second half of the 17th century the palazzo became a lively center for musical and theatrical life, featuring the most important artists of the time, and one room was used as a theater. The palazzo incorporates the basilica of **S. Lorenzo in Damaso,** which in the late 15th century replaced the church established in 380 by Pope Damasus to house various relics. ☒ *Piazza della Cancelleria 1.*

Palazzi dei Massimo

3 F3. For centuries, the ancient Massimo family owned an entire block, and the most important building on that block was the **Palazzo Massimo "alle Colonne,"** rebuilt by Baldassarre Peruzzi (1532–1536) after the sack of Rome. It was one of the first and most significant attempts to restore the devastated city. The curved line of the facade follows the shape of Domitian's *Odeon,* over which the building was erected. The most celebrated of the sumptuous interiors is the chapel, in which Paolo Massimo is said to have been recalled from the dead by St. Philip Neri on March 16, 1584; on that day every year the chapel is open to the public. The **Palazzo Massimo di Pirro** gets its name from a statue of Mars, now in the Capitoline Museums. In the Piazza dei Massimi, which lies behind, is the oldest of the palaces, known as **Istoriato** and decorated with historical scenes; in 1467, this became the site of the first printing office in Rome. The facade is one of the few surviving examples of the painted decorations that were common in Rome during the Renaissance. ☒ *Corso Vittorio Emanuele 141; Corso Vittorio Emanuele 145; Piazza dei Massimi 1–3.*

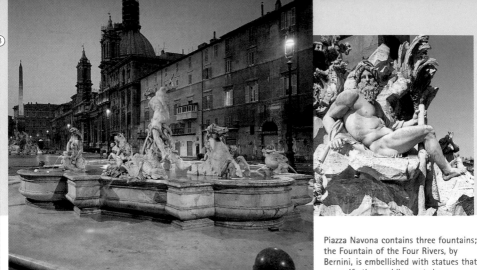

Piazza Navona contains three fountains; the Fountain of the Four Rivers, by Bernini, is embellished with statues that personify the world's great rivers.

Pasquino

3 F3. Leaning against a corner of the Palazzo Braschi is a marble statue in great disrepair. It was discovered a short distance away and placed here in 1501 by Cardinal Oliviero Carafa. The statue is a Roman copy of a Greek sculpture (Menelaus supporting the corpse of Patroclus), but the people of Rome gave it the name of a local tailor, Pasquino, famous for his invective against those in power. From the time of its discovery, anonymous authors attached to it sarcastic comments and political denunciations, generally against the papal government (thus our word "pasquinade"). For centuries, the statue was the most famous and loquacious of Rome's "talking statues" (the others were the Madama Lucrezia in Piazza Venezia and the Marforio, formerly in Via del Campidoglio, now in the Capitoline Museums). The papal administration generally ignored these expressions of popular discontent, but there were cases when those considered guilty of having spoken through Pasquino had to pay harshly for their temerity. The area came to be populated by printers, booksellers, and publishers, and the piazza became known as the Piazza dei Librai. ⊠ *Piazza di Pasquino.*

Piazza Navona ③

3 E3–F3. Along with S. Pietro and the Campidoglio, this is one of Rome's most well known attractions, and for centuries it has been one of the most animated spaces in the city. It stands above the ancient Stadium of Domitian (AD 81–96) and echoes that site's unusual plan and dimensions. The piazza's dramatic setting is the work of

Innocent X Pamphilj (1644–1655), who wanted to transform it into a place for the glorification of his own family and entrusted its execution to the great masters of the Baroque. The result was the palazzo, the church of S. Agnese, and the fountains, the most spectacular of which is the **Fontana dei Fiumi,** in which Gian Lorenzo Bernini expressed all his theatrical talents: a carved rock, with personifications of the major rivers of the four continents, holds up an obelisk surmounted by the dove of the Pamphilj coat of arms. The piazza's ancient function was echoed in its use as a place for tournaments, processions, jousts, and the extraordinary spectacle of a mock naval battle that concluded with the appearance of a gilded ship in the piazza, which had been transformed into a lake and was framed by fireworks. The adjacent **Piazza di Tor Sanguigna** contains both the ruins of Domitian's stadium and one of the most magnificent shrines from the 18th century, attached to the facade of the Palazzo Grossi Dondi. It depicts an Assumption of the Virgin, painted on canvas and surrounded by putti, with two angels below pointing up to the image.

Piazza di Ponte S. Angelo

3 E1. Located at the end of the Ponte S. Angelo and for centuries the principal access route to the Vatican, the piazza was an important junction and busy commercial and banking center. Because of its location, it was chosen as the site for capital executions, the most famous of which was that of Beatrice Cenci and her accomplices in 1599 (☞Palazzo Cenci Bolognetti, 74).

S. Agnese in Agone

3 E3. In the early Middle Ages an oratory was built on the ruins of an ancient Roman stadium, in memory of the martyrdom of St. Agnes. Here, according to tradition, the young Christian, dragged naked to her death, was covered by her hair, which grew miraculously (the event is immortalized in a marble relief by Alessandro Algardi in one of the spaces belowground). Innocent X wanted to rebuilt the church in more majestic form. The structure bears Borromini's unmistakable touch, and the concave facade, tall side towers, and tilt of the dome create a powerful image from every point in the piazza. The church's interior presents a vast panorama of Roman sculpture from the second half of the 17th century, with works of the most significant artists in Bernini's circle. ⊠ *Piazza Navona.*

S. Andrea della Valle ④

5 A5. S. Andrea, modeled on the Chiesa del Gesù, is one of the most solemn and characteristic churches of the Counter-Reformation. The stateliness of the church's dimensions and wealth of its ornamentation express the triumphant reality of Catholicism. It was built between 1591 and 1665 for the Theatine congregation, which played a primary role in this period of ecclesiastic history. Carlo Maderno created one of his greatest works in the majestic, soaring dome, second in size only to that of St. Peter's. The young Borromini collaborated with Maderno and invented the unusual capitals for the lantern of the dome, with cherubim that echo the Iconic volutes. The facade is by Carlo Rainaldi, who accentuated

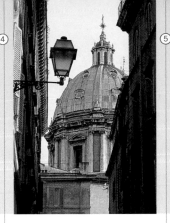

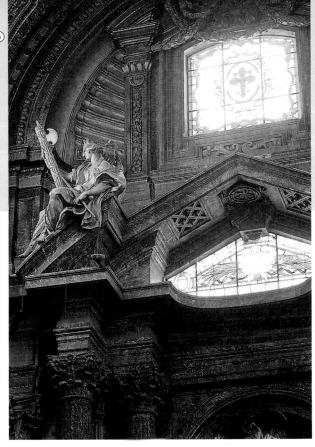

S. Andrea della Valle's magnificent dome is second in size only to the dome of S. Pietro.

vertical and plastic effects in accordance with accepted principles of the Baroque. Artists of note contributed to the church's sumptuous pictorial decoration, including Domenichino, who frescoed the bowl-shaped vault of the apse with *Scenes from the Life of St. Andrew,* and Giovanni Lanfranco, who painted the *Heavenly Glory with the Assumption of the Virgin,* which marked the beginning of a taste for illusionistic effects, culminating in the clamorous success of 17th-century painting. ⊠ *Piazza S. Andrea della Valle.*

S. Apollinare
⊞3 E3. The present-day church is the result of a renovation (1741–1748) by Ferdinando Fuga of an early medieval church that was also dedicated to the bishop-saint of Ravenna. The entrance vestibule has a venerated fresco of the Madonna (15th century). From 1574 to 1773 the adjacent **Palazzo di S. Apollinare** was the headquarters of the Collegio Germanico, established by St. Ignatius of Loyola and restored by Fuga in the sober, monumental style that is characteristic of Jesuit architecture. ⊠ *Piazza S. Apollinare 49.*

S. Giovanni dei Fiorentini ⑤
⊞2 E5–E6. Beginning in the 15th century, a sizable Florentine colony developed along the initial portion of the Via Giulia. The area had warehouses, residences, and a consulate that governed the district's activities. Leo X built a church there for his fellow townsmen and dedicated it to the patron saint of Florence, St. John the Baptist. The construction of the church had the strong support of the Compagnia della Pietà, a confraternity of Florentines established to aid and bury plague victims. Jacopo Sansovino began the building in 1519, and work was continued by Carlo Maderno, who created the unusual elongated dome. The facade was built in 1734 by Florentine Alessandro Galilei, who was asked to design the facade for S. Giovanni in Laterano two years later and who received both commissions from Clement XII Corsini, also from Florence. ⊠ *Via Acciaioli 2.*

S. Maria dell'Anima
⊞3 E3. This is the national church for German-speaking Catholics. It was founded, along with a hospice, after the Jubilee of 1350 by two wealthy German pilgrims, and it was completely rebuilt in its current form on the occasion of the 1500 Jubilee. The tall Renaissance facade is surmounted by the coats of arms of the empire and Hadrian VI, who was teacher and counselor to Charles V. Hadrian was also the last non-Italian pope until the election of John Paul II in 1978. German models inspired the church interior, conceived as a large hall with three naves of equal height, separated by tall, slender cruciform pillars. Impressive funerary monuments attest to the secular presence of Germans in Rome. ⊠ *Via S. Maria dell'Anima.*

S. Maria della Pace
⊞3 E2. The church, built at the behest of Sixtus IV during a period of political and social unrest, has its origins in a miraculous event, when an image of the Madonna (kept in an earlier church and now on the high altar) was struck by a stone and issued forth blood. The pope proclaimed it the Madonna della Pace (Madonna of Peace) and ordered a church built as an offering for peace in Italy. It was completed in 1656 by Pietro da Cortona, who designed a convex facade preceded by a semicircular portico, and it is one of the most typical and harmonious examples of the Roman Baroque. The interior contains the Chigi Chapel, with four figures of sibyls painted by Raphael, who was clearly influenced by Michelangelo's Sistine Chapel sibyls. Baldassare Peruzzi frescoed the Ponzetti Chapel, and the choir and high altar are by Carlo Maderno. The adjacent cloister, Donato Bramante's first work in Rome (1500–1504), is noteworthy for the harmony of its proportions and the compact

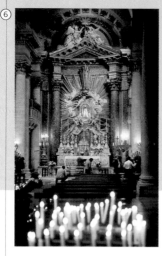

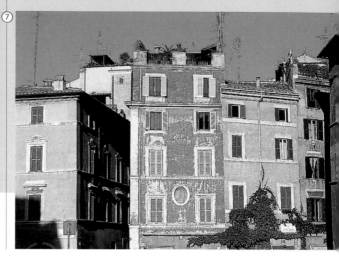

The beautiful interior of the church of S. Salvatore in Lauro, considered the most successful work by Mascherino.

structure of its space. It is close in spirit to the classical models that are its principal sources of inspiration, and like S. Pietro in Montorio (the "Tempietto"), it seems solemn and monumental, despite its modest size. ⊠ *Via della Pace 5.*

S. Nicolò in Agone
(Nicola dei Lorenesi)
⌗3 E3. This is the national church of the Lorrainers, who, breaking away from S. Luigi dei Francesi, obtained the church of S. Caterina in 1622. They rebuilt that church (1636) and changed its name to S. Nicolò di Mira (3rd century), after the figure who, in addition to being the patron saint of Lorraine, is also the protector of marriages. Roman couples often pray at this church on the eve of their nuptials. ⊠ *Via S. Maria dell'Anima.*

S. Pantaleo
⌗3 F3. A small church dating from the Middle Ages, S. Pantaleo acquired a certain importance when Paul V granted it to St. Joseph Calasanctius (1557–1648). This Spanish priest and theologian was transferred to Rome, where he found many homeless and derelict children, who had been in many cases orphaned by epidemics. He founded the first free public school in Europe (located in S. Dorotea, in Trastevere) and the congregation of the Scolopi, or Piarists, whose schools are to this day attended by thousands of children throughout the world. Construction of the present church began in 1681 and was completed

with a simple Neoclassical facade by Giuseppe Valadier (1806); St. Joseph Calasanctius's remains are beneath the ornate high altar. The church's namesake is Pantaleon, a 4th-century martyr who was a physician of exceptional talent. He is the patron saint of doctors, midwives, and wet nurses. ⊠ *Piazza S. Pantaleo.*

S. Salvatore in Lauro ⑥
⌗3 E2. The name "in Lauro" may refer to bay trees that were planted along the Tiber embankment at the time the church was built. The original building, known as far back as the 12th century, was destroyed by fire in 1591 and rebuilt according to the plan of Ottaviano Mascherino; the Neoclassical facade was added in 1857. At one time entrusted to the Celestines, in 1669 the church passed into the hands of the Confraternity of the Piceni, who dedicated it to the Madonna of Loreto. The luminous interior, inspired by Palladian models, has a Latin cross plan with 34 grand travertine columns along the walls. The church contains a *Nativity* by Pietro da Cortona. The monastery complex adjacent to the church includes an elegant Renaissance cloister, and the refectory has a large painting by Cecchino Salviati depicting *The Wedding at Cana* (1550). ⊠ *Piazza S. Salvatore in Lauro 15.*

Via dei Banchi Nuovi
⌗3 E1–E2. This was once part of the ancient Papal Way, the itinerary newly crowned popes followed from the Vatican to the Lateran residence. The street was opened by Sixtus IV and got its name from the 16th-century "new" bank of

Agostino Chigi, the wealthy owner of the Farnesina Villa (a counterpoint to the offices of the 15th-century banking offices, know as the *banchi vecchi,* or old banks). As soon as the street was opened, it became a desirable address for members of the curia, which explains the homogenous character of the residential buildings.

Via dei Banchi Vecchi ⑦
⌗3 F1. Along with Via del Pellegrino, Campo de' Fiori, and Via dei Giubbonari, this was part of the ancient Via Peregrinorum and takes its name from the numerous bankers' offices once located here. The street is lined by various notable Renaissance structures. At number 123 is the 16th-century **Palazzo degli Accetti,** with a rusticated ground floor and a top floor with a loggia; at number 22 the so-called **Palazzo dei Pupazzi** (Palace of the Dolls, 1538–1540), built by the Milanese jeweler Giovan Pietro Crivelli, has refined stucco cupids and female nudes, explaining the building's unusual name. The **Palazzo Sforza Cesarini,** built in 1458–1462 by Cardinal Rodrigo Borgia (later Pope Alexander VI), overlooked this street before the construction of the 19th-century facade on the Corso Vittorio Emanuele (number 282). It housed the papal chancellery until that office was transferred to the Palazzo Riario; in 1536 the building passed into the hands of the Roman branch of the Sforza family from Milan. During the Middle Ages the church of **S. Lucia del Gonfalone,** at 12 Via dei Banchi Vecchi, was the national church of the Bohemians, who had their ancient hospice nearby. It took on great importance after the

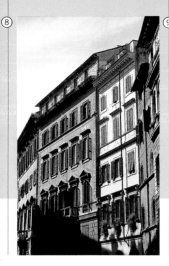

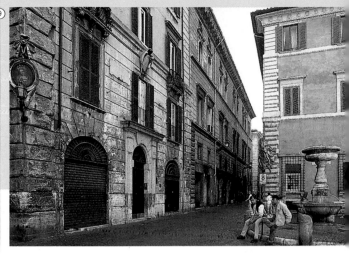

installation in the late 15th century of the Archconfraternity of the Gonfalone. Founded by St. Bonaventure in the 13th century, this group worked zealously to aid hospitals and pilgrims. Made up of members of the aristocracy and the highest social classes, it wielded considerable economic and political power. The nearby oratory (☞ 74) also belonged to the confraternity.

Via dei Coronari ⑨
⊞**3 E2.** The *coronari*, sellers of rosaries (*corone*), were once quite numerous along this street, which for centuries was thronged with pilgrims. After the opening of the Corso Vittorio Emanuele, it lost much of its traditional character. The street bears vestiges of the Roman Via Recta, which was reorganized by Sixtus IV as part of his extensive building program. It preserves its Renaissance and Baroque appearance almost intact, despite the deteriorated state of many of the buildings. The **Palazzo Lancellotti,** from the late 16th century, has a lovely main entrance with columns and a balcony designed by Domenichino. The sides of the facade have two stucco shrines, one with an image of Christ the Redeemer surrounded by a sunburst and supported by an angel and cherubs' heads, the other with an image of the Madonna. At the corner of the Vicolo Domizio is a famous **Immagine di Ponte,** a shrine by Antonio Giamberti da Sangallo the Younger (1523–1527) with a *Coronation of the Virgin* by Perine del Vaga, in great disrepair. It is the oldest of the once numerous sacred shrines that ornament the streets of Rome. The number, variety, and decorative wealth of

A shrine in Via dei Coronari; the street once housed shops where rosaries were sold, resulting in the name.

the shrines impressed travelers throughout the ages. For the most part dedicated to the cult of the Virgin, they also influenced local custom. They were outfitted with oil lamps that lit the streets at night, and people made a habit of placing small altars nearby, decorated with flower and candles, a practice that led to popular open-air celebrations and novenas, often with musical accompaniment.

Via del Banco di S. Spirito
⊞**3 E1.** This street takes its name from the **Palazzo del Banco di S. Spirito** (number 31), designed in 1521–1524 by Antonio Giamberti da Sangallo the Younger. It served as both an elegant backdrop for those coming from Castel S. Angelo and a dividing point between the Via dei Banchi Vecchi and the Via dei Banchi Nuovi. The building housed the mint until 1541 and, after 1666, the Banco di S. Spirito, founded by Paul V in 1605 to support the numerous welfare, religious, and social activities of the hospital of the same name. The slightly concave facade has a triumphal arch on a rusticated base, with windows on the sides and, on the pediment, Baroque statues of *Charity* and *Thrift.* The church of **Ss. Celso e Giuliano** (entrance at 12 Vicolo del Curato), which dates from the 5th century but was rebuilt in the 18th century, contains a beautiful altar by Pompeo Girolamo Batoni (*Christ in Glory,* 1738). The **Palazzo Gaddi** (1430), at number 42, has a harmonious

courtyard embellished with niches with statues and a stucco decorative scheme.

Via del Governo Vecchio ⑧
⊞**3 E2–F2.** The street gets its name from the presence, at number 39, of the **Palazzo del Governo Vecchio,** which has an elegant marble entrance with diamond point rustication. It was built by Cardinal Stefano Nardini (1473–1477), governor of Rome, and it was initially called Via del Governo. When government offices were moved to Palazzo Madama, the street acquired its current name. Like the Via dei Banchi Nuovi, it was part of the medieval Papal Way between St. Peter's and the Lateran; today it is known for its antiques shops. Both noble and simple buildings, most of which date from the 16th or 17th century, flank the street. Some of the facades preserve traces of frescoes and stucco decorations. The street also houses the church of **S. Tommaso in Parione** (entrance at 33 Via Parione), built in 1582 and known to Romans as the site of St. Philip Neri's ordination.

4

Regola

⊞ 3

⊞ 5　Regola

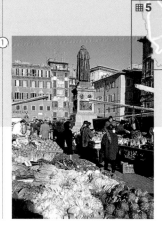

Bordered for a long stretch by the Tiber, from the Mazzini Bridge to the Lungotevere Cenci, this district takes its name from deposits of river sand, or arenula *(corrupted to* reula, *then* regola*). Like Ponte and Parione, it experienced considerable urban development and building between the 16th and 17th centuries, when new streets were opened, piazzas designed, and luxurious palaces erected, such as those for the Farnese and Spada families. But traces of the medieval fabric remain, linked to the path of the Papal Way and the pilgrims' route, such as S. Paolo's picturesque complex of 13th-century houses, near S. Paolo alla Regola.*

Lively Campo de' Fiori is the site of a daily food market; by evening it is a popular gathering place for the young people of Rome. In times past it was the designated site for capital executions.

Campo de' Fiori ①
⊞5 A4. Until the 15th century this area was covered with flower-filled fields, most likely the origin of the name. In addition to being the site of a market (still held daily), many inns and bookstores, and residences of famous courtesans, it was also a place for public executions. In 1600, Giordano Bruno was accused of heresy by the Inquisition and burned at the stake; he was later honored with a statue, which, in its severe expression, recalls the sternness of his denunciations against corruption and vice. The installation of the monument in 1889, nearly three centuries after Bruno's death, provoked violent polemics between Republicans and partisans of the pope.

Oratorio del Gonfalone
⊞3 F1. The powerful Confraternity of S. Lucia del Gonfalone, which also held the nearby church of

S. Lucia (☞ 73), established the oratory (1544–1547). All institutions of this type had both a public church and a private oratory set aside for prayer, worship, and meetings. The building has a modest facade and a sumptuous interior, embellished with a painting cycle (1572–1575) depicting *Scenes from the Passion of Christ,* one of the most interesting examples of Roman Mannerism. The room is surrounded by choir stalls and has a wooden ceiling. ✉ *Vicolo della Scimmia 1/B.*

Ospizio dei Cento Preti
(Hospice of the Hundred Priests)
⊞5 B4. After the construction of the Tiber embankment, very little remained of this structure, which was built by Domenico Fontana in 1587 for Sixtus V. It was erected to accommodate an ambitious welfare project, which placed all the city's beggars in a single institution. The hospice was dedicated to St. Francis of Assisi and was administered by a congregation of 100 priests. At the beginning of the 18th century, Clement XI decided to transfer the facility to the apostolic hospice of S. Michele, after which this structure housed an institution for girls and an ecclesiastic hospital. ✉ *Via dei Pettinari.*

Palazzo Cenci Bolognetti
(Piazza delle Cinque Scole)
⊞5 B5. The mound on which the palazzo of the famous Roman Cenci family rises probably rests atop the ruins of the Statilio Tauro Amphitheater, the first one in Rome built of brick (29 BC). The palazzo is made up of various ele-

ments, unified in the 16th century by flat stucco rustication. Across from the palazzo is the aristocratic chapel of **S. Tommaso ai Cenci,** known as far back as the 12th century but rebuilt during the second half of the 16th century and chosen by Francesco Cenci as the family's burial site. Francesco and his family were protagonists in the darkest event of the time: Having molested his daughter, Beatrice, Francesco was killed by her, with the help of her brother and lover. The following year (1599) the murderers were publicly beheaded in Piazza di Ponte. ✉ *Piazza delle Cinque Scole 23.*

Palazzo Farnese ②
⊞5 A4–B4. In 1514, Cardinal Alessandro Farnese began work on his new palazzo. After he became Pope Paul III, his plans for the building became much more solemn and grand and involved Antonio Giamberti da Sangallo the Younger (principal and side facades), Michelangelo (the impressive cornice and much of the courtyard), and Giacomo della Porta (the rear facade and large loggia facing the Via Giulia). The result is perhaps the most beautiful palazzo in Rome, characterized by the perfect equilibrium of its majestic mass. An array of artists contributed to the drawing rooms' magnificent decoration, which includes the barrel vault of the gallery, frescoed by Annibale and Agostino Carracci (1597–1600) with *The Triumph of Love over the Universe,* which advances beyond Renaissance equilibrium and initiates the spatial illusionism of

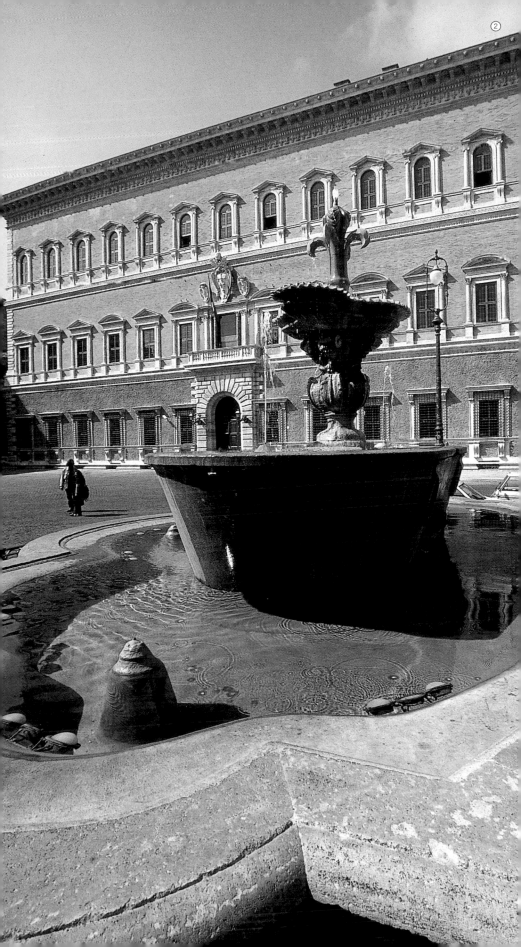

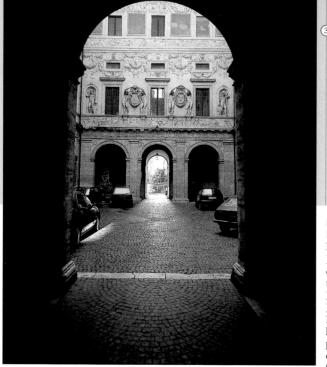

Baroque art. Today the building houses the French Embassy and the French School, a prestigious institute of historical and archaeological studies. In the past the piazza hosted numerous spectacles: a weekly horse market; bullfights; and a festival celebrating the presentation by the king of Naples to the pope of the *chinea*, a white mule, symbol of vassalage. During the 19th century it was also a gathering place for people from the countryside and a place for hiring laborers. At number 96 Piazza Farnese is the church of **S. Brigida,** erected by Boniface IX on the site of a house where the mystic Swedish saint had stayed; it was rebuilt in the 18th century. Until the Protestant reformation it was the location of a Swedish hospice. ✉ *Piazza Farnese 67.*

Palazzo del Monte di Pietà

5 B5. Monte di Pietà was established in 1539 by a friar, Giovanni Mattei de Calvi, as a public lending institution to combat the usury practiced by Jewish lenders of the time. Working-class borrowers secured loans at extremely modest rates of interest against personal possessions left as collateral. Patrons repossessed their property upon repayment of the loan. Private citizens or confraternities often cancelled debts as an act of charity. The Palazzo del Monte di Pietà thus carried out a function of primary importance during times

of economic crisis and in the absence of sufficient welfare institutions. The 16th-century palazzo, acquired by the Monte and later expanded, has an extremely simple facade that is embellished only by a shrine depicting Christ in the tomb and four coats of arms. ✉ *Piazza del Monte di Pietà.*

Palazzo Spada ③

5 B4. This is one of the most refined and celebrated Roman residences, because of both its elaborate stucco decorative scheme on the facade and courtyard (by Giulio Mazzoni, 1556–1560), and the extraordinary contribution of Francesco Borromini. Built for Cardinal Girolamo Capodiferro in the mid-16th century, it was later acquired and renovated by the Spada family. The courtyard contains the gallery designed by Borromini in 1653, an exceptional example of perspectival illusionism. Although it is only 30 feet long, it simulates a length four times greater, and the statue that stands at the back, which appears very tall, is in reality quite small. The **Galleria Spada,** created in the 17th century by Cardinal Bernardino Spada (1594–1661), is a rare intact example of small patrician gallery. The room, which has its original furnishings, frescoes, and brick floors, contains predominantly Italian and Flemish paintings from the 17th century. ✉ *Piazza Capo di Ferro 13,* ☎ *06/686–1158.*

Ponte Sisto ④

5 B4–C4. In the wake of the collapse of Ponte S. Angelo during the Jubilee of 1450, when it was crowded with pilgrims, Sixtus IV decided to restore an ancient bridge to the Janiculum in time for the 1475 Jubilee. The bridge was built during Roman times and probably collapsed during the flood of 589. This project was one of the cornerstones of the urban renewal program of Sixtus IV and his successor, Julius II. Until the late 19th century the bridge was the only one in the city remaining from the time of the Roman Empire. The structure, which links Trastevere to the Regola and Parione districts, incorporates part of the ancient bridge and is made up of four arcades and a large circle for runoff in the central pier, which for centuries was used as a water gauge.

S. Biagio della Pagnotta

3 F1. The church was erected in the 12th century, rebuilt in the 18th century, and restored during the following century. The name is derived from the custom of distributing a roll that has been blessed to the faithful on St. Blaise's feast day, February 3. The church is in the care of Armenian Catholic priests. ✉ *Via Giulia 64.*

S. Caterina da Siena

5 A4. Erected between 1766 and 1776 by the Sienese Archconfraternity, this church is located on the site of a 16th-century oratory. The entire block was set aside for the welfare and hospitality of Sienese citizens. Two orders of columns modeled on Borrominian motifs decorate the building's concave facade. ✉ *Via Giulia.*

S. Eligio degli Orefici ⑤

5 A3. St. Eligius (588–600), a talented goldsmith and counselor to the French kings, was bishop of Noyon and devoted himself to

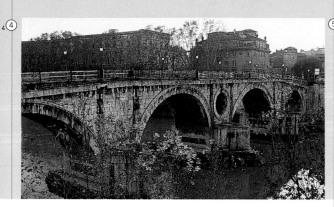

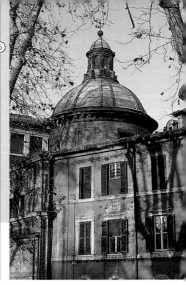

spreading the faith among the people of Flanders. As patron saint of goldsmiths and blacksmiths, his veneration quickly spread from France and Flanders throughout the west (there is a second Roman church dedicated to him: S. Eligio dei Ferrari, near Piazza Bocca della Verità). The design of this church (1509–1575) is attributed to Raphael; the facade was completed in the 17th century. The interior, on a Greek cross plan, is somber and harmonious, punctuated by gray pilaster strips against a white backdrop, and clearly reveals Bramante's influence. The noteworthy hemispherical dome probably was designed by Baldassarre Peruzzi. ⊠ *Via S. Eligio 8/A.*

S. Girolamo della Carità

⊞**5 A4.** The building (1654–1660) is closely linked to the memory of St. Philip Neri, who lived in the adjacent monastery and established his institutions here. To the left of the high altar is a chapel designed by Filippo Juvarra (1705) and dedicated to the saint. Inside the church are a refined marble decorative scheme, an intricate coffered ceiling, and an unusual chapel by Borromini that was commissioned by the Spada family in 1660. It is a shallow space, separated from the nave not by the usual balustrade, but by a pair of angels that support a faux drapery of jasper (one of the wings revolves on a hinge, allowing access to the chapel). The small alcove feels like a domestic space, with two chests topped with statues of the reclining figures of Spada family members, flowered tapestries, family portraits, and images of saints. Marble inlays on the walls mimic damask, and the floor is designed with a floral motif that alludes symbolically to the inexorible passage of time. ⊠ *Via Monserrato 62/A.*

S. Maria in Monserrato

⊞**5 A4.** The church was begun in 1518, following the design of Antonio Giamberti da Sangallo the Younger, for the Confraternity of S. Maria di Monserrato (Montserrat is a famous sanctuary near Barcelona), which was established by Alexander VI in 1495. It was the national church, first for the people of Aragon and Catalonia, then for all Spaniards, replacing the church of S. Giacomo (now Our Lady of the Sacred Heart). Many of the church's most beautiful works come from S. Giacomo, including the statue of *St. Jerome* by Jacopo Sansovino, funerary monuments, and the marble flooring. The building also contains Annibale Carracci's *St. Diego di Alcantara* and the funerary monuments of two popes, Callistus II and Alexander VI, both Spaniards, transferred here from the Vatican grottoes. Above the 18th-century entrance is a group of the *Madonna and Child Sawing the Rock,* which refers to the serrated shape of the mountain on which the Catalonian sanctuary is located. ⊠ *Via Monserrato at Via di Montoro.*

S. Maria dell'Orazione e Morte

⊞**5 B4.** The strange name—St. Mary of the Oration and Death—has its origins in the charitable activity of the Company of Good Death, established in 1535 to gather unburied corpses. This group built a church in 1576, and rebuilt between 1733 and 1737 according to a design by Ferdinando Fuga. The elaborately decorated interior has an elliptical plan surmounted by a high dome. Two winged skulls over the central doorway allude to the builders' profession, and beneath the church is a subterranean cemetery in which approximately 8,000 bodies were buried over the course of three centuries (from 1552 to 1896). ⊠ *Via Giulia at Via del Mascherone.*

S. Maria del Pianto

⊞**5 B5.** The church was established in 1616 to house an image of the Madonna from the nearby Portico di Ottavia that was said to have cried following a deadly brawl on the site. The fresco is located on the high altar. The building was designed along a Greek cross plan, with large pilasters and a dome on pendentives decorated in stuccowork; its facade has remained unfinished. During the Counter-Reformation the church hosted a popular catechism competition among boys from various parishes, which concluded with the proclamation of an "emperor of Christian doctrine." The victor was carried in triumph before the pope, from whom he could request a favor. ⊠ *Via S. Maria dei Calderari 29.*

S. Maria della Quercia ⑥

⊞**5 B4.** The church has the same name as the important Renaissance sanctuary located near Viterbo. Dating from the early 16th century, the building was erected for the populous colony of Viterbo natives in the district; the project had the backing of Julius II, whose heraldic symbol was the oak tree or *quercia.* The building's appearance is the result of a 1727 reconstruction that introduced a Greek cross plan surmounted by a hemispherical dome and a convex facade crowned by a high attic. ⊠ *Piazza della Quercia 27.*

S. Paolo alla Regola

⊞**5 B5.** This church was built in the late 17th century on the site of a house where, according to tradition, St. Paul had lived. The street of the same name bears traces of an important medieval street called Strada della Regola (from

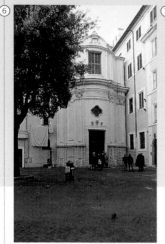

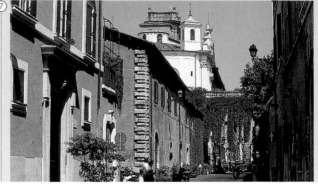

the name of the district), which, prior to modern demolitions, preserved much of the original residential fabric. Still standing are some 13th-century buildings (in great disrepair), known as the **Case di S. Paolo,** with porticos, loggias, and towers. A short distance away is the church of **S. Maria in Monticelli** (at number 28 of the street of that name), perhaps named for the ruins that lie below. An extremely ancient structure, it was restored by Paschal II (1101) and again transformed during the 18th and 19th centuries. The interior has a fragment of mosaic in the apse, with the head of Christ the Redeemer (12th century) and a 14th-century crucifix. ⊠ *Via S. Paolo alla Regola 6.*

S. Salvatore in Onda
⊞**5 B4.** The name of this church, which refers to the flooding of the Tiber, is mentioned as far back as the 12th century, but numerous later restorations have completely altered its original appearance. Attached is a monastery that has housed the Hermits of St. Paul, the Augustinians, and the Conventual Friars. During the early 19th century, the church was the base for the pastoral activity of St. Vincent Pallotti, who Romans consider the second Philip Neri because of his tireless works of charity and welfare, particularly with prisoners, the sick, and the young. In 1835 he founded a society for Catholic missionary work, the members of which were called Pallottines. Initially the order was made up of only 12 priests, but later the order expanded to include laypersons and spread worldwide. Pius XI called the saint a precursor of Catholic Action, the lay apostolic

movement. The present-day church is within the Pallottine motherhouse. ⊠ *Via dei Pettinari 51.*

S. Spirito dei Napoletani
⊞**5 A3.** Founded in 1619 by the Confraternity of Neapolitans, this church was rebuilt between 1701 and 1709 by Carlo Fontana. The two-story facade with a sculpted entry and rose windows was reconstructed in 1853. Inside the building is a painting by Luca Giordano (1705): *The Martyrdom of St. Gennaro,* patron saint of Naples. In 1630, the adjacent hospice became the site of the Collegio Ghislieri, founded by Roman physician Giuseppe Ghislieri for the instruction of the poor, and, like the many other city institutions, made possible through private philanthropy. ⊠ *Via Giulia 34.*

S. Tommaso di Canterbury
⊞**5 A4.** This church is located in a renovated (1864) earlier church, SS. Trinità degli Scozzesi, an 8th-century edifice that itself was rebuilt in 1575 to repair damage inflicted during the sack of Rome. The building is contained within the Collegio Inglese, founded by Gregory XIII in 1579 to strengthen unstable ties between the Catholic Church and England. This initiative, like the creation of the Greek and German colleges, was part of the ecumenical approach that guided the policies of this pope, who wanted cosmopolitan Rome to be a tangible symbol of the opening of the Catholic Church to the world. But Gregory's projects failed, and many of the priests who were educated in the college were killed in England during 17th- and 18th-century persecutions. ⊠ *Via Monserrato 45.*

Ss. Giovanni Evangelista e Petronio dei Bolognesi
⊞**5 B4.** In 1575 the Bolognese community in Rome acquired the complex of S. Giovanni Calibita on the Tiber Island. With the support of Pope Gregory XIII, who was from Bologna, they abandoned the first church and established a new church on this site (1582), dedicated to St. John and to St. Petronius, the patron saint of their own city. The Bolognese community was quite large, particularly during the 16th and 17th centuries, and ties between Rome and Bologna were very close. Many Bolognese artists contributed to the city of the popes, including Guido Reni, Domenichino, the Carracci, and the sculptor Alessandro Algardi, who is buried in this church. ⊠ *Via del Mascherone.*

SS. Trinità dei Pellegrini
⊞**5 B4.** In 1548, St. Philip Neri founded a community of priests to tend the growing crowds of pilgrims, particularly during Holy Years, and the sick. This group took the name of the Archconfraternity of Pilgrims and Convalescents. It was one of the most significant manifestations of the desire for strong religious renewal in Rome during the second half of the 16th century. The group's activities had incredible results, and during the 1575 Jubilee alone, approximately 170,000 pilgrims were offered assistance and hospitality, with additional help from numerous laypersons. Paul IV gave this church to the confraternity in 1558; it was rebuilt in between 1603 and 1616, and the facade was completed in 1723. The high altar has a *SS. Trinità* by Guido Reni. ⊠ *Via dei Pettinari 36/A.*

Via dei Giubbonari
⊞**5 B5.** The numerous clothing shops that line this street follow a

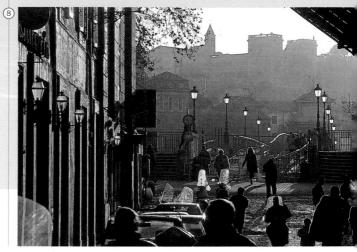

An evocative section of the Via Giulia ⑦, the 16th-century street laid out for Pope Julius II by Donato Bramante.

The final section of the Via dei Pettinari ⑧ and, at the end, the Ponte Sisto, built in 1473.

secular tradition that is perpetuated in its name (*giubbonari* are jacket-makers). It has always been a thriving area, thanks in part to the fact that the street was part of the Via dei Pellegrini. Midway the street opens into the Largo dei Librari with the little church of **S. Barbara dei Librari,** founded in the 11th century on the ruins of the Theater of Pompey and under the aegis of the Università dei Librari, a corporation of printers, bookbinders, and scribes that rebuilt the church in 1680.

Via Giulia ⑦
▦5 A3–B4. Continuing the urban renewal projects of his uncle Sixtus IV, Julius II decided to replace the narrow, winding medieval streets that led to the Vatican with broad, rectilinear stretches that were more elegant and also more easily traveled by pilgrims. The pope commissioned Bramante (1508) to design two parallel streets on the opposite banks of the Tiber, the Via della Lungara and the Via Giulia, which were linked by the Ponte Sisto and by another bridge, never built, opposite the Hospital of S. Spirito. According to Julius II's plans for the street that bears his name, the principal public buildings of the papal state were to face each other, but this never came to fruition. Despite the demolitions of the modern era, the Via Giulia has preserved a certain stylistic homogeneity and is now one of the most harmonious streets in Rome and one of the most popular, thanks to its galleries and antiques shops. Many notable palazzi line the street, such as the **Palazzo Falconieri** (number 1), designed by Borromini, with large Baroque sculptures at the sides of the facade and a magnificent loggia facing the Tiber. The memorable **Palazzo Sacchetti** (number 62) was erected in 1552 and has a reception hall decorated

with scenes from the life of David by Cecchino Salviati (1554) and a gallery with Pietro da Cortona's *Holy Family* and *Adam and Eve.* Near the **Carceri Nuove** (number 52), the prisons built by Innocent X (1655), are part of what was meant to be the grand **Palazzo dei Tribunali,** planned by Julius II and designed by Bramante, but never completed. Vestiges of the rusticated foundation, with projecting benches that have long been known as the Via Giulia sofas, remain.

Via di Monserrato
▦5 A3–A4. The street assumed this name immediately after the construction of the church of S. Maria di Monserrato, which in its turn was named after a famous Catalan sanctuary. In earlier times the street contained the houses and prisons of the powerful Savelli family and was know as the Via di Corte Savella. It is distinguished by elegant buildings and churches, including the **Casa di Pietro Paolo della Zecca** (Paul II's superintendent of coinage), which dates from the late 15th century and has traces of frescoes on its facade. The 16th-century **Palazzo Incoronati de Planca** (number 152) has the Planca family coat of arms over the entrance. The two facades of the **Palazzo Ricci** are covered with frescoes (from ca. 1525), representative of a fashion that was popular during the Renaissance, but which has very few surviving examples in Rome.

Via del Pellegrino
▦5 A4. The name refers to the ancient Via Peregrinorum, which took pilgrims from the Tiber Island area and the market of

S. Angelo in Pescheria toward Ponte S. Angelo. Alexander VI expanded the street in 1497, following an urban reorganization plan begun by Nicholas V and Sixtus IV. Near the **Arco di S. Margherita** is one of the most original and decorative shrines in the city. It depicts a *Madonna and Child* against an architectural background; the image is surmounted by a sunburst "glory" interwoven with a crown supported by putti; the figure of St. Philip Neri appears below. The sculpture also depicts in stucco the so-called procession "machines" that were widely used during the 17th and 18th centuries. These wooden, cardboard, or plaster structures reproduced altars, temples, or statuary compositions of sacred subjects, and they were transported through the streets of the city during the religious processions of the Baroque era, along with hundreds of crucifixes, candlesticks, and banners painted with religious scenes.

Via dei Pettinari ⑧
▦5 B4. Sixtus IV renovated this street at the time of the rebuilding of the Ponte Sisto to link Trastevere to the commercial zones of the Ponte, Parione, and Regola districts. Like many others the area—such as Via dei Cappellari (hat-makers), Via dei Giubbonari (jacket-makers), Via dei Chiavari (key-makers), Via dei Baullari (chest-makers), Via dei Chiodaroli (nail-makers), Via dei Falegnami (carpenters), Via dei Funari (rope-makers) , and so forth—this street's name refers to one of the commercial activities that was carried out here (in this case the making and selling of combs).

5

S. Eustachio, Pigna, and S. Angelo

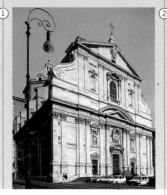

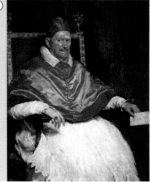

During the Roman period this area had many significant public buildings and sites, including the Pantheon, the Theater of Marcellus, and the sacred zone of Largo Argentina. Many other sites were destroyed or incorporated into later buildings. Throughout the Middle Ages the quarter remained inhabited, preserving much of the ancient road network. Beginning in the 13th century it experienced new vitality as the center of various artisan and commercial activities. Traces of that era are still present in place names, in the winding lanes, and in some buildings that escaped Renaissance and Baroque expansion. This is particularly evident in the district of S. Angelo, where, in 1555, the Jewish Ghetto was established. When the popes returned from Avignon, the three districts, like others contained within this bend of the Tiber, received crowds of pilgrims making their way toward the Ponte S. Angelo. Many palaces and churches (some of the city's most famous) testify to the monumental urban development that took place between the 15th and 18th centuries. The continuity of the area's urban fabric was damaged by interventions carried out between the 19th and 20th centuries, including the opening of the Corso Vittorio Emanuele and the Corso Rinascimento and the expansion of the Palazzo Madama.

Chiesa del Gesù ①
▦**5 A6.** The original appearance of the church, which was built for the Jesuits between 1568 and 1584, was quite different. The designs of Giacomo da Barozzi (know as Vignola) and Giacomo della Porta were completely in keeping with the principles of sobriety and austerity expressed by the Council of Trent and were also in accordance with the evangelical poverty preached by St. Ignatius of Loyola, founder of the order. The magnificent Baroque decoration dates from the second half of the 17th century, when the order decided that the church should offer a more explicit demonstration of the triumphs of the Catholic Church and the Jesuit order, then at the height of its power. Giovanni Battista Gaulli, called Baciccia, frescoed the vault of the nave with *The Triumph of the Name of Jesus,* one of the most majestic and original attempts at dominion over infinite space, typical of Baroque art. The altar of St. Ignatius (who is buried here) is the largest and most ornate in Rome; conceived by Andrea Pozzo, it was created by more than 100 artists and craftsmen and is made up of a profusion of white and colored marble, gilded bronze, silver, lapis lazuli, and semiprecious stones. Opposite is the altar of St. Francis Xavier, a Jesuit missionary who performed significant work in India and Japan. Designed by Pietro da Cortona, it contains a reliquary with the saint's arm.
✉*Piazza del Gesù.*

Collegio Romano
▦**3 F4–F5.** The austere edifice was built in 1582 to house the oldest and most prestigious Jesuit scholastic institution, which the order's founder, St. Ignatius of Loyola, called the "universal seminary." Internationally famous instructors teach here, and during

Velázquez's portrait of Innocent X hangs in the Galleria Doria Pamphilij, established by that same pontiff.

its history important cultural institutions have been located on the premises, including the Astronomical Observatory, the Museo Kircheriano, the Spezieria, and an extensive library. After 1870 the first state high school (Ennio Quirino Visconti) of the new Italian capital was established here. In 1930 the Jesuit university moved to the Palazzo della Pontificia Università Gregoriana, in Piazza della Pilotta. ✉*Piazza del Collegio Romano.*

Galleria Doria Pamphilj ②
▦**3 F5.** The Palazzo Doria Pamphilj, one of the grandest in Rome, is one of the few that is still inhabited by the family from which it takes its name. It houses an extraordinary art gallery, established by Innocent X in 1651, that displays works from the 16th and 17th centuries and two splendid portraits of Innocent by Diego Velázquez (1650) and Gian Lorenzo Bernini. When Camillo, the pope's nephew, married Olimpia Aldobrandini, the original collection was enriched with important works by Raphael, Titian, Beccafumi, and Parmigianino, as well as outstanding paintings from the Ferrara school. Camillo patronized the most famous artists of his time (Bernini, Borromini, Algardi, Pietro da Cortona, and Caravaggio) and acquired numerous paintings by Bolognese artists and landscapes by Claude Lorrain. The union with the Doria family (1760) brought to the gallery masterpieces by Sebastiano del Piombo and Bronzino, as well as some tapestries. The magnificent drawing room of the private apartment is also open to visitors. On the

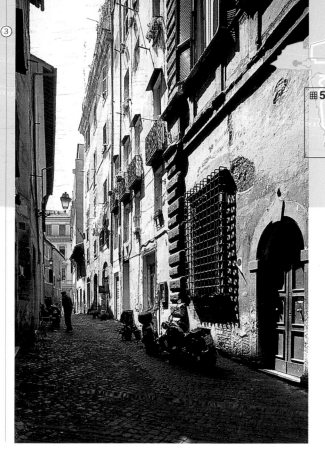

facade along the Via del Plebiscito is a magnificent 18th-century shrine that contains a group of angels and cherubs above a dense sunburst shape and supporting an oval frame with an image of the Madonna. ⊠*Piazza del Collegio Romano 2*, ☎*06/679-7323.*

Ghetto ③
⊞**5 C6.** The Jewish community in Rome, originally established in Trastevere, began to move into the S. Angelo district, near the Tiber Island, during the 13th century. A papal bull by Paul IV in 1555 established the Ghetto, imitating the one created in Venice shortly before. The area was surrounded by walls and became the obligatory and exclusive place of residence for the Roman Jews, who lived here in overcrowded and demeaning conditions. In 1848 the walls were taken down, and beginning in 1888 the Ghetto was demolished and replaced with four blocks completely disconnected from the surrounding urban fabric. The **Synagogue** (1899–1904), which replaced an earlier edifice destroyed by fire in 1903, stands out amid the city's architecture, with its pavilion-roof dome on a square drum and its Assyrian-Babylonian decorative motifs that recall the original land of the Jewish people. The facade on the Via del Tempio has Jewish symbols (a seven-arm candelabrum, the tablets of the Ten Commandments, a star of David, a palm branch). The building houses the **Museo d'Arte Ebraica,** which contains archaeological remains, sacred objects, vestments, liturgical furnishings, manuscripts, and documents. ⊠*Synagogue and Museum: Lungotevere dei Cenci,* ☎*06/684-0061.*

Palazzo Madama
⊞**3 E3–F3.** Built in 1503 as the Roman residence of the Medici family, the palazzo takes its name from "Madama" Margaret of Austria, widow of Alessandro de' Medici, who had lived here. The building changed hands many times and experienced many architectural transformations over the centuries. In 1871 it became the seat of the Italian Senate. ⊠*Piazza Madama.*

Palazzi dei Mattei
⊞**5 B6.** In the 15th century the large block defined by Via Caetani, Via Paganica, Via delle Botteghe Oscure, and Via dei Funari was occupied by the Mattei family, The family gradually built a series of palaces that bore the names of the estates of the various family branches. The oldest is the **Palazzo di Giacomo Mattei** (17–19 Piazza Mattei), erected in the mid-15th century and expanded in the 16th century. The **Palazzo Mattei Paganica,** at 4 Piazza dell'Enciclopedia Italiana, was begun in 1541 and houses the National Encyclopedia Institute. Beneath the building are the remains of the Theater of Balbo (13 BC). Behind these ruins was a large portico, the vestiges of which housed, in medieval times, various commercial and manufacturing activities, giving the street the name *botteghe oscure,* or "dark shops." The impressive **Palazzo Mattei di Giove** (31 Via dei Funari), designed by Carlo Maderno (1598–1618), has a courtyard richly decorated with ancient sculptures and stuccowork. The building houses various cultural institutions. On the facade is a simple shrine with an image of the Virgin enclosed in an oval frame decorated with stars and stuccowork flowers. ⊠*Piazza Mattei.*

Palazzo di Venezia
⊞**6 A1.** This building is the first important expression in Rome of the Renaissance canons for civil architecture theorized by Leon Battista Alberti. It was constructed in 1455 for the Venetian cardinal Pietro Barbo, who later became Paul II. It was designed as a block on a rectangular plan, with corner towers and a central courtyard with portico and loggia. The basilica of S. Marco became the Palatine Chapel, and the piazza, which was designed to complement the palace and as the monumental end for the road, became the famous end

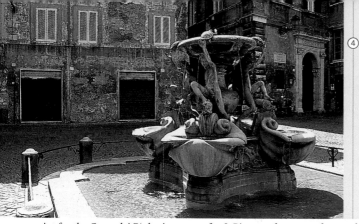

Piazza Mattei: the Fontana delle Tartarughe, a masterpiece by Giacomo della Porta (1581–1584), was embellished in 1658, perhaps by Bernini.

The dome of the Pantheon ⑤ (AD 118–AD 125), a majestic realization of imperial architecture, summarizes Romans' knowledge of building; it was used as a model by Brunelleschi for the Duomo in Florence.

point for the Corsa dei Bàrberi, a riderless horse race held at Carnival. The designer of the complex still has not been identified, but Alberti's influence is clear, both in the overall design, in the vault of the entrance hall off the piazza, and in the extremely beautiful courtyard. The name is derived from the fact that the building was given to the Venetian Republic in 1564 to house its embassy. Today it contains the **Museo di Palazzo di Venezia,** which includes paintings from the 13th to the 18th centuries, sculptures in marble and wood, bronzes, porcelain, glasswork, ivories, and tapestries. ⊠ *Via del Plebiscito 118,* ☎*06/699–94319.*

Pantheon ⑤

▥**3 F4.** This is the best preserved monument from ancient Rome, thanks to its transformation into a church (S. Maria ad Martyres) in 609. It is said that the day the building was consecrated, 28 wagons of martyrs' bones were transported here, taken from various city cemeteries. This event is the origin of All Saints' Day (November 1), instituted by Gregory IV in the 9th century. The ancient temple was built by the emperor Hadrian (AD 118–AD 125) on the site of a temple from the Augustan age (AD 27–AD 25) that was dedicated to the worship of all the gods (thus the name). It is a wonderful example of the technical skill of the Roman architects. The dome is the largest ever built in brick (142 feet in diameter; St. Peter's is 139 feet), and because the height of the dome from the floor is equal to the diameter, it defines a spherical space inserted into a cylinder, producing a sensation of perfect and simple harmony. During the Middle Ages the building was used as a fortress; in 1625, Pope Urban VIII gave Gian Lorenzo Bernini the bronze from the portico to make the baldacchi-

no for S. Pietro and cannons for Castel S. Angelo (provoking the famous pasquinade: "What the barbarians didn't do, the Barberini did"). After Raphael was buried here, during the Renaissance, the Pantheon became a burial site for artists, and in 1878 it was chosen as the site for the tombs of the kings of Italy. The **Piazza della Rotonda,** which opens up in front of the Pantheon, is one of the most popular and liveliest in Rome. In addition to the splendid, ancient monument, it is noted for its fountain, designed by Giacomo della Porta. ⊠*Piazza della Rotonda.*

Piazza Mattei ④

▥**5 B6.** This small piazza is like a jewel box, surrounding one of the most beautiful fountains in Rome, the **Fontana delle Tartarughe,** designed by Giacomo della Porta (1581–1584), with the tortoises added later, perhaps by Gian Lorenzo Bernini. The piazza is flanked by the **Palazzo Costaguti** (number 10), which dates to the mid-16th century. Its rooms, which cannot be visited, are famous for the number and quality of paintings and the richness of the furnishings. Some of the greatest 17th-century artists worked here, including Guercino, Domenichino, and the Zuccari.

Piazza della Pigna

▥**3 F4.** The name is derived from the large bronze pinecone that adorned one of the many Roman monuments in the area (it is now in the Cortile della Pigna in the Vatican). The small church of **S. Giovanni della Pigna** (51 Vicolo della Minerva) was known in the 10th century and given by Gregory XIII to the Company of Piety Toward Prisoners (1577), which had it rebuilt in 1624. Inside are tombs of two members of the aristocratic Porcari family. In 1453, Stefano Porcari was put to death

here by Pope Nicholas V for organizing a plot to install a republican government. The remains of the Porcari houses are incorporated into a 19th-century building at the back of the piazza, on the Via della Pigna.

S. Agostino

▥**3 E3.** Built in 1420, this is one of the first Renaissance churches in Rome, although it was later expanded and altered. It contains many artworks, and the high altar, designed by Gian Lorenzo Bernini, includes a Byzantine icon of the Virgin, which was brought from Constantinople after the Turkish conquest (1453). Romans venerate Jacopo Sansovino's *Madonna del Parto* (1521), and numerous ex-votos surround the sculpture. The church also has a painting of *The Prophet Isaiah* by Raphael (1512), a sculpture group of *St. Anne and the Madonna with Child* by Andrea Sansovino (1512), and a 15th-century panel depicting *God the Father.* But the church's most famous work is the *Madonna dei Pellegrini* by Caravaggio (1605), which caused an uproar from the start because of the lowly and domestic setting it portrays and the realism of its dirty and tattered pilgrims. To the side of the church is the **Biblioteca Angelica** (8 Piazza S. Agostino), the first public library in Rome, established in 1614 by the Augustinian Angelo Rocca and specializing in ecclesiastical and historical-literary studies. It contains more than 1,000 books, manuscripts, incunabula, and prints, as well as two globes, celestial and terrestrial, from 1599–1603, the only ones of this type in Italy. ⊠*Piazza S. Agostino.*

S. Carlo ai Catinari ⑦

▥**5 B5.** The name of this church refers to both St. Charles Borromeo and to the bowl-makers who worked in the district. It was

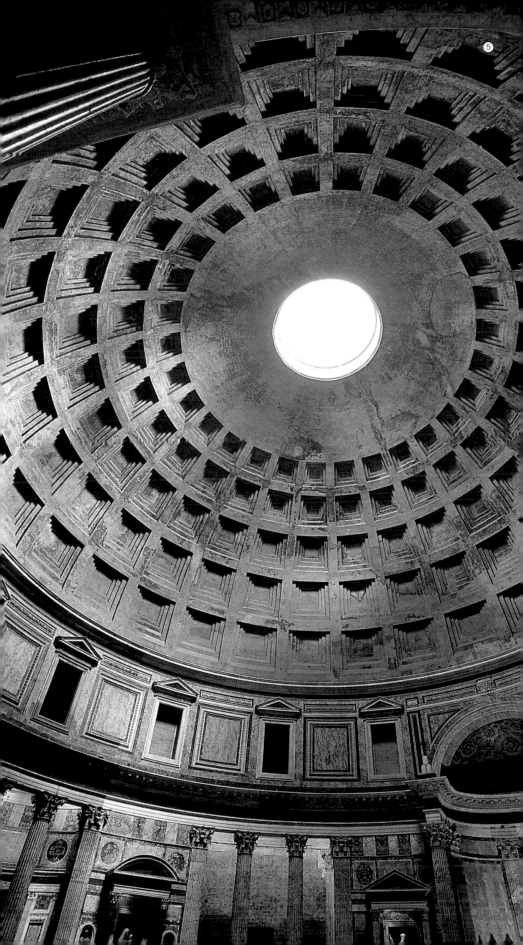

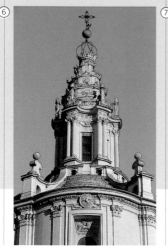

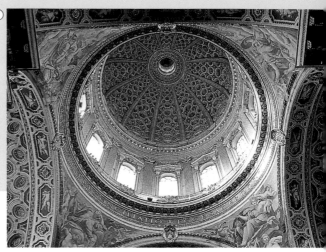

built for the Barnabites in 1610–1620, in honor of the most important figure of the Catholic Reformation and the inspiration for the political and apostolic action of Pius IV. The architect was Rosato Rosati, and the soaring dome is one of the most beautiful in the city. The church has many paintings inspired by the life and works of the titular saint, including works by Domenichino, Pietro da Cortona, and Guido Reni. ⊠ *Piazza Cairoli*

S. Caterina dei Funari
▦ **5 B6.** The church's name refers to the rope-makers who worked in the ruins of the portico of the Theater of Balbo, vestiges of which were discovered in the area behind the church. An earlier medieval church, given by Paul III to St. Ignatius of Loyola (1537), became the seat of the Confraternity of the Miserable Virgins and was rebuilt in 1564. The beautiful travertine facade has two rows of Corinthian pilasters, festoons, and other relief ornamentation. ⊠ *Via dei Funari*

S. Eustachio
▦ **3 F3.** According to one of the many legends related to his life, Eustace was a valiant general in the troops of the Emperor Trajan (2nd century AD). He converted to Christianity after encountering a stag with a cross on its head during a hunting party. A stag's head with a cross can be seen on the tympanum of the church, which Constantine founded, supposedly on the site of the saint's martyrdom. The church was restored in the 12th century (the bell tower belongs to this phase) and partially rebuilt during the 18th century. The interior has a notable high

altar in bronze and polychrome marble by Nicola Salvi (1739), surmounted by a baldacchino by Ferdinando Fuga (1746). ⊠ *Via S. Eustachio 19.*

S. Gregorio della Divina Pietà
▦ **5 C6.** Legend has it that the church stands on the site of the birthplace of St. Gregory the Great (ca. 540–604). The church's current appearance dates from 1729, when Benedict XIII renovated it and gave it to the Congregazione degli Operai della Divina Pietà, which assisted aristocratic families that had fallen upon hard times. A plaque on the facade has a biblical passage in Hebrew and Latin that reproaches the Jews for persevering in their faith. The church stands near one of the entrances to the Ghetto and was used for the compulsory sermons to the Jewish community. ⊠ *Piazza Monte Savello 9.*

S. Ivo alla Sapienza ⑥
▦ **3 F3.** This church is incorporated within the **Palazzo della Sapienza,** which was the site of the University of Rome until 1935 and now houses the State Archives. Urban VIII wanted to transform the ancient university chapel and entrusted the work to Borromini, who best expressed his talent in the church of S. Ivo (1642–1660). As in S. Carlino, the architect adopted a central plan, but one based on a hexagon, unusual in Italian architecture. The same motif is repeated in the light-filled dome and, on the exterior, in the multifoiled drum. Most amazing, however, is the twisting spire surmounted by an aerial structure in iron. The structure must have looked disconcerting and almost

scandalous in a city filled with serene, rotund domes. It is no accident that there is nothing else like it in Rome. With its powerful vertical thrust and the blinding whiteness of the interior, S. Ivo is one of the most accomplished expressions of the period's quest for spiritual renewal. ⊠ *Corso Rinascimento 40.*

S. Luigi dei Francesi ⑧
▦ **3 E3.** In the late 15th century the French colony acquired a small church and made it the center of their public assistance services. They planned a renovation, which was carried out in 1589. All the figures on the facade are French: below, Charlemagne and St. Louis (Louis IX, king of France, who died during the Eighth Crusade in 1270); above, St. Clotilde (5th-century queen of the Franks and patron saint of women) and St. Joan of Valois (daughter of Louis XI, founder of the Order of the Nuns of the Annunziata in 1500). St. Louis is honored in the fresco at the center of the vault (1756). The high altar has an *Annunciation* by Francesco Bassano, and one of the chapels has Domenichino's *Scenes from the Life of St. Caecilia* (1616–1617). The church's principal attraction is the chapel painted by Caravaggio for the French cardinal Mathieu Cointrel (1599–1602, ☞ *151*), also known as the Cantarelli chapel. The three canvases (*Martyrdom of St. Matthew, The Calling of St. Matthew,* and *St. Matthew with the Angel*) reveal miracles occurring in the midst of everyday reality, an event shared by all and perennially relevant. Light plays a new and decisive role in these paintings, which later artists could not ignore. Numerous tombs testify to the continuous French

S. Carlo ai Catinari's ⑦ wonderful dome, from 1620, has pendentives with paintings by Domenichino depicting the *Cardinal Virtues*.

The broad and solemn 16th-century facade of S. Luigi dei Francesi ⑧, created in travertine; one of the numerous masterpieces contained within is Caravaggio's canvas of *St. Matthew with the Angel*.

⑧

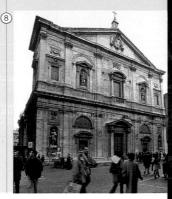

presence in Rome, and the painter Claude Lorrain (1600–1682), who spent decades lovingly studying the Roman countryside, is buried here. Next to the national French church is the **Palazzo di S. Luigi**, the facade of which, on the Via di S. Giovanna d'Arco, has a theatrical entrance surmounted by a loggia. For centuries it was the principal institution offering assistance to French pilgrims and residents of the city. ✉ *Piazza S. Luigi dei Francesi 5.*

S. Marco
⊞**6 A1.** Completely renovated by Paul II during the second half of the 15th century, this basilica became the private chapel for the pope's newly built Palazzo di Venezia. But its origins are much earlier; it was founded in the 4th century by Pope St. Mark in honor of the evangelist of the same name. It was rebuilt by Gregory IV in the 9th century, and the mosaics in the apse are from this period. They depict a standing Christ, flanked by various saints including the evangelist Mark and Pope Mark, as well as the donor, Pope Gregory, holding a model of the church. The solemn facade, with a three-arch portico surmounted by a loggia, was constructed with materials from the Coliseum and the Theater of Marcellus. The gilded and blue coffered ceiling is one of two 15th-century ceilings that survive in Rome (the other is in S. Maria Maggiore). The church's outstanding artistic patrimony includes works by Palma the Younger, Melozzo da Forlì, and Antonio Canova. The granite tomb in the presbytery contains the remains of Pope Mark and the Christian martyr saints Abdon and Sennen. ✉ *Piazza S. Marco 48.*

S. Maria sopra Minerva ⑨
⊞**3 F4.** The church gets its name from the ruins of the Roman temple of Minerva Calcidica, believed to lie below. Entrusted to the Dominicans, it was rebuilt beginning in 1280 and was altered and expanded many times over the centuries, up to an unfortunate Gothic-style renovation in the 19th century. The Dominicans, always firm supporters of the church, particularly in matters of doctrine, became especially powerful during the Counter-Reformation, when they dominated the Inquisition Tribunal. This explains the importance assumed by this church, its sumptuous aristocratic chapels, and the extraordinary wealth of its artistic patrimony. The statue of the *Resurrected Christ* by Michelangelo (1519–1520), the frescoes by Filippino Lippi (1488–1493) in the Carafa Chapel, the funerary monuments of Clement VII and Leo X by Antonio Giamberti da Sangallo the Younger (1536–1541), and the funerary monument of Francesco Tornabuoni by Mino da Fiesole (1480) are some of the many works of art in this church. Two famous Tuscans are also buried here: St. Catherine of Siena (☞ 51), patron saint of Italy, who died in Rome in 1380, and Fra Angelico, Dominican painter of the monastery of S. Marco in Florence, who died in 1455. The monastery contains the **Biblioteca Casanatense**, which specializes in theology and church history. ✉ *Piazza della Minerva.*

S. Maria in Monterone
⊞**3 F3.** The name derives from the Sienese Monterone family, who founded a hospice next to the church for their compatriots. The building, mentioned as far back as 1186 and entirely rebuilt in 1682, has eight Ionic columns in the interior. In 1728, the Mercedari, then in possession of the church, had the adjacent monastery built with an elegant rococo facade. ✉ *Via Monterone 75.*

S. Maria in Via Lata
⊞**3 F5.** According to ancient tradition, the church stands on the spot where Sts. Peter and Paul and the evangelists John and Luke stayed. Storerooms from the Roman Empire were discovered beneath the edifice and were transformed into an oratory during the 5th century. When an upper level was added to the church in the 9th century, these structures were enclosed. The building was renovated in the 17th century, when Pietro da Cortona created the elegant facade and portico. The interior is decorated with frescoes and Baroque-era marble and stuccowork. The high altar, attributed to Gian Lorenzo Bernini, has a 13th-century panel with an image of the *Vergine Advocata,* which is kept in a case adorned with precious gems. The painting is venerated by pilgrims and Romans alike because of the numerous miracles attributed to it. The name of the church derives from the name of the ancient Roman street, which corresponds to the present-day Via del Corso, the urban portion of the Via Flaminia. ✉ *Via del Corso 306.*

S. Nicola in Carcere
⊞**5 C6.** This church has ancient origins (perhaps 7th century) and stands on the ruins of three Roman temples. It was rebuilt in 1128 and renovated numerous times during subsequent centuries. It was probably attended by the Greek colony that resided in the district, which may explain its dedication to a Greek saint; "in carcere" refers to a prison that existed on the site during the 8th century. The simple facade, which incorporates two ancient columns, is by Giacomo della Porta (1599).

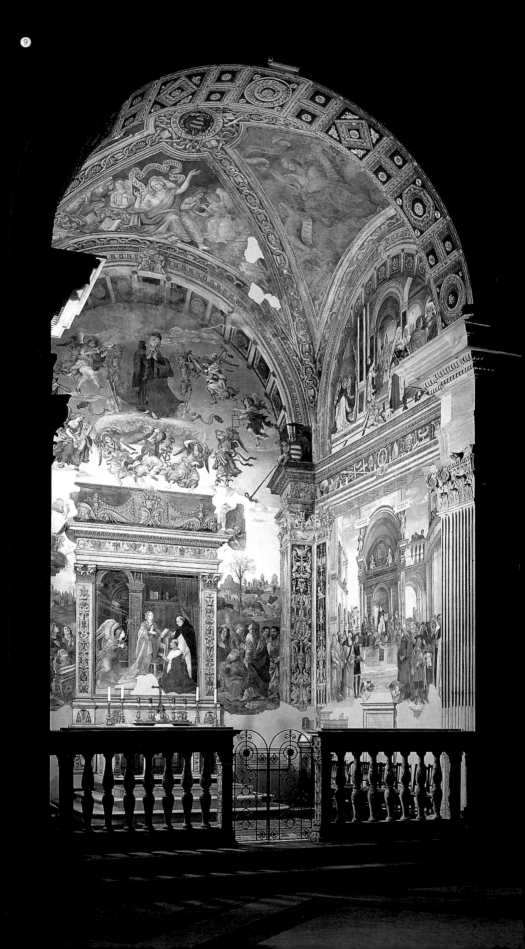

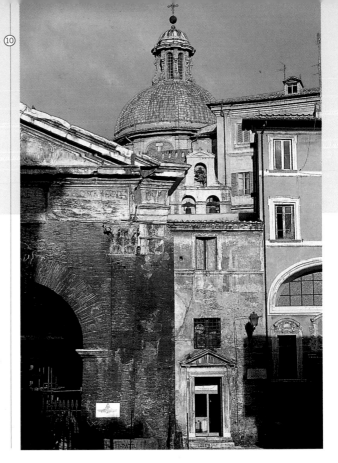

The Carafa Chapel, entirely covered with frescoes by Filippino Lippi (1488–1493), is one of the treasures of S. Maria sopra Minerva ⑨, which is extraordinarily rich in outstanding masterpieces.

Part of the elegant front of the Portico d'Ottavia ⑩, a monument from ancient Rome and, in the back, a view of the dome of S. Angelo in Pescheria.

In Roman times this area was bounded by the slopes of the Campidoglio, the Theater of Marcellus, and the Tiber port, where the vegetable market (Foro Olitorio) was located. Vestiges of the three ancient temples are visible both outside and inside the church; these have been identified in ancient writings as the temples dedicated to Hope, Janus, and Juno the Deliverer. ⊠ *Via del Foro Olitorio*

S. Stefano del Cacco
⊞**5 A6.** The church was built on the ruins of the Temple of Isis, the most important sanctuary of the Egyptian cult in ancient Rome. A statue of an Egyptian divinity with the head of a monkey (a *macaco*, or croo monkey) was discovered nearby, hence the name of the church. Already known in the early Middle Ages, the church was restored many times (the bell tower and apse are from the 12th century). In 1607, it was renovated by the Sylvestrine monks to whom the church had been granted in 1563 and who still serve here. ⊠ *Via S. Stefano del Cacco 26.*

Via delle Coppelle
⊞**3 E3–E4.** The street takes its name from the barrel-makers who worked in the area during the Middle Ages. The **Palazzo Baldassini** at number 35 was designed by Antonio Giamberti da Sangallo the Younger (1514–1525) and is organized around a courtyard with a portico and loggia; some traces of Renaissance frescoes, grotesques, and stuccowork remain. Today it houses the Luigi Sturzo Institute, which promotes studies in the political, historical, and social sciences. The institute has a specialized library and extensive archive with documents relating to the working-class Catholics who played a decisive role in founding the Christian Democratic

Party and in postwar Italian politics. Since 1663 **S. Salvatore alle Coppelle** (72b Piazza delle Coppelle), rebuilt over an older church in the 18th century, has been the headquarters for the Confraternity of Perseverance, which was established to assist foreigners who are taken ill.

Via del Portico d'Ottavia ⑩
⊞**5 B6–C6.** The Portico d'Ottavia was an enormous square portico, built in the 2nd century BC and rebuilt by the emperor Augustus (23 BC), who dedicated it to his sister Octavia. During the Middle Ages it was the site of a busy commercial center; a fish market, which dated to that time, functioned until 1880. The only trace of the Roman building that remains is the majestic propylaea, which function as the entrance to the church of **S. Angelo in Pescheria** (6 Via di Tribuna Campitelli), built in the 8th century but restored on numerous occasions. Next to the church is the **S. Andrea dei Pescivendoli** oratory (1689), which has a beautiful facade decorated in stuccowork. The street has some medieval and Renaissance buildings, such as the

13th-century **Torre dei Grassi** (at number 25), the 15th-century **Case dei Fabi** (at numbers 8 and 13), and the **Casa di Lorenzo Manilio** (1468), which is decorated with ancient sculptures and epigraphs.

6
Campo Marzio

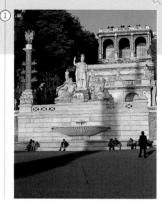

In ancient times this district was dominated by large public monuments, and it remained sparsely inhabited for a long time thereafter. During the 15th century it began to be more densely populated when the commercial mooring on the Tiber, near the tomb of Augustus, attracted groups of foreign merchants (Dalmatians, Illyrians, Bretons, and others), and numerous sites were established to assist the growing influx of pilgrims and foreigners who arrived in the city at Porta del Popolo. The creation of the trident, formed by Via del Corso, Via del Babuino, and Via di Ripetta, during the 16th century initiated a period of gradual urbanization, which increased over the next two centuries. In addition to churches and aristocratic palazzi, the district was embellished with various infrastructures to accommodate foreigners making the grand tour (including many artists and writers), who increasingly made Rome one of their stops. Numerous inns were opened, then hotels, cafés, artists' studios, and artisan workshops, which soon turned the Campo Marzio into a center of international tourism for the city.

Ara Pacis Augustae
⊞3 C3. The peace established by Augustus after a century of bloody civil wars was celebrated with this monument, erected between 13 BC and 9 BC in the Campo Marzio. The remains of the altar were discovered in various stages, begin-

ning in the 16th century. The monument consists of a marble enclosure, entirely decorated in reliefs that, high above a flight of steps, surround the actual altar. The reliefs on the long sides depict a procession of figures from the imperial family and allude to the dynastic continuity necessary for the stability of the empire. Four panels on the short sides show the majestic figures of *Pax*, portrayed as a woman in a luxuriant landscape, and the goddess *Roma*. Two other mythological scenes (*Aeneas Making a Sacrifice* and *Lupercalia*) evoke the origins of the capital city. The Altar of Peace has been protected inside a glass pavilion since the 1930s. ⊠ *Piazza Augusto Imperatore*.

Chiesa di Gesù e Maria
⊞3 B4. Both the church and the adjacent convent were built in between 1672 and 1675 by the Discalced Hermit Monks of St. Augustine as a monastery for contemplatives and mendicants. The sober facade reflects the austerity of the order's life, while the magnificent interior, rich in polychrome marble, stuccowork, and paintings, expresses the Baroque taste for theatricality and sumptuous decoration. The single barrel-vaulted nave houses four funerary monuments of the Bolognetti family (1678–1690), conceived as theater stages for the figures. The confessionals below are masterpieces of cabinetmaking. ⊠ *Via del Corso 45*.

Chiesa del Divino Amore
⊞3 D4. During the 12th century a church was erected here, dedicated to St. Caecilia, on the site where, according to tradition, the house of the saint's father stood. In 1729, the structure, which was also dedicated to St. Blaise, was rebuilt by the mattress-makers' guild, following a design by Filippo Raguzzini that preserved the ancient bell tower with two stories of three-mullioned windows. In 1801 the church was given to the Confraternity of the Madonna del Divino Amore, hence its current name. The confraternity, founded in 1744, was previously located in a sanctuary of the same name on the Via Ardeatina. ⊠ *Vicolo del Divino Amore*.

Chiesa della Trinità dei Monti
⊞3 C5. The church was financed by the sovereigns of France, who were overwhelmed by the sanctity and miracles worked by Francis of Paola, the famous Calabrian hermit who was sent by Sixtus IV to the bedside of Louis XI, king of France, and was for many years an advisor to Louis's son, Charles VIII. The latter provided the saint with the means to establish a monastery for his order, the Minim Friars, with a church dedicated to the Trinity. Its position atop the Pincio, overlooking the city, and its soaring facade flanked by two bell towers have made it one of the most well-known sites in Rome. The church houses a wealth of artwork, including one of the most famous frescoes in Rome, Daniele da Volterra's *Deposition*, which shows the strong influence of Michelangelo. The monastery refectory was decorated by Andrea Pozzo (1694), the cloister by other Mannerists, who painted scenes from the life of St. Francis of Paola. The piazza of the same name, with the obelisk of Sallust at its center, marked the beginning of the Strada Felice, the long, straight street conceived by

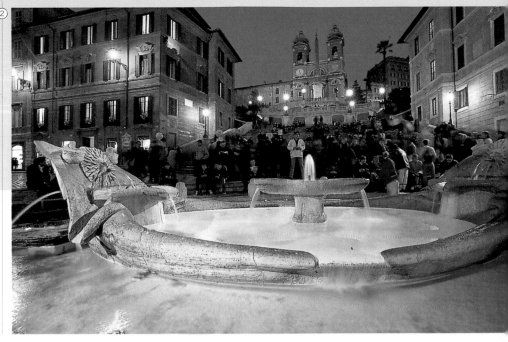

Sixtus V, linking Trinità di Monte with S. Croce in Gerusalemme. ✉ *Piazza Trinità dei Monti 3.*

Colonna dell'Immacolata Concezione

⊞ **3 C5.** In 1845 Pius IX proclaimed the dogma of the Immaculate Conception of Mary, after centuries of study and debate on the subject. To celebrate this event, a monument was erected that incorporated a column of marble that was discovered in the Campo Marzio a century before. A broad octagonal base embellished with statues of the prophets Moses, Isaiah, Ezekial, and David supports the column, which in turn is surmounted by a bronze statue of the Virgin. Since 1929 there has been a tradition to leave flowers at the column on the Feast of the Immaculate Conception (December 8), which is marked with popular celebrations and the participation of the pope. ✉ *Piazza di Spagna.*

Palazzo Borghese

⊞ **3 C4–D4.** In 1596 Cardinal Camillo Borghese purchased this palazzo, which had been built a few years earlier. After he became Paul V, he had the building enlarged by Flaminio Ponzio, who transformed it into a palace for the Borghese family. The Largo della Fontanella Borghese leads to the majestic courtyard with two-story arcades decorated with ancient statues. At the back of the courtyard is a magnificent pool, called the Bath of

Venus, embellished with Baroque statues and fountains. The palace used to house a famous art gallery, which was moved to the Villa Borghese in 1891. The large building opposite the main facade of the palazzo was set aside for employees and stables. For approximately 50 years, Piazza Borghese has been the site of a famous stamp and rare book market. ✉ *Piazza Borghese.*

Palazzo Ruspoli

⊞ **3 C4–D4.** Built by Bartolomeo Ammannati (1556–1586) for the Ruccellai family, the building passed into the hands of the Caetani, and then, in 1776, the Ruspoli family. Martino Longhi the Younger designed the famous grand staircase (1640), considered one of the jewels of civil Roman architecture, and the Mannerist Jacopo Zucchi frescoed the gallery of the piano nobile. The ground-floor rooms used to house the Caffè Nuovo, a favorite meeting place in 19th-century Rome. ✉ *Piazza S. Lorenzo in Lucina.*

Piazza del Popolo ①

⊞ **3 A3–A4.** In medieval times, well before the piazza took on its current theatrical appearance, this was the principal entrance point to the city for pilgrims and travelers from the north, who arrived along the Via Flaminia near the church of S. Maria del Popolo. The piazza's appearance began to take shape when Sixtus V erected the Egyptian obelisk of Ramses II in 1589 to

punctuate the junction of the trident made up of the Via di Ripetta, Via del Corso, and Via del Babuino. The growing influx of visitors necessitated further reorganization of the space, which was designed by Giuseppe Valadier in the early 19th century and completed with the creation of two large semicircles and ramps that climb to the Pincio belvedere. For centuries the piazza was the point of departure for solemn processions of sovereigns and ambassadors; it was also the site of Carnival festivals, games, and fairs. The **Porta del Popolo**, the ancient Porta Flaminia in the Aurelian Wall, has a majestic interior facade by Gian Lorenzo Bernini, created on the occasion of the arrival of Queen Cristina of Sweden (1655). When she converted to Catholicism, Pope Alexander VII gave her a triumphal welcome to the city, in part because the event represented a Catholic victory after the humiliation the church suffered in the Peace of Westphalia.

Piazza di Spagna ②

⊞ **3 C5.** The name dates from the 17th century (it was previously called Piazza della Trinità), when the Spanish Embassy was installed in the Palazzo Monaldeschi. This period also marked the beginning of a violent rivalry for possession of the piazza between Spain and France, which owned the church overlooking the space. In 1629, an unusual fountain in the form of a semisubmerged boat (the

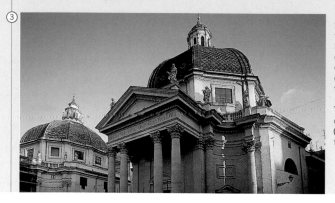

S. Maria dei Miracoli, in foreground, and S. Maria di Montesanto ③, the twin churches of Piazza del Popolo, were commissioned by Alexander VII and designed by Carlo Rainaldi to mark the beginning of Via del Corso.

The soaring interior of S. Maria della Concezione in Campo Marzio ④ contains numerous works of art from Eastern Rite churches.

Barcaccia) was erected at the center of the piazza at the behest of Urban VII, who wanted to commemorate the disastrous flood of 1598. The fountain design was entrusted to Pietro Bernini, but the clever solution of the street-level basin (to get around the difficulty of poor water pressure) reveals the imagination of Pietro's son, Gian Lorenzo. The finishing touch to the piazza's theatrical design is the **scalinata,** the stairway leading up to the church (on axis with the Barcaccia and the Via Condotti). It was built in between 1723 and 1726, after decades of proposals, and was designed by Francesco De Sanctis, who replaced two existing tree-lined streets. Triumphal and yet simple, the stairway of Piazza di Spagna is one of the most magnificent and characteristic creations of the early 18th century. On the right is the **Casina Rossa,** where the poet John Keats died in 1821 and which now houses the Keats-Shelley Memorial House, one of the most complete libraries of the English Romantic period. ✉ *Casina Rossa: 26 Piazza di Spagna,* ☎ *06/678–4235.*

S. Antonio dei Portoghesi
▦**3 D3.** The church was built around the mid-17th century in a district with a Portuguese community, on the site of a hospice for Portuguese pilgrims. The fanciful Baroque ornamentation of the church's facade includes two virile figures that support the side volutes and two angels with trumpets on the tympanum. ✉ *Via dei Portoghesi 2.*

S. Giacomo in Augusta
▦**3 B4.** This was the church of the ancient hospital of S. Giacomo degli Incurabili; its name comes from its location near the tomb of Augustus. The church was rebuilt in 1592–1600 by Francesco da Volterra and Carlo Maderno, on an elliptical plan with an imposing facade and, for the first time in Rome, two bell towers to the sides of the apse, instead of flanking the facade. In the 16th century the **Ospedale di S. Giacomo,** founded in 1338, specialized in incurable diseases, particularly syphilis, which was known as the French disease because it was introduced to Roman citizens by the troops of Charles VIII. The great need for shelters at the time necessitated a partial renovation of the hospital, which became one of the most important charity and welfare institutions in the city. The hospital pharmacy became famous for the preparation of an infusion known as Holy Wood, which was thought to be particularly effective for alleviating the effects of syphilis. ✉ *Via del Corso 499.*

S. Girolamo degli Illirici
▦**3 C3.** A community of immigrants from Illyria and Croatia, threatened by the Turks, moved to Rome in the 14th century. In 1453, they obtained from the pope the little church of S. Marina, near the port of Ripetta, and they rededicated the building to their national saint. Sixtus V had the church rebuilt by Martino Longhi (1588) the Elder, with a Renaissance facade in travertine, with two orders of pilaster strips and a small bell tower. ✉ *Piazza Porto di Ripetta.*

S. Ivo dei Brettoni
▦**3 D3.** The present-day church is the result of a 19th-century renovation of an older house of worship, given by Callistus III to the French community from Brittany, to which it still belongs. It became a center of hospitality and assistance for pilgrims from that region. St. Ivo Hélory (1253–1303), patron saint of Brittany, was particularly dedicated to the legal protection of the poor, and the future confraternities of St. Ivo were inspired by his example. ✉ *Vicolo della Campana*

S. Maria della Concezione in Campo Marzio ④
▦**3 E4.** This is an Eastern, Antiochene rite Catholic church, founded around 750 by Pope Zacharias for a group of nuns from the Convent of St. Anastasia in Constantinople. The nuns had been forced to flee the persecutions of Emperor Leo III (717–741), who forbade the making and worship of holy images. The church housed a great number of Byzantine icons, one of which— the 12- to 13-century *Madonna Advocata*—still adorns the high altar; it depicts the Virgin in a gesture of intercession, her right arm raised and her left on her chest. During later years, the church and convent complex were taken over by Benedictine nuns and gained the support of various Roman aristocratic families. The building was completely redesigned in its current Baroque form between 1668 and 1685. The former Convent of S. Maria encompasses the medieval church of **S. Gregorio Nazianzeno** (3 Vicolo Valdina), which has frescoes dating from the 11th and 12th centuries and a beautiful Romanesque bell tower (12th–13th century) with four rows of mullioned windows. ✉ *Piazza Campo Marzio 45.*

S. Maria di Montesanto and S. Maria dei Miracoli ③
▦**3 A4.** These "twin" churches act as monumental entrances to the Via del Corso and are essential elements in the theatrical design of Piazza del Popolo and the trident (Via del Corso, Via di Ripetta, Via del Babuino) that radiates out from the piazza. Alexander VII understood the urban necessity for these two structures, which were begun by Carlo Rainaldi and

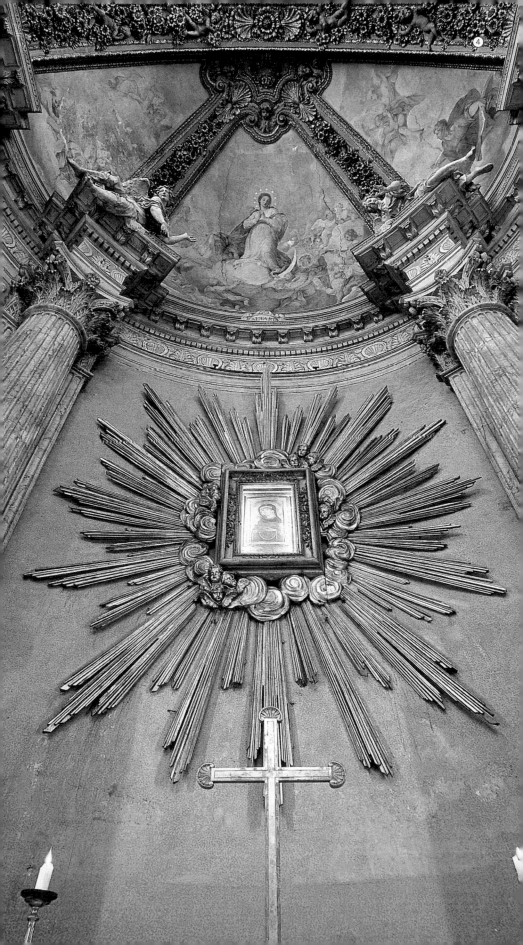

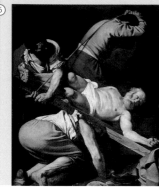

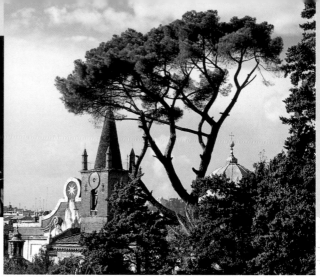

completed by Gian Lorenzo Bernini and Carlo Fontana in the late 17th century. Both churches have a central plan and are preceded by an open vestibule with four columns with statues, but their appearances differ. S. Maria di Montesanto has an elliptical plan and a dodecagonal dome; S. Maria dei Miracoli has a circular plan and an octagonal dome. The former church has statues of saints (1674) on its facade, perhaps conceived by Bernini, and houses a late 14th-century panel depicting the Virgin of Montesanto, as well as bronze portraits of various popes. S. Maria dei Miracoli takes its name from a painting of the Madonna over the high altar. The facade has statues of saints that show the influence of Bernini and an extremely elegant 18th-century bell tower. ⌧ *Piazza del Popolo.*

S. Maria del Popolo ⑤
⊞**3 A4.** The current building was preceded by a chapel erected by Paschal II in 1099, at the end of the First Crusade. The name most likely reflects the fact the Roman people financed the construction. Reconstruction, which began in the late 15th century, involved numerous illustrious architects. Bramante redesigned the choir, Raphael designed the Chigi Chapel, Carlo Fontana the Cybo Chapel, and Gian Lorenzo Bernini made various contributions to the structure and furnishings. The interior is a treasure trove of works of art. The choir contains monuments of Cardinals Ascanio Sforza and Girolamo Basso della Rovere (1505–1507), masterpieces by Andrea Sansovino; above these are precious painted windows by Guillaume de Marcillat (*Childhood of Christ* and *Scenes from the Life of the Virgin*, 1509). Pinturicchio painted the beautiful frescoes on the vault (*Coronation of Mary, with Evangelists, Sibyls, and Doctors of*

the Church, 1508–1510), and Raphael provided the drawings for the mosaics in the dome (*God, Creator of the Firmament, with Symbols of the Sun and the Seven Planets*, 1516). The church's most famous artworks are Caravaggio's two masterpieces, in the first chapel in the left transept: *The Crucifixion of St. Peter* and *The Conversion of St. Paul* (1601–1602). Luther stayed at the Augustinian monastery attached to the church. ⌧ *Piazza del Popolo 12.*

S. Maria Portae Paradisi
⊞**3 B4.** The origin of this church's name (St. Maria of Heaven's Gate) is uncertain. It was rebuilt in 1523 by Antonio Giamberti da Sangallo the Younger. Above the entrance is a marble relief of a *Madonna and Child* by Andrea Sansovino. The octagonal interior beneath the dome has rich decorative frescoes and stuccowork and includes, among other things, notable funerary monuments of Matteo Caccia (1645) by Cosimo Fancelli and of Antonio di Burgos by Baldassarre Peruzzi (1526). ⌧ *Via Canova 29.*

S. Rocco
⊞**3 C3–C4.** Built in 1499 by the Confraternity of the Porto di Ripetta, the church was rebuilt in the 17th century and underwent a later Neoclassical restoration. The hospital of the confraternity, adjacent to the church, was transformed in 1517 into a lying-in hospital that welcomed "honest but unmarried women." Women were assisted in absolute confidentiality, so their pregnancies were never known to the world outside. Inside the church, to the left of the presbytery, an elegant chapel has a venerated image of the *Madonna*

delle Grazie (17th century). ⌧ *Largo S. Rocco 1.*

Ss. Ambrogio e Carlo al Corso ⑥
⊞**3 C4.** St. Ambrose and St. Charles Borromeo were, respectively, the bishop of Milan in the 4th century and the archbishop of the same city in the 16th century. The two saints, who played a defining role in the history of the church, are the most venerated in Lombardy, and the community from that region was responsible for the building of this house of worship, beginning in 1612. The project was entrusted to Onorio Longhi and to Martino Longhi the Younger, then to Pietro da Cortona, who designed the dome (one of the most beautiful in the city) and the interior decoration. The floor plan is unique in Rome, with a continuation of the side naves in an ambulatory, within the presbyteryan— obvious reference to Gothic models, such as Milan's cathedral. The magnificent interior has an extremely rich Baroque decorative scheme, much of which celebrates St. Charles. The most noteworthy artwork is the high altar by Carlo Maratta (1685–1690), which has a *Glory of Sts. Ambrose and Charles*. In the ambulatory, in a niche behind the high altar, is a fine 17th-century reliquary containing the heart of St. Charles. ⌧ *Via del Corso 437.*

Via del Babuino
⊞**3 A4–B4–B5.** The straight line that joins Piazza del Popolo to Piazza di Spagna was laid out by Clement VII and Paul III during the first half of the 16th century and takes its name from an ancient statue of a silenus, now next to the church

The *Crucifixion of Peter*, a masterpiece by Caravaggio, is one of two splendid canvases by the artist in S. Maria del Popolo ⑤. The church is adjacent to the beautiful park on the Pincio that is filled with pine trees.

Ss. Ambrogio e Carlo al Corso ⑥, dedicated to two major Lombard saints, is surmounted by a late Baroque dome of great interest. It was built in between 1668 and 1669 by Pietro da Cortona.

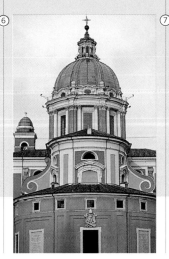

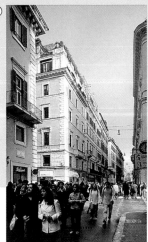

of S. Atanasio. Along with the nearby Via Margutta, the new street was soon inhabited by out-of-towners (predominantly Neapolitans) and by artists. It then became well known for its art and antiques trade, which still makes it one of most popular streets in the historic center. At number 149 is the Greek Catholic church of **S. Atanasio** (1580–1583), with an unusual and charming interior; at number 153b is the interesting English evangelical church of **Ognissanti** (All Saints), one of the few neo-Gothic structures in Rome (1882–1887).

Via dei Condotti
▦3 C4–C5. This is one section of the long Via Trinitatis, laid out by Paul III (1534–1549), which linked the church of Trinità dei Monti to the Tiber. The street takes its name from the important waterlines (*condotti*) that ran beneath, supplying the entire Campo Marzio. Today the street is famous for its luxury clothing and jewelry shops, but during the 18th and 19th centuries it was the heart of the city, with the most exclusive and renowned hotels and cafés frequented by artists, intellectuals, and travelers. Of these, the oldest (1760) and most famous is the **Caffè Greco** (number 86), which over the years was patronized by Gogol, Stendhal, Modigliani, and Toscanini, and which still has some of the original furnishings. The street has other elegant buildings, including the **Palazzo dell'Ordine di Malta** (Palace of the Knights of Malta, number 68), built in the 17th century and expanded in the 19th century, with some original wooden ceilings still visible. Nearby is the church of the **SS. Trinità dei Spagnoli** (at number 441 of the street of the same name) and the adjacent monastery, built in 1741–1746. The church has various paintings

depicting Giovanni di Matha and Felice di Valois, the two French priests who, in the late 12th century, founded the Trinitarians. The order worked devotedly, first in Europe, then throughout the world, for the liberation of prisoners and slaves.

Via del Corso ⑦
▦3 A4–F5. This is a section of the ancient Via Flaminia and was for centuries the principal access route to the city for visitors and pilgrims from the north. During the early centuries of Christianity, the street was lined some of the most ancient churches in the city, including S. Marcello, S. Lorenzo in Lucina, S. Maria in Via Lata, S. Maria in Aquiro and S. Silvestro in Capite. The **Ospedale di S. Giacomo** (1339) was instrumental to the street's subsequent development. The Renaissance and Counter-Reformation popes made the street more uniform, with the transformation of the modest existing houses into aristocratic palazzi; they also built numerous new churches (S. Giacomo in Augusta, Ss. Ambrogio e Carlo al Corso, Gesù e Maria). During this time the street became a setting for festivals, parades, and spectacles, particularly the famous Carnival races, from which the street gets its name and which, until the late 19th century, were the most widely attended events in the city. Artists, writers, and musicians from throughout Europe popularized an extremely lively image of Roman Carnival, contributing to the widespread image of the extroverted, boisterous Roman.

Via dei Prefetti
▦3 D4. During medieval times, prefects (citizen governors) had their offices on this street. The most important building today is the 16th-century **Palazzo di Firenze** (number 27), so-called because of the Medici family from Florence. The building now houses the Dante Alighieri Society, dedicated to the dissemination of Italian language and culture throughout the world. Midway down the street is the small **Chapel of the Madonna della Pietà** also known as the Chapel of Divino Amore, because of its proximity to the church of the same name. It is dominated by an impressive 17th-century Madonna and child.

Via di Ripetta
▦3 A4–D3. Laid out at the behest of Leo X in 1518, the street was called Via Leonina until the 18th century, when it was renamed for its proximity to the Ripetta embankment. The design of the Tiber embankment, which entailed the destruction of the Porto di Ripetta (one of the most important examples of 18th-century Roman architecture) and the isolation of the tomb of Augustus, eliminated a precious portion of the ancient building fabric along the street. There are, however, still significant buildings to be seen. In addition to two imposing monuments erected by the first Roman emperor (the Ara Pacis and the tomb of Augustus), there are also the churches of S. Girolamo degli Illirici, S. Maria Portae Paradisi, and S. Rocco.

7
Trevi and Colonna

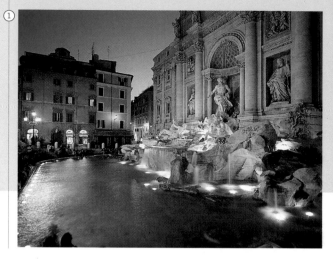

With the excepftion of the areas adjacent to the Trevi and SS. Apostoli piazzas, the Trevi district was sparsely inhabited until the Renaissance. Urbanization began during the papacy of Sixtus V, with the opening in 1585 of the Strada Felice. During the two subsequent centuries the area was enriched with new churches and palazzi, both in the lower zone, near Piazza SS. Apostoli, and around the papal residence on the Quirinal Hill. Rome's new function as a capital city brought transformations, such as the construction of government buildings on the Quirinal and the opening of the Via del Tritone, Via Barberini, Via Bissolati, and the King Umberto I Tunnel. The Colonna district, which in medieval times had many residences and churches along the Via del Corso, continued to develop, thanks to the interventions of Gregory XIII and Sixtus V. Between the 18th and 19th century, the area adjacent to Via del Corso became the social heart of the city, the site of popular celebrations, cafés, and the first political demonstrations. The area at the foot of the Pincio has preserved its original character, but the zone around Montecitorio underwent profound transformations after 1870. This became the political city (Palazzo di Montecitorio, Palazzo Chigi) that replaced entire city blocks and continues to expand.

Chiesa del SS. Nome di Maria
6 A2. Built in 1737 for the Confraternity of the Most Holy Name of Mary, the church was founded as a sign of gratitude to the Virgin for the victory over the Turks in Vienna (1683). The architecture, clearly inspired by the nearby church of S. Maria di Loreto, is complex and laden with decorative elements. The high altar has a venerated panel with an image of the Virgin and child (13th century), which comes from an earlier, small church, S. Bernardo della Compagnia. ✉ *Foro Traiano 89.*

Fontana di Trevi ①
3 E5. The Trevi Fountain, the most spectacular and majestic of Rome's fountains, was created at the behest of Clement XII over a 30-year period (1732–1751). The fountain's water comes from the Aqua Virgo, the aqueduct built in 19 BC, which is fed from a source that, according to legend, was pointed out to some thirsty soldiers by a young girl (*virgo*). At the center of the fountain is the ocean god, whose shell-shaped chariot is drawn by seahorses guided by Tritons. The statues in the side niches represent Abundance and Salubrity, and the entire sculptural group rests on jagged rocks rising out of the sea (represented by the basin with raised edges). This fountain is linked to a great many legends and popular traditions, including the belief that those who throw a coin in its waters are sure to return to Rome. It is possible that this derives from the extremely ancient custom of pilgrims leaving coins on St. Peter's tomb. ✉ *Piazza di Trevi.*

Galleria dell'Accademia di S. Luca
3 E5. The National Academy of S. Luca continued the activity of the University of Painters, which was founded in the 15th century and whose members met in a church dedicated to St. Luke, on the Esquiline Hill (the evangelist saint is the patron of painters and artists in general, as well as notaries, butchers, and doctors). Since 1932 the academy and the art gallery of the same name have been located in Palazzo Carpegna (redesigned by Borromini in 1643–1647). The gallery houses sculpture and a collection of important paintings by Italian and foreign artists from the 16th to the 19th centuries. The works are gifts or bequests from patrons and artists, following a tradition, begun in the the 17th century, for academy members to donate at least one of their works to the institution. The academy houses a notable collection of members' portraits, prize-winning canvases, and the controversial *Madonna with St. Luke*, begun by Raphael and perhaps completed by another artist. ✉ *Piazza dell'Accademia di S. Luca 77,* ☎ *06/679–8850.*

Galleria Nazionale d'Arte Antica ②
4 D2. Pope Urban VIII wanted his new family palazzo to be near his Quirinal residence. This building was begun in 1625 by Carlo Maderno, who designed a structure with a central element and open wings that combined aspects of an urban palazzo and a garden villa. Gian Lorenzo Bernini designed the garden facade and the staircase, and Francesco Borromini is responsible for the spiral stair-

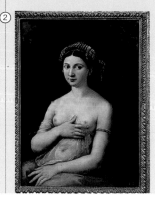

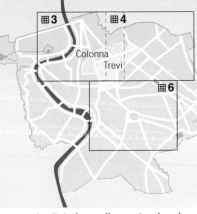

Raphael's *Fornarina*, which, according to tradition, is a portrait of the artist's beloved. The portrait hangs in the Galleria Nazionale di Arte Antica in the Palazzo Barberini.

case in the right wing. The luxurious residence was built to accommodate official functions and entertainments of the Barberini family. The palazzo included a theater and ball court, and the broad space in front of the building was used for cavalcades and tournaments. Most rooms have frescoed ceilings, the most famous of which is the main drawing room, painted by Pietro da Cortona with *The Triumph of Divine Providence,* a dramatic and theatrical celebration of the pope and his family. At the center, Divine Providence triumphs over Time and gives the Barberini coat of arms to Immortality. The side scenes illustrate the virtues of Urban VIII and the projects accomplished during his papacy. Acquired by the state in 1949, the Palazzo Barberini now houses the Galleria Nazionale d'Arte Antica, established in the late 19th century as a repository for works from various private collections (Corsini, Torlonia, Sciarra, Chigi, Barberini, and others), legacies, and acquisitions. The collection, one of the most important in Rome, includes paintings by the most famous Italian and foreign masters from the 13th to the 18th centuries. The most admired paintings are Raphael's *Fornarina,* Hans Holbein's *Portrait of Henry VIII,* and Caravaggio's *Judith and Holofernes* and *Narcissus.* The collection also includes Filippo Lippi's *Madonna and Child;* Tintoretto's *Adulteress;* Titian's *Venus and Adonis;* Il Bronzino's *Portrait of Stefano Colonna;* and El Greco's extraordinary sketches, *The Adoration of the Shepherds* and *The Baptism of Christ.* The apartment has an extensive collection of majolica, porcelain, glass, furniture, and clothing from the 17th and 18th centuries. ✉ *Via Quattro Fontane 13,* ☎ *06/481–4591.*

Galleria Colonna

▦3 E5. The foremost private collection in the city, along with the Doria Pamphilj, is housed in one of the largest residential complexes in Rome. Pope Martin V built the Palazzo Colonna in the early 15th century, on the ruins of a medieval castle. It was expanded and rebuilt in 1730 by Filippo Colonna, incorporating a palazzo built in 1484 for Cardinal Giuliano della Rovere (the future Julius II), first a rival but later related to the Colonna family. The sobriety of the exterior contrasts with the sumptuous scale and decorations of the interiors, which include the splendid gallery that has often been compared to Versailles. The ceilings are sumptuously decorated with frescoes that celebrate the glories of the Colonna family, particularly Marcantonio, victor over the Turks in the Battle of Lepanto. Large mirrors, chandeliers, gilded stuccowork, inlaid floors, and antique statues create a magnificent frame for the painting collection, which was begun in the 17th century and offers works from the 14th to the 18th century. The high points of the gallery and adjoining spaces are the ornate great hall, the hall of landscapes (which contains two jewel caskets and 17th-century French and Flemish landscapes), a room with a ceiling fresco of *The Apotheosis of Martin V,* and the throne room, designed to receive visits from the pope. ✉ *Via della Pilotta 17,* ☎ *06/679–4362.*

Oratorio del Crocifisso

▦3 E5. Built in 1568 by Giacomo della Porta for the Order of the Confraternity of the Crucifix, this building was established to venerate the famous crucifix in the nearby church of S. Marcello al Corso. The chapel of the **Madonna dell' Archetto** (1851) is located on the adjacent Via di S. Marcello, at number 41B. Despite its very small size (it is the smallest votive chapel in Rome), the chapel is a space of extraordinary architectural and decorative harmony. It was built by Marchese Alessandro Papazzurri (owner of the palazzo next door, now known as the Palazzo Balestra) to accommodate a revered holy image of the Madonna (*Madonnae Causa Nostrae Letitiae*) painted on majolica-covered stone in 1690. ✉ *Piazza dell'Oratorio.*

Palazzo Capranica

▦3 E4. One of Rome's first Renaissance-style palazzi, this was built before Bramante's arrival in the city. It was begun in 1451 by Cardinal Domenico Capranica to house an ecclesiastical college (the first of its type in Rome) that he established. Most of the building is taken up by the Capranica Cinema, one of the oldest theaters in the city, that began as a private theater built by the Capranica family in 1694. According to tradition, the palazzo stands on the site where St. Agnes once lived, and a chapel within the Collegio is dedicated to her. ✉ *Piazza Capranica.*

Palazzo Chigi

▦3 E4. It took more than a century to complete this grand palazzo, which has housed government cabinet offices since 1961. Begun in 1580 by the Aldobrandini family, the work continued during the papacy of Clement VIII (a member of that family), and the building was considerably expanded in the following century during the papacy of Alexander VII, a member of the wealthy Tuscan Chigi family known for their patronage of the arts. The solemn entrance on Piazza Colonna, the courtyard fountain, and the rich decoration of the interior spaces date to the 18th century. An elegant and original decorative scheme in stucco squares adorns the courtyard, and

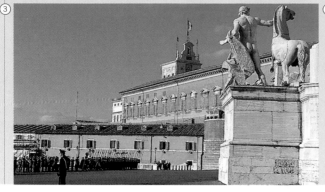

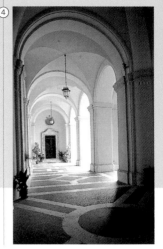

a grand staircase adorned with antique sculptures rises to the second floor, which houses the Cabinet Room. On the third floor is the sumptuous Gold Room, decorated in Neoclassical style. Between the 17th and 18th centuries, when the palazzo was one of the liveliest centers of Roman social life, the general populace was involved in the festivities held here and received generous donations of food, wine, and money. ⊠ *Largo Chigi/Piazza Colonna.*

Palazzo di Propaganda Fide ④
⊞**3 C5.** The Congregation of Propaganda Fide, established by Gregory XV in 1622, is the church's central agency for missionary work. Established during a period of great excitement about geographic discoveries and grave spiritual crisis caused by the Reformation, the Propaganda Fide represented a milestone in the history of Catholicism and a turning point in the evangelical process. The 16th-century palazzo was transformed gradually, with successive interventions by various architects, including Bernini (1644). But the most innovative contribution was made by Borromini (1646–1667), whose design was one of his last and most significant creations. The facade on Via di Propaganda Fide looms over the narrow street, and the walls seem animated by an uncontainable internal pressure that pushes and compresses the window frames, which are barely held back by the tall pilaster strips. The same intense vibration, although attenuated by diffused light, is found in the **church of the Re Magi,** inside the palazzo. ⊠ *Piazza di Spagna 48.*

Palazzo del Quirinale ③
⊞**3 E6.** A cornerstone of Baroque Rome, this palazzo has always been a seat of political power. First it was the summer residence of the popes, then the papal palace, the royal palace, and finally the official residence of the president of Italy. The construction of the building, begun under Gregory XIII, was completed during the papacy of Clement XII (1730–1740). The most celebrated architects of the Counter-Reformation and Baroque periods participated in its construction. The solemn facade is animated by Carlo Maderno's entrance (1615), with statues of St. Peter and St. Paul, and by the Loggia of Benedictions above, designed by Bernini (1638), who was also responsible for the circular tower on the left. The inner courtyard, which has a severe Counter-Reformation appearance, is used for receiving heads of state. The rooms contain works by Botticelli, Pietro da Cortona, Claude Lorrain, Lorenzo Lotto, Melozzo da Forlì, and Guido Reni, who executed the wonderful frescoes for the private chapel of Paul V, the so-called Chapel of the Annunciation. The spacious gardens in the back of the palazzo have an unusual Organ Fountain, built for Clement VIII, and an elegant Coffeehouse, erected at the most scenic point for Benedict XIV (1741). The Palazzo Quirinale overlooks a piazza of the same name that dominates one of the most beautiful views of the city. Numerous popes were involved in the planning of this piazza, from Gregory XIII to Pius IX. The focus of activity in the piazza is the **Fontana di Monte Cavallo,** with the **Dioscuri,** two colossal statues of Castor and Pollux holding back their horses, which came from the Baths of Constantine, and, at the center, an **obelisk** that was once graced the facade of the tomb of Augustus. ⊠ *Piazza del Quirinale.*

Piazza Barberini
⊞**4 D2.** The piazza assumed its modern urban character toward the end of the 19th century, with the building of the Via del Tritone and Via Vittorio Veneto, which intersect here. Before that time, the area was dominated by fields, with scattered houses, workshops, and inns populated by artists. Since 1625 the piazza has borne the name of the Barberini family, whose palazzo and gardens extended as far as Via XX Settembre. The family of Urban VIII commissioned Gian Lorenzo Bernini to create two well-known fountains. At the center of the piazza is the spectacular **Fontana del Tritone,** created for the pope in 1642–1643, with four dolphins with the Barberini heraldic bees raising up a shell on which the Triton stands. At the corner of the Via Veneto is the **Fontana delle Api** (Fountain of the Bees, 1644), which also sports the Barberini coat of arms.

Piazza Colonna ⑤
⊞**3 E4–E5.** Until the late 19th century the piazza was the center of the papal city. Its monumental development resulted from its position at an important intersection of two streets traveled by pilgrims, one linking Porta Salaria to Ponte S. Angelo, the other going from Porta del Popolo to the Campidoglio. In the late 16th century Sixtus V began the demolition of the modest houses that faced the piazza, and these were replaced with patrician palaces. Later this was the site of the papal post office, as well as the location of numerous popular cafés. The central **column** that gives the piazza its name was erected in AD 180–AD 193, to celebrate the victories of Emperor Marcus Aurelius against the barbarians at the eastern boundaries of the empire. The

The Palazzo di Propaganda Fide ④, on which both Bernini and Borromini worked, is the site of the historical congregation of the same name that is in charge of the coordination of various missionary activities of the church.

The column of Marcus Aurelius stands at the center of Piazza Colonna ⑤; it was erected in 180–193 to celebrate the eastern victories of the emperor against the Marcomanni, the Quadi, and the Sarmatians and depicts his military undertakings.

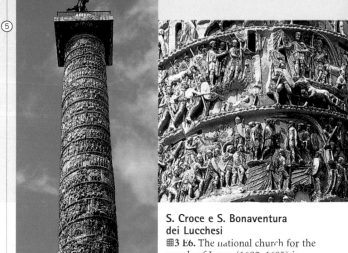

imperial statue that originally topped the monument was lost in medieval times, and Sixtus V replaced it with a bronze statue of St. Paul (1588–1589). The late Baroque church of **Ss. Bartolomeo e Alessandro** was built by an 18th-century confraternity of the people of Bergamo, who dedicated it to the patron saints of their city.

Piazza di Montecitorio
⊞3 E4. The piazza was laid out by order of Clement XII Corsini (1730–1740) to create a suitable urban space in front of the palace of the same name. Innocent X (1653) commissioned Gian Lorenzo Bernini to design the **Palazzo di Montecitorio,** which was later converted into law courts and was known as the Curia Innocenziana; today the building houses the Chamber of Deputies. The structure's legal function made it significant in people's lives, particularly because during the 19th century, its largest bell rang out to indicate the beginning of the school day and the opening of offices. In front of the palazzo is an Egyptian **obelisk** from the 4th century BC, which the emperor Augustus used as the gnomon of a sundial. It was moved here in 1796 by Pius VI, who restored its function. The pierced bronze globe, embellished with heraldic symbols of the pope, is traversed by the sun's rays, which indicated the hours on special fillets inserted into the pavement of the piazza.

Pontificia Università Gregoriana
⊞3 E6–F6. The impressive palazzo of the Pontificia Università Gregoriana was erected in 1927–1930 to accommodate the prestigious institution founded by St. Ignatius of Loyola in 1551 and previously located in the palazzo of the Collegio Roman and in the Palazzo Borromeo. Today it is an active center for research and study

in religion and philosophy. The facade, which has a wealth of classical motifs, recalls the architectural lines of the Collegio Romano. The corner house between Via dei Lucchesi and Via dell'Umiltà has a **17th-century shrine** with a painted image of a crucifix, perhaps related to the nearby Capuchin monastery. ✉ *Piazza della Pilotta.*

S. Andrea delle Fratte
⊞3 D5. The name of the church recalls the original rural location, on the periphery of the city (*fratte* means "thickets"). The present-day church was begun in 1612 for the Marchese Paolo Del Bufalo, on the site of an older church that had belonged first to the Scottish community, then to the Minim Friars of St. Francis of Paola. The church's most interesting features are the creations of Francesco Borromini, who worked here from 1653 until 1665. The unusual bell tower conveys a measure of his inspired invention of new forms. Several architectural orders, each different, are superimposed, culminating in the complex crowning element with volutes that support the insignia of the saint (the diagonal cross) and the donor family (the buffalo), surmounted by a metal crown. Inside the church are two marble statues of angels made by Gian Lorenzo Bernini for the Ponte S. Angelo. These are the only statues for the bridge that the artist personally executed, and they were never located there because Clement IX wanted to protect them from the elements. Like all the other angels in the series, they carry symbols of Christ's Passion: the scroll and the crown of thorns. ✉ *Via S. Andrea delle Fratte 1.*

S. Croce e S. Bonaventura dei Lucchesi
⊞3 E6. The national church for the people of Lucca (1682–1695) is sober on the exterior but has a surprising interior similar to a drawing room, with exuberant furnishings in marble and gold, and stucco friezes. It was erected over the ruins, still visible below, of the church of S. Nicola de Portiis (9th century), which belonged to the Minorite Capuchin Friars and was given to the people of Lucca by Urban VIII in 1631. In the courtyard is the **Palazzo di S. Felice,** which takes its name from St. Felix of Cantalice, a humble Capuchin friar and friend of St. Charles Borromeo and St. Philip Neri. For more than 40 years St. Felix wandered the streets of Rome, begging for contributions for his order, singing praises to the Madonna, and telling edifying stories. ✉ *Via dei Lucchesi 3.*

S. Ignazio ⑥
⊞3 E4–F4. The piazza (1727–1728) on which the church stands is a refined urban Rococo creation. The facades of three buildings feign the presence of symmetrical streets converging in the wide space, defining a sort of theatrical backdrop. The church (1626–1685), commissioned by Gregory XV to honor the founder of the Jesuits, imitates, in its facade and interior, the Chiesa del Gesù. The pictorial decoration was for the most part created by the Jesuit Andrea Pozzo, a mathematician, set designer, and student of perspective who was extremely well versed in the use of optical devices to create fictitious spaces. Because there were no funds to construct a dome, he resorted to an ingenious trompe l'oeil, a gigantic canvas depicting a sumptuous dome with a broad drum on columns, in place of the dome that had been planned. The *Entry of St. Ignatius*

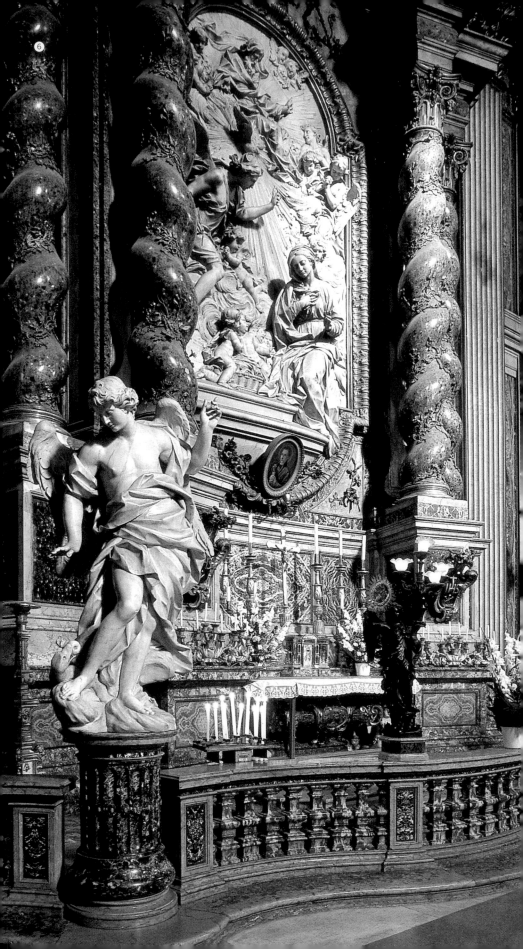

The ornate altar in the left transept, a precious creation from the Baroque period, includes the *Annunziata*, a marble altarpiece by Filippo della Valle, one of the most notable of the many works in S. Ignazio ⑥.

An evocative view of S. Maria di Loreto, SS. Nome di Maria, and Trajan's Colum ⑦, three well-known monuments that form a fascinating corner of Rome, between Piazza Venezia and the Forum of Trajan.

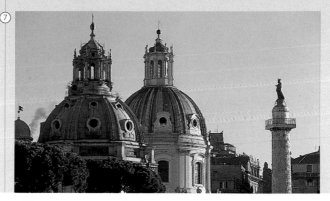

into Paradise in the vault of the central nave is a masterpiece of illusion and the culmination of the Baroque use of pictorial means in the service of religious propaganda. The painted columns seem to extend the walls of the church to the sky, creating a faux space that seems as believable as the actual space. It is the realm of the divine, contiguous to the human realm, miraculously perceivable beyond the terrestrial experience. ⊠*Piazza S. Ignazio.*

S. Lorenzo in Lucina
⌗3 D4. The name may derive from the house that stood here in Roman times and that belonged to a rich matron named Lucina. The building was later transformed into a church. It was rebuilt by Paschal II in the 12th century (the portico and bell tower remain) and radically redesigned in the 17th century for the Order of Minorites. There is a particularly interesting chapel designed by Gian Lorenzo Bernini for Innocent X's physician, Gabriele Fonseca, whose vivid portrait is by the same master. The high altar has a famous *Crucifixion* by Guido Reni, and behind it, a marble throne with an inscription that recalls the placement by Paschal II (1112) of relics of St. Laurence in the altar, including a fragment of the martyr's gridiron. ⊠*Via in Lucina 16/A.*

S. Marcello al Corso
⌗3 F5. The church was erected over a 4th-century building dedicated to Pope Marcellus I (308–309), who, according to legend, was forced by the emperor Maxentius to work in the stables of the central post office until he died of exhaustion. Between the 16th and 17th centuries the church was rebuilt, with contributions by Jacopo Sansovino, Antonio da Sangallo the Younger, and Carlo Fontana, who is responsible for the

notable two-story concave facade. Above the entrance is a beautiful medallion relief supported by angels that depicts St. Philip Benizi rejecting a tiara; according to legend, the saint, who lived in the 13th century and was a member of the Order of Servants of Mary, refused to become pope. Outstanding amid the church's ornate furnishings is a funerary monument for Cardinal Giovanni Michiel by Jacopo Sansovino. The cardinal was a nephew of Paul II and was poisoned by the Borgia family in 1503. ⊠*Piazza S. Marcello 5.*

S. Maria in Aquiro
⌗3 E4. No convincing explanation has come to light for the title "in Aquiro," and there is no information about the origins of this church, although it is quite ancient and is mentioned in relation to a restoration carried out by Gregory III (731–741). In 1389 Urban VI called it S. Maria della Visitazione, recalling the biblical episode of Elizabeth's visit to Mary. In the 16th century it was granted to the Confraternity of Orphans and was rebuilt. In addition to 17th- and 19th-century paintings, the church contains a highly regarded detached fresco (*Madonna and Child with St. Stephen*), dating from the 14th century. ⊠*Piazza Capranica 72.*

S. Maria di Loreto ⑦
⌗6 A2. Begun in 1507 by order of the Confraternity of Bakers, this church combines Bramante's classic style with the new Mannerist tendencies inaugurated by Michelangelo. The two styles are clearly evident in the facade, where a square base punctuated by Corinthian pilaster strips and niches is surmounted by a large dome on an octagonal drum, culminating in a fanciful empty lantern. The sculptural group on the entrance

tympanum, depicting *The Virgin and the Blessed House of Loreto*, may be by Andrea Sansovino (1550). The most admired works in the church are the two angels by Stefano Maderno and the *St. Susanna* by François Duquesnoy (1629–1633), the Flemish sculptor who collaborated with Bernini on the baldacchino and various statues for S. Pietro. In this work he expressed his artistic ideals, which were based on the rigorous study of nature and antiquity; the substantial and harmonious forms and the grace of the figure of St. Susanna became a model for much 17th- and 18th-century sacred statuary. ⊠*Piazza Madonna di Loreto 26.*

S. Maria Maddalena
⌗3 E4. The church was built in the 17th century at the behest of the Ministers of the Sick, an order founded by St. Camillus de Lellis in 1582 to minister physically and spiritually to the sick. The facade (added in 1735), which has a concave silhouette and a wealth of statues, niches, and ornamentation, and the sacristy, with its extremely refined decorative scheme, are among the most representative examples of the Rococo style in Rome. Many of the paintings in the church depict scenes from the life of St. Camillus, whose order acted heroically during various epidemics of plague and cholera in Italy. The order also deserves great credit for improving health care, along the lines achieved earlier in Spain by St. John of God. St. Camillus and his followers isolated those with contagious diseases, studied their diets, improved hospital structures, and worked to aid the dying. The church contains the tomb of St. Camillus and his death mask. ⊠*Piazza della Maddalena 53.*

S. Maria dell'Umiltà
⌗3 E5. The church was built in the early 17th century for Francesca

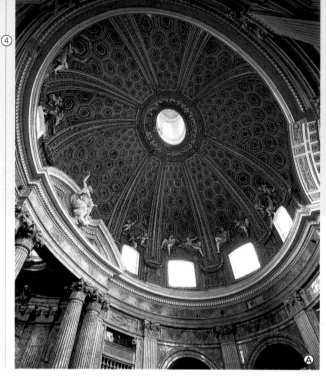

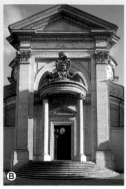

Kingdom of Italy with Rome as the capital. ⊠*Piazza S. Giovanni in Laterano,* ☎*06/698–86386.*

Palazzo Pallavicini Rospigliosi
⊞4 F2. Cardinal Scipione Borghese, nephew of Paul V, the first pontiff to reside at the Quirinal Palace, decided to build a residence in the immediate vicinity of the new papal see. The building, completed by Carlo Maderno in 1616, changed hands numerous times before passing to the Rospigliosi family in the late 17th century. The new owners enlarged the building and embellished it. The wedding of Gian Battista Rospigliosi (1646–1722) with Maria Carmela Pallavicini brought the palace into the possession of the Pallavicini family, its current owners. In 1614, Guido Reni painted the ceiling fresco of the Casino Pallavicini with a splendid *Aurora,* the result of his passionate study of Raphael and classical statuary; it is a fundamental work in the history of the classical ideal. The **Galleria Pallavicini,** one of the few galleries of the great families that still survives, contains paintings by Botticelli, Signorelli, Pietro da Cortona, Lorenzo Lotto, Paul Bril, Luca Giordano, Rubens, Tintoretto, the Carracci, and Velásquez. ⊠*Via XXIV Maggio 43,* ☎*06/474–4019.*

S. Agata dei Goti
⊞6 A3. Founded in the 5th centu-

ry, this church was the center of an Arian cult in the Goth community in Rome, the only evidence of such practice in the capital. In 593, Gregory I reconsecrated the church to the Catholic religion and gave it its present name. A porticoed atrium leads to the facade, which was rebuilt during the 18th century. The interior preserves part of the original structure and has Baroque and 19th-century additions. The church has three naves, divided by 16 granite Ionic columns. In 1933, a 12th- to 13th-century mosaic canopy was reinstalled in the presbytery. Agatha was born in Catania and martyred there around 251; her breasts were cut off and she was placed on burning coals. She is venerated as a protector against breast cancer and fires. ⊠*Via Mazzarino 16.*

S. Andrea al Quirinale ④
⊞4 E2. Gian Lorenzo Bernini designed this jewel of Baroque architecture (1658–1661), which was commissioned by Cardinal Camillo Pamphilj for the Jesuit novitiate. The artist adopted an elliptical plan, one of his favorite schemes, with the main axis parallel to the entrance. Inside, the compelling rhythm of the large piers draws your eye toward the central altar niche, which contains an image of St. Andrew borne aloft to heaven. The intense colors of the marble and the light of the stuccowork and gilding enhance

the spectacular nature of the miraculous event. The facade's two curved wings, which invite and welcome passersby, is equally brilliant. It is said that Bernini's sole payment for his work was a donation of daily bread, sent to him from the novitiate's oven. In the adjacent monastery are the rooms of St. Stanislaw Kostka, who came to Rome as a Jesuit novice and died here at the age of 17, in 1568. The beautiful statue in polychrome marble by Pierre Legros (1703) shows him lying on his deathbed. Stanislaw is the patron saint of novices and of university students throughout the world. The Jesuits still place flowers in the rooms where he lived and died. ⊠*Via del Quirinale 29.*

S. Carlo alle Quattro Fontane
⊞4 E2. Commissioned by the Spanish Trinitarian fathers, this was Rome's first church dedicated to St. Charles Borromeo after his canonization in 1610. Francesco Borromini was the talented architect, and this, his first autonomous project, gave proof of the revolutionary power of his art. The small size of the space forced him to devise ingenious building plans. Vigorous columns that emphasize the undulating line of the walls punctuate the elliptical interior space. An oval dome, a fanciful geometric lacework of cross-shaped, hexagonal, and octagonal coffers, soars above. The coffer shapes diminish as the ceiling rises, creating the illusion of exaggerated height, and the abundant light from the lantern highlights the compact unity of the space and the complexity of its internal tensions. The facade's concise juxtaposition of concave and convex walls, largely unfettered by decorative elements, creates an effect of heightened tension. This facade was completed some years later and was the last work by the great mas-

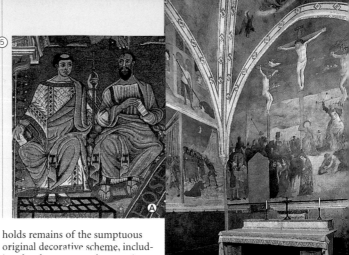

⑤

(A) Under the spectacular dome of S. Andrea al Quirinale ④, the faithful gather at the center of the liturgical celebration in a triumph of light; (B) the facade's sinuous forms, which invite visitors to enter, are by Bernini.

S. Clemente ⑤ (upper church): (A) detail of the mosaic decoration of the bowl-shaped apse vault and (B) the Chapel of St. Catherine (1428–1431), frescoed by Masolino da Panicale, probably in collaboration with Masaccio.

ter, who in his youth had been deeply affected by the austere piety of St. Charles, and who wanted to conclude his career by returning to this, his first creation. In 1667, exhausted and isolated, Borromini committed suicide by throwing himself upon his sword. ⊠ *Via del Quirinale 23.*

S. Caterina a Magnanapoli

⊞6 A2. This church was founded around 1575, along with the convent of Dominican nuns, who brought with them some relics of St. Catherine of Siena. Rebuilt between 1628 and 1641, the facade has two architectural orders of the same width. A 20th-century double staircase leads to a portico with three arches surmounted by the second row, with a large window and niches. The interior, with a single nave and three side chapels, has ornate 17th- and 18th-century decorations. Carlo Marchionni's monumental high altar (1787) has a tabernacle in agate, lapis lazuli, and gilded bronze, and a sculptural group by Melchiorre Caffà, made from colored marble and stucco, depicting the *Ecstasy of St. Catherine.* Caffà, one of the most successful interpreters of Bernini's vocabulary, was in this case clearly inspired by the *Ecstasy of St. Teresa* in S. Maria della Vittoria. The convent, which in 1619 also included the nearby **Torre delle Milizie,** was demolished in 1924. ⊠ *Largo Magnanapoli.*

S. Clemente ⑤

⊞6 D5. Named after Peter's third successor (88–97), this basilica offers a a centuries-long collection of monuments that traverses most of the city's history, from the 1st century AD to the threshold of the modern era. According to tradition, the upper church, commissioned by Pope Paschal II (1099–1118), was built over the house where the saint was born. It

holds remains of the sumptuous original decorative scheme, including the altar canopy, the mosaic floor, and the gleaming apse mosaic, which incorporates a cross within an exuberant plant motif. The political significance of the image is clarified by the inscription, which says that law alone withers vines, which, instead thrive beneath the sign of the cross. The image is also a container for relics, and it holds fragments of the cross from Golgotha. Masolino da Panicale (perhaps with Masaccio) painted the frescoes (1428–1431) in the Chapel of St. Catherine, one of the most venerated Christian martyrs in the capital. Some 18th-century frescoes in the central nave depict significant episodes from the life of St. Clement. In AD 97 Clement was condemned to exile and forced labor in the famous marble quarries of Chersoneso, in the Crimea, where he continued his missionary work. There was no water in the quarries, and prisoners risked dying of thirst. Clement, having seen a lamb scraping the earth with its hooves, began to dig at that spot, from which a spring burst forth. Trajan had Clement thrown into the Black Sea with an anchor around his neck. Clement is also the subject of most of the frescoes in the lower church (4th century), executed between the 9th and 11th centuries. This group of work includes, among others, the *Legend of Sisinius*, prefect of Rome, who ordered his soldiers to arrest the pope. Blinded by God, they instead imprisoned a column (the scene is well known thanks to the inscriptions in crudely realistic vernacular, to which Clement replies in formal Latin). Another miracle immortalized here has always attracted popular devotion. It recounts how the sea waters opened up once each year, to allow the faithful to pray at the martyr's watery grave. According to legend,

one year a widow lost her only son, and returning in the procession a year later, she found the child unharmed. Saints Cyril and Methodius, who evangelized the Slavic peoples, brought the saint's relics to Rome in 868. A altar dedicated to them later held the remains of St. Cyril. Beneath the apse of the lower basilica, vestiges of Roman buildings and a sanctuary dedicated to the cult of Mithras (3rd century AD) are visible. ⊠ *Piazza S. Clemente.*

S. Francesco di Paola

⊞6 B3. Francis of Paola (ca. 1436–1507), a hermit saint, came from Calabria. In 1632, a wealthy believer from the same region donated the funds for the construction of this church, which was set aside for the order of Minim Friars, who dedicated themselves to a rigorously ascetic life. The church became the national church of the Calabrians. The ornate lower portion of the travertine facade, articulated by pilasters, contrasts with the simplicity of the upper order, which was refinished in plaster in the 18th century. Inside is Giovanni Antonio de Rossi's dramatic high altar (ca. 1655), a magnificent stucco drapery made to look like bronze and supported by angels, is noteworthy. The nearby **Torre dei Margani** (12th century), in Piazza S. Pietro in Vincoli, was transformed into the church bell tower. It is a massive, square structure that terminates in a balustrade and still has a medieval coat of arms. ⊠ *Piazza di S. Francesco di Paola 10.*

S. Giovanni in Laterano ⑥

⊞7 E1–F1. As cathedral of the bishop of Rome, S. Giovanni in

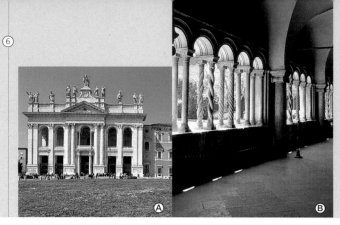

(A) The monumental facade of S. Giovanni in Laterano, the cathedral of Rome, is an elegant, solemn creation by Florentine architect Alessandro Galilei (1732–1735); (B) a view of the cloister, created in the early decades of the 13th century; (C) the tabernacle, built in 1367, is decorated with frescoes. The silver reliquaries contain the heads of the Apostles Peter and Paul.

Laterano is called the mother of all churches. It was built in the 4th century over the barracks of the Equites Singulares (the emperors' mounted guards), in the area that Constantine donated to Pope Miltiades. According to medieval legends, the Lateran was the place where Pope Sylvester baptized the emperor, ill with leprosy, who, when he was healed, converted to Christianity. Pope Gregory I, who consecrated the basilica to St. John the Baptist and St. John the Evangelist, performed the dedication of the church. The basilica is also known as the Redeemer, because of both the icon preserved in the nearby chapel of the Sancta Sanctorum and the legend of the apparition of the face of Christ on the day of the consecration. Thanks in part to Constantine's donations, the church has always had precious ornaments, and it is popularly believed to contain exceptional relics. The most important are those related to St. John the Evangelist: the chalice from which he drank poison, the chain with which he was bound, and the miraculous tunic he used to raise three people from the dead. Some of the many other relics are the sackcloth of John the Baptist, the cloth Jesus used to dry the feet of his disciples, and the red garment Jesus was given by the soldiers of Pontius Pilate. In 1370, the remains of the heads of Peter and Paul were brought from the Sancta Sanctorum. The church then acquired a prestige even greater than that of the basilicas of Sts. Peter and Paul and was considered the true heart of Christendom. The original structure underwent numerous and radical transformations over the course of the centuries, up to the Baroque renovations by Borromini. The central entrance on the facade has bronze doors from the Curia (the site of the Roman Senate) in the Forum,

while the last door on the right is the Porta Santa, or Holy Door, and is opened only during Jubilee years. The long history of the building is manifested in the extremely rich interior decoration, and the cloister is a masterpiece of mosaic art. ⊠ *Piazza S. Giovanni in Laterano 4.*

S. Lorenzo in Fonte

⊞6 A4. This small church, also known as Ss. Lorenzo e Ippolito, is linked to the imprisonment of the martyr St. Laurence. Because of the presence of underground structures from Roman times and a well, this was believed to be the place where the saint was incarcerated and where he baptized his jailer, Hippolytus (the painting on the high altar depicts this legend). The current structure, which dates from a 1656 renovation, is very simple, with a Neoclassical facade. ⊠ *Via Urbana 50.*

S. Lorenzo in Panisperna

⊞6 A4. According to tradition, the church was built in the time of Constantine, on the site of the saint's martyrdom, but the current building is the result of a 1576 renovation. The adjacent Convent of the Poor Clares at one time distributed bread and ham on the saint's feast day (August 10), in remembrance of deacon Laurence's distribution of the church's treasures to the poor of Rome before his death. It is probably that custom that gave the street its name, "panisperna," from the words for bread (*pane*) and ham (*perna*). The outer gate leads to a courtyard, in which stands a rare example of a medieval house with an exterior staircase. In the presbytery, a dramatic painting depicts the martyrdom of St. Laurence. ⊠ *Via Panisperna 90.*

S. Lucia in Selci

⊞6 B5. Enclosed within a 17th-century Augustinian convent, the church of S. Lucia in Selci was built, certainly no later than the 8th century, over an ancient Roman building (the portico of Livia, none of which is still visible). Reconstructed by Carlo Maderno in 1604, it has a rectangular interior space with a barrel vault, two altars, and paintings depicting the *Martyrdom of St. Lucy* and the *Vision of St. Augustine.* The altar canopy in polychrome marble and gilt and alabaster statues are attributed to Maderno, the choir to Francesco Borromini. ⊠ *Via in Selci 82.*

S. Martino ai Monti

⊞6 B5. The church, located in an area rich in archeological finds from Roman times (partially visible in the vicinity and belowground), was founded in the early 6th century by Pope Symmachus, who dedicated it to St. Sylvester and St. Martin of Tours (ca. 316–397). The latter was known for his ascetic and missionary life, particularly for the episode where he gave his cloak to a beggar. It is not certain if this was the location of the ancient *titulus Equitii,* where the early Christians of the quarter used to meet. The building has been restored many times, and its current appearance is the result of a 17th-century renovation. The interior has three naves divided by ancient columns. The side naves have precious 17th-century wooden ceilings and noteworthy paintings. A central staircase descends to the dramatic crypt, animated by a great number of columns that contain the remains of various martyrs. The crypt leads to spaces that still have structural elements and architectural fragments from Roman and medieval times and frescoes from the 9th century. ⊠ *Via Monte Oppio 28.*

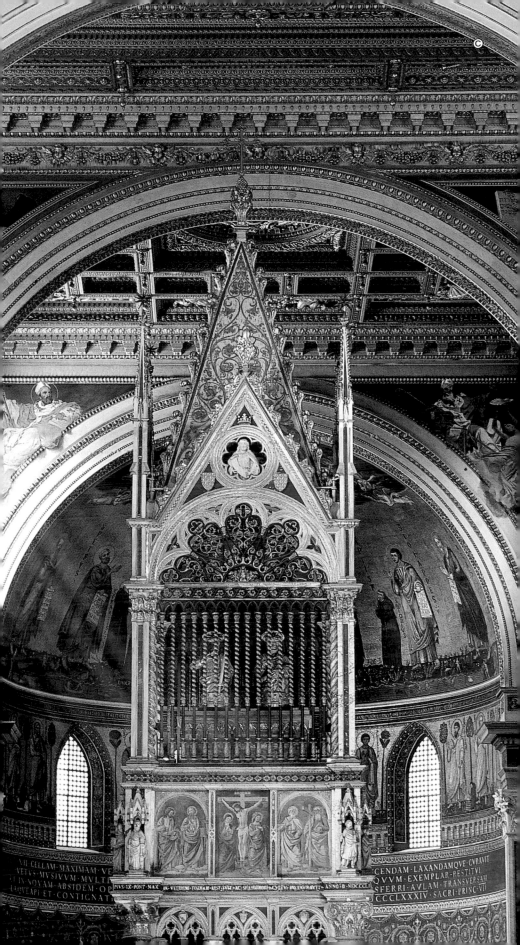

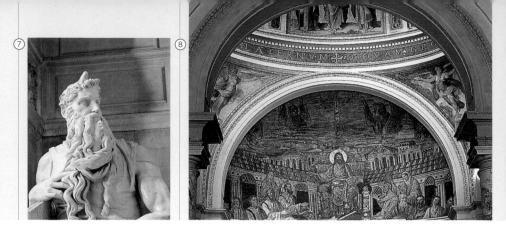

⑦ ⑧

S. Pietro in Vincoli ⑦

⊞**6 B4.** In the 5th century Pope
Sixtus III ordered a church to be
built to hold a precious relic: the
chains (*vincula* in Latin, from
which the name "in Vincoli" is
derived) that bound St. Peter in the
prisons of Jerusalem. According to
legend, the chains were found adjacent to those of the apostle's
Roman imprisonment, and they
miraculously welded together,
forming a single chain, which is
kept here, beneath the high altar.
Cardinal Giuliano della Rovere, the
future Pope Julius II, made radical
changes to the church (1471–
1503), and other alterations were
made in the 18th century. The
basilica's many works of art include
an early Christian sarcophagus (in
the crypt), paintings by Guercino
and Domenichino, and a Byzantine
mosaic from the 7th century that
depicts St. Sebastian with a beard.
These works are eclipsed, however,
by Michelangelo's renowned *Moses*,
the only work the artist completed
for the tomb of Julius II. The original project called for a much more
opulent presentation (a structure
on many levels, crowded with biblical figures) and a more prestigious
and momentous location that was
selected by Julius II himself:
beneath the dome of St. Peter's and
above the tomb of the apostle.
✉*Piazza S. Pietro in Vincoli 4/A.*

S. Prassede ⑨

⊞**6 A5.** According to tradition,
Praxedes was the sister of St.
Pudentiana and the daughter of
Senator Pudens, in whose house
the apostle Peter stayed. Legend
has it that St. Praxedes collected
the remains and the blood of martyrs, and the legend is recounted in
an inscription on a round porphyry well cover in front of the
entrance. The 5th-century church
was completely rebuilt in 822 by
Pope Paschal I, on the occasion of
the transfer of the relics of 2,300
martyrs from the catacombs. In
the apse a mosaic depicts *Christ
Offering a Benediction, Surrounded
by Saints,* above a frieze showing
12 lambs (the apostles) and the
two celestial cities, Jerusalem and
Bethlehem. Paschal I built the
Chapel of S. Zeno (called the
"Garden of Paradise") as a mausoleum for his mother, Theodora.
It is entirely covered with mosaics,
which portray the Virgin and
child, Sts. Praxedes and
Pudentiana, and Christ with the
apostles. The dome contains an
image of Christ supported by four
angels, and medallions with busts
of male and female saints frame
the door. Another chapel contains
the so-called Column of the
Flagellation, brought from
Jerusalem in 1223. A reliquary
contains three thorns, said to be
from Christ's crown. ✉*Via
S. Prassede 9/A.*

S. Pudenziana ⑧

⊞**4 F4.** Tradition states that the
church dedicated to Pudentiana,
the sister of St. Praxedes, was built
over the house of their father,
Pudens, and that he himself transformed it into a place of worship.
The current building, which dates
from the late 4th century but has
been altered many times, has an
apse decorated with the oldest
Christian mosaics that survive
from a place of worship. They
almost certainly can be dated from
the papacy of Innocent I
(401–417), according to an inscription, now lost. In the solemn central image, Christ is seated on a
jewel-studded throne, surrounded
by the 12 seated apostles, and two
women place crowns of martyrdom on the heads of Peter and
Paul. It is likely that the women
symbolize the two essential components of the early Christian
community, one stemming from
Judaism and the other from
paganism. The scene is surmounted by an impressive jeweled cross,
next to which are the symbols of
the four evangelists, the so-called
"tetramorph," inspired by the
Apocalypse of St. John, which
appears here for the first time.
Here, as in the church of St.
Praxedes, popular myth spread the
belief of the existence of a well, in
which St. Pudentiana was thought
to have gathered the blood of
3,000 martyrs. In 1610, a eucharistic miracle, similar to the one in
Bolsena, where blood spilled from
a consecrated vessel to rekindle the
faith of a doubting priest, is said to
have occurred in the Caetani
Chapel. ✉*Via Urbana 160.*

S. Stefano Rotondo

⊞**6 F5.** The church was built in the
5th century to hold the remains of
St. Stephen, the first Christian
martyr, who was the object of
widespread veneration after the
discovery of his tomb near
Jerusalem in 415. The word
"Rotondo" refers to the church's
circular plan, modeled on the
church of the Holy Sepulchre in
Jerusalem and utilized here for the
first time in a church in Rome.
Two centuries later, Pope Theodore I
transported the remains of the
martyrs Primus and Felician to the
church and had a mosaic created
with their images on either side of
a jeweled cross. According to tradition, they were two Roman brothers who renounced their pagan
faith and were baptized at the time
of the terrible persecutions under
Diocletian. They tirelessly
preached their new faith and aided
imprisoned Christians, until they
were put to death publicly in 305,
after enduring atrocious tortures.
The outer wall of the church is
frescoed with 34 moving scenes of
Martyrology (1572–1585), commissioned by Pope Gregory XIII.
✉*Via di S. Stefano Rotondo 7.*

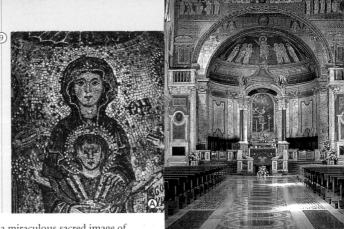

The mosaic apse in the church of S. Pudenziana ⑧ dates from the founding of the present–day building in the late 4th century.. The mosaic depicts Christ enthroned with the apostles and Sts. Pudentiana and Praxedes.

(A) Detail of the early Christian mosaics of the Chapel of S. Zeno, the principal Byzantine monument in Rome, located in the right nave of the basilica of S Prassede ⑨; (B) a view of the central nave of the same church.

S. Vitale

⊞4 E2. The church was founded by Pope Innocent I in 402, thanks to the generosity of Vestina, widow of a Roman notable. It was built to hold the remains of Sts. Gervase and Protase and their father, Vitalis, which were removed from Bologna and Milan after the discovery of their tombs by St. Ambrose. In the 6th century, Pope Gregory the Great established a procession of widows, in memory of the church's benefactress. The building originally had three naves, but was reduced to a single nave by Sixtus IV on the occasion of the Jubilee of 1475. In 1598, Clement VIII ceded the church to the Jesuits, who linked it to the church of S. Andrea al Quirinale and carried out a complete restoration. The interior is decorated with scenes from the lives of martyrs and prophets and from the martyrdom of St. Vitalis. ⊠ *Via Nazionale 194/B.*

Scala Santa

⊞7 E2. While he was overseeing the construction of the new Lateran Palace, Pope Sixtus V decided to save the private chapel of the popes (dedicated to St. Laurence), which was part of the ancient Patriarchate, the papal residence during the Middle Ages. The building was also called the Sancta Sanctorum, because of the relics it contained, connected to Christ, the apostles, and to significant figures of the Christian faith. The old palace's staircase was also salvaged and moved to the chapel. According to a 15th-century tradition, the stairs are identified with those ascended by Christ during his Passion, in Pontius Pilate's palace, and since that time worshippers have climbed them on their knees. The restored mosaics and frescoes in the chapel date from the 13th century. The most important of the many treasures is

a miraculous sacred image of Christ, thought to be "not painted by human hands." The 5th- to 6th-century panel is now in the Museo Sacro in the Vatican. ⊠ *Piazza S. Giovanni in Laterano 14.*

Ss. Domenico e Sisto

⊞6 A3. The Baroque-era church was preceded by a small house of worship from the first millennium, known as S. Maria a Magnanapoli, which housed the Dominican nuns of the Convent of S. Sisto at the baths of Caracalla. At the behest of Pope Pius V, a Dominican, an opulent monastic complex was built on the site of and encompassed the small ancient church. This new structure was given the name of Ss. Domenico e Sisto, in remembrance of the old convent. Some of the most famous architects of the time were involved in the century-long building project (1569–1663), which concluded with the creation of the elegant facade, dramatic in its height and staircase. The interior has a single nave covered with a barrel vault and three altars on each side. Gian Lorenzo Bernini designed the first altar on the right and the high altar. ⊠ *Largo Angelicum 1.*

Ss. Marcellino e Pietro

⊞6 D6. This structure, built in 1751, replaced a 4th-century church that stood near the Via Labicana Catacombs. In 1256, the remains of the two martyrs to whom the building is consecrated were brought to the church. Even earlier it was an important destination for pilgrims, because of the presence of a hospice, entrusted in 1276 to the Confraternity of those Commended to the Savior. The cube-shaped exterior, divided by pilaster strips, presages neoclassicism, and the stepped dome and the interior are clearly inspired by Borromini. ⊠ *Via Merulana 162.*

Torre de' Conti

⊞6 B3. This is one of the most imposing remnants of medieval Rome, a city crowded with the towers and fortresses of the nobility, often erected, as in this case, on the solid remains of ancient edifices. The tower was built by Innocent III in 1203, over part of the Forum of Vespasian. It then passed into the hands of Innocent's family, the Conti di Segni, one of the most prominent families in the history of the church, to which it contributed 12 popes and 25 cardinals. Conceived not only as a private building, but also as a symbol of papal power, the tower was part of an extensive fortification system that was partially destroyed by the earthquake of 1349 and partially collapsed in 1644. ⊠ *Largo Ricci.*

Torre delle Milizie

⊞6 A2. According to legend it was from this tower that the emperor Nero watched Rome burn, while he composed verses and songs. In reality its construction is much more recent, and it represents an important example of civic architecture from medieval Rome. Built in the early 13th century by the powerful Conti di Segni family, it passed into the hands of the Annibaldi and then Boniface VIII. Boniface turned it into a stronghold in the struggle between the Caetani and Colonna families. In the 17th century it was incorporated into the Dominican Convent of S. Caterina a Magnanapoli. Damaged by lightening numerous times, the tower lost its third floor during the earthquake of 1348, which also caused the ground to sink and the tower to tilt markedly, a characteristic that is still visible. ⊠ *Largo Magnanapoli.*

9

Campitelli and Celio (Campitelli and the Coelian Hill)

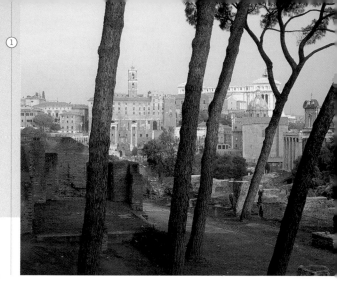

The Campitelli includes the most important archaeological zones in the city: the Campidoglio, the Palatine, and the Roman Forum. In postclassical times the district was predominantly occupied by ancient ruins. The slopes of the Campidoglio, which was the principal commercial center of the city during the early Middle Ages, had the area's only residential concentration. During the 20th century, this disctrict was terribly scarred by fascist demolition, which led to the isolation of the Campidoglio from the rest of the neighborhood and the opening of the Via del Mare (now the Via del Teatro di Marcello). The Coelian Hill and district were also long ignored and sparsely populated. Even during ancient times there were few patrician residences or public buildings here, and the district was animated only when the Coliseum hosted spectacles. During the Middle Ages and Renaissance the hill became depopulated; some villas and small farms remained, but the only significant buildings were Christian places of worship, some of the most ancient in the city (Ss. Giovanni e Paolo, Ss. Quattro Coronati, S. Maria in Domnica). In the 20th century, the area's relative proximity to the center made it a site for considerable urban development.

Arco di Costantino ②
(Arch of Constantine)
⊞**6 D3.** Located on the ancient Via Trionfale, which was traveled by victorious generals and emperors, the Arch of Constantine is Rome's grandest and best-preserved ancient arch. It was dedicated to the emperor by the Roman senate and people to celebrate the victory over Maxentius (312), achieved, as the epigraph reads, "by divine inspiration": legend tells of the appearance of the cross to Constantine before his decisive battle. The arch is a miscellany of sculptures and reliefs from earlier monuments, juxtaposed with those made during the time of Constantine. During this historical period in Rome, which had lost its position as capital to Constantinople, it must have been very difficult to find sufficient skilled labor to create the decoration for a large public monument. Thus started the practice of reusing ancient materials, a custom that lasted throughout the Middle Ages and made the Arch of Constantine a precious gallery of official Roman sculpture. The composite nature of the monument did not escape Raphael, whose harsh judgment of the reliefs from the Constantinian era ("very silly, without any good art or design") remained the prevailing opinion about late-ancient art until a few decades ago.
✉*Piazza del Colosseo, corner of Via di S. Gregorio.*

Carcere Mamertino
(Mamertine Prison)
⊞**6 B2.** This is part of the ancient state prison, where many illustrious enemies of Rome met their deaths. The medieval legend, according to which the apostle Peter was imprisoned here and baptized his jailers with water from a source that sprang from underground, seems to be without basis. In 1726, the building was transformed into a house of worship, S. Pietro in Carcere. Above the prison is the church of **S. Giuseppe dei Falegnami,** created for the association of carpenters in 1598. The Chapel of the Crucifix, which has a venerated 16th-century wooden crucifix, is located in a space excavated between the floor of the church and the ceiling of the prison. ✉*Clivio Argentario 1.*

Colosseo
⊞**6 C4–D4.** The largest amphitheater in the Roman world (it could hold more than 70,000 spectators) was built by the emperors of the Flavian dynasty between AD 72 and AD 80, on a site earlier occupied by the artificial lake of Nero's immense Domus Aurea. Indeed its ancient name was the Amphitheater of Flavius, and the present name, which dates from the 8th century, derives from the colossal bronze statue of Nero, no longer in existence, that was more than 114 feet high. Here ancient Romans attended gladiator combats and hunts of wild animals. Romantic tales about the sacrifice of Christians to wild beasts have no historical basis. But the Coliseum has always provoked a number of legends and popular fantasies, making it a symbol of the city and its rule. The Venerable Bede's prediction (8th century) is well known: "As long as there is the Coliseum, there will be Rome; as long as there is Rome, there will be the world." The last Coliseum spectacle we know of took place in 523, a date that marks the beginning of the monument's abandonment and deterioration. During subsequent centuries it was used as a quarry

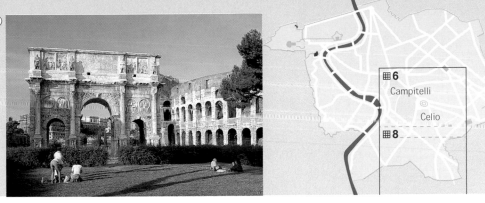

The Arch of Constantine, with three barrel vaults, and, on the right, the Amphitheater of Flavius, universally known as the Coliseum.

for building materials. During the baronial struggles of the Middle Ages, it was transformed into a fortress and later occupied by various institutions (hospitals, confraternities, and artisan associations) that profoundly altered its structure. The popes were the greatest exploiters of its stones, and between the 15th and 17th centuries the travertine of the ancient amphitheater provided material for major building projects, from S. Giovanni in Laterano to S. Pietro, from the Palazzo Venezia to the Palazzo della Cancelleria, from the Palazzo Barberini to the Porto di Ripetta. In light of this merciless plunder, Bernini took a remarkable stance in opposition to the practice, and planned the overall renovation of the complex for the 1675 Jubilee. These plans called for the construction of a church at the center of the arena, to be consecrated to the martyred saints who supposedly died on this site (there was already a chapel here). The project was never built, but the 1675 Jubilee decreed the sanctity of the site, an act confirmed by Benedict XIV in the mid-18th century, with the building of the 14 stations of the Via Crucis and with an edict prohibiting the monument's desecration. During the 19th century there was an increase in restoration, consolidation, and excavation work, and the Coliseum gradually was cleared of the vegetation that had covered it and structures that had been added over the course of time. ⊠ *Piazza del Colosseo.*

Foro Romano ①

⊞**6 C2.** Throughout the entire republican period the Roman Forum was the center of the city's political, commercial, and religious activity; the repository of its mythological and historical traditions; and, with home to its statuary, edifices, and commemorative monuments, a site of celebration of Rome's power. The long history of the Forum begins with the origins of the city (8th century BC) and ends in the 7th century AD, when the area was abandoned and decayed into an accumulation of ruins outside the medieval city. The only architectural elements to survive were the few temples that were transformed into churches, beginning in the 6th century, including S. Adriano, Ss. Cosma e Damiano, S. Maria Antiqua, the Oratorio dei Quaranta Martiri, and S. Lorenzo in Miranda. A few other structures were preserved and surrounded by fortified complexes belonging to the nobility. The Forum disappeared from historical memory, and the few literary attempts to reconstruct its ancient appearance (such as the *Mirabilia Urbis Romae,* the principal guide to the city during the Middle Ages) confused the buildings and capriciously mixed Christian and pagan traditions. During the Renaissance, when it was reduced to a grazing site, the Forum was plundered irremediably and utilized as a stone quarry for the rebuilding of the city. The new Rome of the popes destroyed the Rome of the Caesars precisely at a moment when the most cultivated Renaissance courts were harboring a passion for antiquity. The studies of German archaeologist Johann Joachim Winckelmann during the 18th century opened a new era of research, archeological excavations, and laws for the preservation of monuments, all of which have finally allowed the reconstruction of the area's millennial history. ⊠ *Via dei Fori Imperiali and Piazza S. Maria Nova.*

Monastero di Tor de' Specchi

⊞**6 B1.** The convent was founded in 1433 by Roman noblewoman Francesca de Ponziani (St. Frances of Rome), who established a congregation of Benedictine Oblates dedicated to charitable works (oblates dedicate themselves to service and take a vow of obedience from which they may withdraw at any time). The severe building encloses delightful cloisters and rooms, including the Cappella Vecchia, illuminated by Gothic windows, decorated with a fresco cycle (ca. 1468) with 25 scenes from the life of St. Frances, and covered with a fine 15th-century ceiling. Another space, perhaps designed as a refectory, has a green decorative scheme (ca. 1485) depicting the temptations of St. Frances. In 1596, in addition to the already existing **church of S. Maria de Curte,** a church consecrated to the **Ss. Annunziata** was erected. ⊠ *Via della Tribuna di Tor de' Specchi 40.*

Oratorio di S. Giovanni in Oleo

⊞**8 D6.** This small octagonal structure, perhaps a martyrium, was built in the 5th century on the site where the saint was thought to have suffered immersion in a cauldron of boiling oil, from which he emerged unharmed. Francesco Borromini, who designed an unusual coping for the circular drum, restored the building in 1658. The interior decoration (with *Scenes from the Life of St. John the Evangelist*) is dated 1716. ⊠ *Via di Porta Latina.*

Orti Farnesiani
(Farnese Gardens)
⊞**6 C2–D2.** The gardens were created by Cardinal Alessandro Farnese, nephew of Paul III, during the mid-16th century in an area of the Palatine rich in symbolic significance because it is tied to the mythical origins of Rome and to

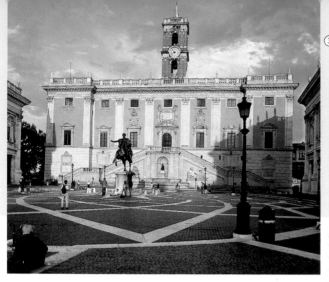

the memory of the emperors who had their opulent residences here. This nearly century-long project was begun by Il Vignola and completed by Carlo Rainaldi. An entrance in the Forum led through a series of ramps to the *Ninfeo della Pioggia* (a grotto) and the *Teatro del Fontanone*, then to an upper terrace with gardens and two aviaries built in the shape of arched pavilions with pagoda-style roofs. Little remains of the original gardens, the most beautiful on the Palatine; the present layout, with rectangular avenues and a variety of rare and exotic plants, is almost entirely the result of 19th-century projects. ⊠ *Archaeological Zone of the Palatine.*

Palatino (Palatine)

⊞6 C2–D2–D3. This is the hill where, according to tradition, Romulus founded Rome in the 8th century BC; here, too, near Romulus's hut, the first emperor, Augustus, constructed his house. His successors followed suit and built increasingly opulent dwellings. In time, the name of the hill, "palatium," became a term associated in all European languages with grand formal buildings. The shift of imperial power to Constantinople marked the beginning of the decline for the Palatine, although it continued to be, at irregular intervals, a location for sovereigns and popes. During the Byzantine domination, when the Dux (leader) of Rome resided here, Christian houses of worship were established over the ancient ruins. In the late 4th century, a space from Domitian's palace was occupied by an oratory dedicated to St. Caesarius, then converted to a monastery of Greek monks; S. Anastasia was founded

during the same period. Subsequently S. Teodoro, S. Maria Antiqua, and the Monastery of S. Maria in Pallara were built; the latter was later dedicated to St. Sebastian. During the 11th and 12th centuries the hill was fortified and became the site of ferocious baronial struggles. In the Renaissance it was occupied by the principal patrician families, who covered it with villas and gardens, the most famous of which belonged to the Farnese (the Orti Farnesiani). Excavations and often vandalism were carried out during the 18th century; in the 19th century there began to be systematic archaeological research, which continues today. The archaeological area of the Palatine, in addition to containing an extraordinary group of masterpieces of ancient art, preserves a crude graffito that is of great importance to the history of Christian iconography: a crucified man with the head of a donkey, and a man at the foot of the cross with his arm raised and a Greek inscription that reads Alexamenos Worships His God. The author of the drawing was clearly making fun of a Christian. Dating from the first half of the 3rd century AD, this is one of the oldest representations of the Crucifixion. ⊠ *Via S. Gregorio.*

Piazza del Campidoglio ③

⊞6 B1. For centuries the Campidoglio was a center and symbol of power. First it was the stronghold of early Rome, then the location of prestigious public buildings, the mint, the state archives and, above all, the Temple of Jupiter, the greatest sanctuary in ancient Rome. It became the site of the most solemn public ceremonies, such as the investiture of the con-

suls and the celebration of military triumphs. Its sacred role endured through subsequent eras. Medieval German emperors came here to formally request the approval of the Roman people, and this is the site where the great poets were crowned with laurel. Beginning in the 12th century, the hill became the center of executive, judicial, and commercial power, and it was the principal site for government offices (the Senatori and Conservatori) and associations of artists and craftsmen. But the growing power of the papacy gradually did away with the municipal authorities centered on the Campidoglio and took over what had been the symbol of Rome's greatness, removing all trappings of civil power from the site. Paul III decided that the Campidoglio should become a site that symbolized the church's supremacy, and he turned the large-scale project over to Michelangelo. The artist came up with a theatrical solution—a trapezoidal terrace, with the senate building at the back, framed by two side palazzi, overlooking the city from a monumental staircase. The fulcrum of the piazza was the **equestrian statue of Marcus Aurelius**, a rare ancient bronze that escaped destruction because it was thought to be a portrait of Constantine, the first Christian emperor. This was the first monumental piazza in modern Rome, and the magnificent stage was the setting for a pause in the solemn papal processions from the Vatican to the Lateran, where the pope received homage from the Capitoline magistrates. Many churches, convents, and houses were built around the piazza and later demolished to make way for the construction of the monument to Vittorio Emanuele. The Campidoglio continues to be a place of power and memory of the ancient world. The senate building houses the offices of the municipal

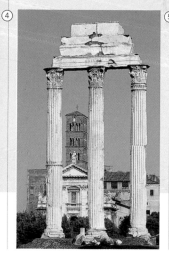

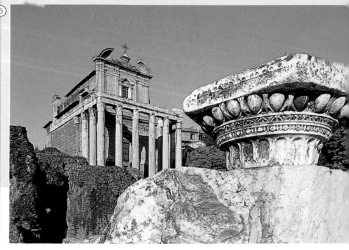

administration, and the buildings on either side contain the **Musei Capitolini** (the Capitoline Museums), the oldest public art collection (which began with a donation from Sixtus IV in 1471) and one of the most magnificent in the world. ⊠ *Musei Capitolini, Piazza del Campidoglio,* ☎ *06/671–03069.*

S. Anastasia
⊞**6 D2.** The church was built at the foot of the Palatine in the 4th century, perhaps through the initiative of a sister of the emperor Constantine, who wanted to dedicate it to the venerated 3rd-century Roman martyr. Some of the saint's relics are in the church. During the Byzantine domination it became the official church of representatives of the Eastern empire who resided on the Palatine. After various renovations over the course of centuries, it was entirely rebuilt in the late 17th century, at the behest of Urban VIII, and the interior was redecorated in the early 18th century. ⊠ *Piazza S. Anastasia.*

S. Francesca Romana ④
⊞**6 C3.** The church was built in the 9th century above the earlier Oratory of Ss. Pietro e Paolo, which in turn had been erected within the ancient Temple of Venus and Rome (2nd century AD). It was called S. Maria Nova to distinguish it from S. Maria Antiqua in the Roman Forum. The church was restored in the 12th century (the bell tower and beautiful apse mosaics depicting the Madonna and child with saints date from this phase) and was rebuilt once again in the 17th century. At the beginning of that century it took its present name, after the body of St.

Frances of Rome was moved here from the Tor de' Specchi Convent. The sacristy contains a 5th-century icon with an image of the Virgin and some interesting paintings from the 16th to the 18th centuries. ⊠ *Piazza S. Francesca Romana 4.*

S. Giovanni a Porta Latina
⊞**8 D6.** Built in the 5th century in the vicinity of the Oratory of S. Giovanni in Oleo, this church was renovated many times over the centuries, until the most recent restoration, which returned it to its Romanesque appearance. The interior, on a basilica plan, has an interesting painting cycle with *Scenes from the Old and New Testaments* dating from the 12th century. ⊠ *Via di Porta Latina 17.*

S. Gregorio Magno
⊞**6 E3.** The church was built on the site of St. Gregory the Great's home, where the saint established a monastery in 575, dedicated to St. Andrew. The present exterior is the result of a 1629–1633 renovation ordered by Cardinal Scipione Borghese. The interior dates from the 18th century. The Salviati Chapel contains an ancient fresco of the Madonna and child, which, according to tradition, spoke to the saint. There is also a beautiful marble altar from the 15th century. At the back of the right nave is another prized altar, decorated with bas-reliefs depicting the so-called *30 Masses of St. Gregory.* Next to the church are three small chapels built in the early 17th century. The one in the center, dedicated to St. Andrew, has frescoes by Domenichino and Guido Reni (1608); the one on the right is the Oratory of St. Sylvia, mother of St. Gregory, and has a lively *Concert of*

Angels by Guido Reni in the apse vault. The third chapel, dedicated to St. Barbara, has a large marble table from the 3rd century, said to be the one where an angel sat next to the poor to whom St. Gregory offered a meal. This legend, one of many connected to this extraordinary figure, is often represented in his iconography. ⊠ *Piazza S. Gregorio 1.*

S. Lorenzo in Miranda ⑤
⊞**6 C2.** The ancient pagan temple of Antoninus and Faustina (AD 141) was transformed in the 7th century into a church, which preserved the solemn vestibule and six columns in front of the Baroque facade. It is dedicated to St. Laurence of Rome, one of the city's most venerated figures, perhaps because it was on this site that the trial took place that condemned him to martyrdom. The name "in Miranda" might derive from the Latin verb *mirari* (to admire), referring to the magnificent panorama of the Roman Forum that opened in front of the building. In 1429, Martin V gave the church to the Collegio degli Speziali (College of Chemists or Herbalists), now the Collegio Chimico Farmaceutico, which retains St. Laurence as its patron saint. The painting on the high altar, by Pietro da Cortona, depicts *The Martyrdom of St. Laurence* (1640). ⊠ *Via in Miranda 10.*

S. Maria Antiqua
⊞**6 C2.** The church was installed in the 6th century in a room of a 1st-century AD building, perhaps part of the ancient imperial palace. It was called "Antiqua" in the 10th century, after a church erected over the temple of Venus and Rome

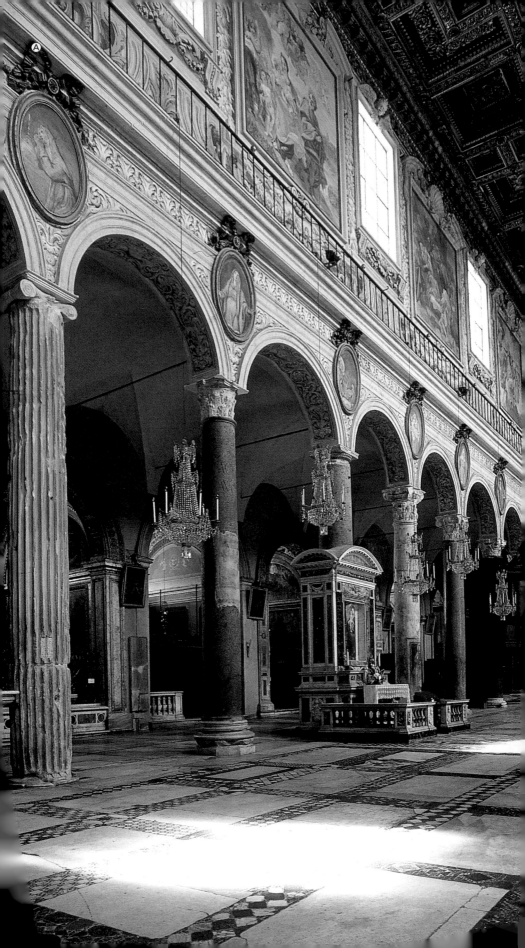

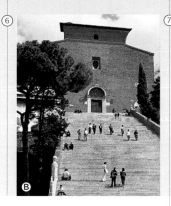

S. Maria in Aracoeli ⑥ has three naves divided by ancient columns made from different types of marble; (A) an ornate coffered wooden ceiling, and (B) a 13th-century brick facade.

The extraordinary Baroque altar in S. Maria in Campitelli's ⑦ was designed by Carlo Rainaldi (1667), who was also responsible for the overall design of the building; at the center, a priceless miraculous image of the Virgin.

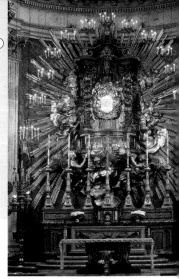

became known as S. Maria Nova (S. Francesca Romana). Pontiffs from the East, who occupied the papacy for more than 150 years, lavished attention on this church, commissioning paintings for its walls many times over. The results are still visible in the exceptional layering of frescoes (at some points up to five superimposed one on top of another), which attest to the different styles in Roman art during the Byzantine period. These range from stiff frontal representations, similar to icons, such as a Virgin and child enthroned, to the right of the apse, to more fluid and naturalistic depictions, as in the fragmentary frescoes of the Annunciation, to the right of the apse (above the aforementioned Virgin) and on the southeast pier. At the time of Pope John VII (705–707), the building became the bishop's church of Rome and the center of Eastern-inspired piety in the city. The nearby **Oratorio dei Quaranta Martiri** (Oratory of the 40 Martyrs) is decorated with 8- and 9th-century frescoes of the torture of 40 soldiers put to death in Armenia because of their Christian faith during the persecutions of Diocletian. ⊠ *Largo Romolo e Remo 1.*

S. Maria in Aracoeli ⑥
▦**6 B1.** The church was erected in the 7th century at the highest point of the Capitoline Hill. It was a Benedictine abbey from the 10th century until the mid-13th century, when it was taken over by the Franciscans. The name of the church (which did not appear before the 14th century) recalls the legend that the emperor Augustus had an altar built here following the appearance of the Virgin and a prophecy announcing to him the birth of the Redeemer. The event is represented in a 12th-century altar in the left transept. During the late 13th century the church assumed its present form, and in 1348 the

monumental stairway leading to the church was added as an offering to the Virgin for the end of the plague. The original austere atmosphere of the Franciscan church was altered over the centuries by the addition of an enormous quantity of ornaments, furnishings, and funerary monuments. The principal works include frescoes by Pinturicchio of *Scenes from the Life of St. Bernardine* (1486); Benozzo Gozzoli's *St. Anthony* (1454–1458); the *Tomb of Luca Savelli*, (ca. 1287), attributed to Arnolfo di Cambio; the tombstone of Giovanni Crivelli by Donatello (1432); and the 14th-century presbytery pulpits. As in all significant Roman churches dedicated to the Madonna, this one has a venerated Marian icon above the high altar; the painting dates from the 11th century. In a chapel next to the sacristy is a statue of the *Holy Child,* sculpted, according to legend, from wood from an olive tree in Gethsemane. The sculpture is an object of secular veneration because of its supposed miraculous powers, including the ability to heal the sick and resuscitate the dead. ⊠ *Piazza del Campidoglio 4.*

S. Maria in Campitelli ⑦
▦**5 B6.** The church was built in 1662–1667, on the site of an earlier church, to house an image of the Madonna to which the people attributed the miracle of the liberation of the city from the plague of 1656. Alexander VII entrusted Carlo Rainaldi with the design, and it is one of the architect's most successful projects. The facade with superimposed niches is enlivened by the skillful use of detached columns, and the interior has an original juxtaposition of a grand Greek-cross space and a narrower space with a dome and apse. The miraculous image of Mary on the high altar is a precious 11th-century work. ⊠ *Piazza Campitelli 9.*

S. Maria della Consolazione
▦**6 C1.** The church has its origins in the last wish expressed by a man condemned to death in 1385. On the site of his execution, beneath the nearby Tarpeian Rock, he asked that an image of the Madonna be placed, to console those who were sentenced to death. Later miracles attributed to this image made this a venerated site, and the church was built, then renovated starting in 1583 by Martino Longhi the Elder. Until 1936 the spacious edifice behind the church was occupied by the Ospedale della Consolazione, a hospital that specialized in trauma care, where physicians worked alongside benefactors and saints, including St. Luis Gonzaga, who died here in 1591 attending to victims of cholera. ⊠ *Piazza della Consolazione 84.*

S. Maria in Domnica
▦**6 F4.** This church is also known as S. Maria della Navicella, because of the presence of a small marble boat (*navicella*) in the piazza opposite, a 16th-century copy of an ancient ex-voto. Built in the 7th century on the site of a Roman barracks, the church and oratory constituted one of the first charitable institutions in the city dedicated to assisting the poor. It was rebuilt under Paschal I between 818 and 822 and restored during the 16th century, when the elegant exterior portico and wonderful inlay and gilded coffered ceiling were executed. The precious apse mosaics date from the time of Paschal I and are an important example of Roman art from the Carolingian period. The triumphal arch is dominated by the figure of Christ between two angels and the apostles, and the lower register

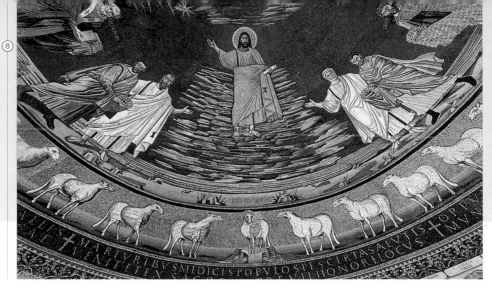

depicts Moses and Elijah. The vault of the apse has an image of the Virgin and child enthroned amid hosts of angels, with Paschal I kneeling and humbly touching her feet. ⊠ *Piazza Navicella 10.*

S. Sebastiano al Palatino

⊞**6 D3.** The entire eastern section of the Palatine (in the area of the churches of S. Sebastiano and S. Bonaventura) is occupied by a gigantic terraced area surmounted by the large temple of the god Elagabalus, who was identified with the sun. It was erected by the emperor of the same name (3rd century AD), who wanted to be worshiped as a god. The most sacred objects in Rome were assembled in this edifice, including the venerated Palladium, the ancient image of Pallas Athena from Troy. This explains the name of the church, **S. Maria in Pallara** (from the Palladium), erected in the Middle Ages in this area and later consecrated to St. Sebastian who, according to tradition, was martyred here. Mentioned in documents as far back as the 10th century, the church preserves some painting fragments from this era in the apse. The rest of the church was destroyed during the renovation ordered by Urban VIII in 1624. A short distance away, at 7 Via S. Bonaventura, is the church and monastery of **S. Bonaventura,** erected in 1625 by St. Bonaventure Grau, on the site of an ancient cistern of the Claudian aqueduct. ⊠ *Via S. Bonaventura 1.*

S. Sisto Vecchio

⊞**8 C4.** This ancient church (mentioned in the 4th century) is consecrated to Sixtus II, a pope and martyr killed during the persecutions

of the emperor Valerian (258), along with many of his companions, including the deacon Laurence, to whom he is closely linked. In the 6th century Sixtus II's remains were moved to the church from the Catacombs of St. Calixtus. The church was rebuilt by Innocent III and in 1219 was given to St. Dominic de Guzmán, who established his first monastery in Rome here. The Romanesque bell tower dates from this period, as do some vestiges in the cloister and an interesting fresco cycle with *Scenes from the New Testament and the Apocrypha.* The entire complex was radically restructured in 1724–1730 by Benedict XIII. ⊠ *Piazzale Numa Pompilio 8.*

S. Teodoro

⊞**6 C2.** This church on a central plan was built around the mid-6th century, during a period of strong Byzantine influence in both art and religious orientation, confirmed by the dedication to St. Theodore of Euchaita, one of the most venerated Eastern martyrs, patron of soldiers and armed forces. The structure was entirely rebuilt by Pope Nicholas V (1453–1554), and the piazza opposite and the two-flight staircase are by Carlo Fontana (1703–1705). The apse mosaics of *The Redeemer with Sts. Peter, Paul, and Theodore* are from the original church. ⊠ *Via di San Teodoro 7.*

S. Tommaso in Formis

⊞**6 E4.** In 1207, Innocent III granted the ancient little church of S. Tommaso to St. John of Matha, who immediately installed the order he had founded in France, which was dedicated to the worship of the Trinity and to freeing slaves and prisoners. Near the church the

Trinitarian fathers built a hospital, which prospered for two centuries, then fell into decline and was destroyed in 1925. The church, restored many times between the 16th and 18th centuries, has lost most of its medieval furnishings and structure. Of the Trinitarian monastic complex and hospital, part of the side facade remains, with a pointed arch door and a broad Romanesque entrance surmounted by a mosaic niche with a depiction of Jesus between two freed slaves. ⊠ *Via S. Paolo della Croce 10.*

Ss. Cosma e Damiano ⑧

⊞**6 C2.** The structure is the result of the unification of two buildings from the imperial period donated by King Theodoric to Pope Felix IV. The pontiff consecrated the buildings to Cosmas and Damian, two Eastern brothers who were physicians and martyrs, perhaps in opposition to the pagan cult of the Dioscuri, which had a temple nearby in the Roman Forum. The total renovation by Urban VIII (1632) saved the precious original mosaics in the apse, which depict Christ with Sts. Peter and Paul presenting the titular saints of the church, who hold their crowns of martyrdom, accompanied by St. Theodore of Euchaita and Felix IV. The grandeur of the figures, the balance of the composition, and the precise characterization are clear reminders of classical art inserted within a typically medieval transcendent atmosphere. Compositions with seven figures were enormously popular in Rome and perhaps had as their model the mosaic apse in S. Giovanni in Laterano, which no longer survives. ⊠ *Via dei Fori Imperiali 1.*

The bowl-shaped apse vault of Ss. Cosma e Damiano ⑧. The unusual 6th- to 7th-century mosaic echoes a Roman compositional scheme with seven figures (Christ; Sts. Peter, Paul Cosma, Damian and Theodore; and Felix IV).

Piazza dei Ss. Giovanni e Paolo ⑨ is dominated by the brick mass of the church of the same name. The original structure is early Christian, and the superb bell tower is Romanesque. This is one of the quietest and most evocative corners in the Celio district.

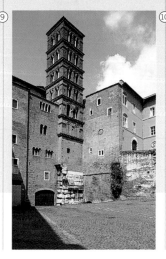

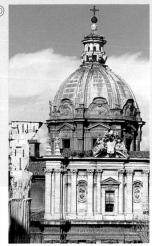

Ss. Giovanni e Paolo ⑨

⊞6 E4. The basilica has its origins in a titular church established in the house of the martyr brothers John and Paul, two Christian officials put to death during the papacy of Julian the Apostate (361–363) after they were discovered donating their wealth to poor Christians. The building was restored in the 12th century with the addition of a portico, a beautiful Romanesque bell tower (erected on the ruins of a Roman temple), and a monastery. In subsequent centuries the building underwent various renovations, and in 1952 the early Christian facade was restored. Excavations have uncovered a complex of 1st- to 5th-century buildings beneath the church, a noteworthy testament to early Christianity's existence within the pagan world. Some of the spaces have frescoes with mythological scenes, while others are decorated with Christian images, including the execution of three people, probably Crispus, Crispinianus, and Benedicta, companions of the titular saints. Next to the basilica is the 19th-century **Chapel of S. Paolo della Croce,** founder of the Passionist fathers (1694–1775), who have cared for the church since 1773. In addition to the three usual vows (poverty, chastity, and obedience), members of the order take a fourth vow to promote the devotion of Christ's Passion. ⊠ *Piazza dei Ss. Giovanni e Paolo 13.*

Ss. Luca e Martina ⑩

⊞6 B2. During the 6th century a church was built here, dedicated to the martyr St. Martina (who lived in the 3rd century). The church was said to be "in three forums" because it is situated at the point where the Roman Forum meets the forums of Cesar and Augustus. Sixtus V gave the church to the Drawing Academy of St. Luke

(1588), which had been established shortly before to offer apprenticeships and theoretical training to young artists. Restoration work directed by Pietro da Cortona, head of the academy, brought to light the bodies of several martyrs, including Martina. This led Urban VIII and his nephew, Cardinal Francesco Barberini, to finance construction of a grander building (the pope's coat of arms crowns the facade, and the heraldic bees of the Barberini appear throughout the church). Working for nearly 30 years (1635–1664), Pietro da Cortona created one of the most refined Baroque churches in Rome. In addition to a statue of the saint in a supine position by Niccolò Menghini (1635), there is a crypt, sumptuously decorated with marble and columns, and a gilded bronze altar above the tomb of St. Martina, another masterpiece by Pietro da Cortona. ⊠ *At the entrance to the Roman Forum.*

Ss. Quattro Coronati

⊞6 D5. The dedication to four "crowned" saints, that is saints conferred with the crown of martyrdom, is somewhat complicated. One tradition speaks of four soldiers condemned for not having recognized the divinity of Asclepiades. These figures were later confused with four other Roman martyrs, Severus, Victorinus, Carpophorus, and Severian. This tale was then layered with a story of Dalmatian sculptors killed by Diocletian for refusing to sculpt a statue of that pagan god, with the result that this church is venerated by an association of stonecutters and marble workers. Erected in the 5th century, the church was transformed into a

basilica by Leo IV (847–855), who was responsible for moving the remains of the martyred saints into the marble arches of the crypt. Between the 12th and 13th centuries a monastery and a charming cloister were added, and in 1246 the complex was transformed into a fortress, which often served as a refuge for pontiffs who did not feel safe in the Lateran. During this period the monastery chapel (the Oratory of St. Sylvester), reserved for private masses of the pope and curia, was decorated with a painting cycle depicting the legend of Sts. Sylvester and Constantine. The cycle was an outright papal manifesto that openly stated the pontiff's supremacy over the imperial power, embodied at that time in the extremely feared Holy Roman Emperor Frederick II . ⊠ *Piazza Ss. Quattro Coronati 20.*

10
Ripa, S. Saba, and Testaccio

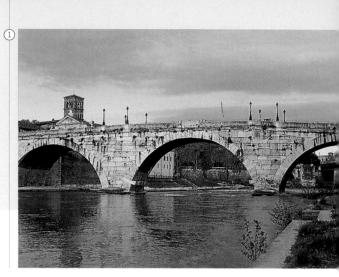

In ancient times this area was populous, animated, and teeming with warehouses and commercial activity connected to the large river port. During the Middle Ages it became solitary and rural, scattered with abandoned ruins and isolated monastic settlements, and often afflicted by swampiness and malaria because of flooding of the Tiber. Urbanization did not come until the late 19th century, but construction tended to be respectful of the landscape and left open broad, unbuilt areas. In modern times, the district has developed various faces: an aristocratic, refined neighborhood on the Aventine; public buildings at the foot of the hill, near the river; and the working-class district of Testaccio.

Aventino

▦**8 A1–A2.** The solitude and silence that characterize this hill perpetuate its isolation, which dates from the most distant days of antiquity, and in fact the Aventine was not included within the urban boundaries until the 1st century AD. The district's archaeological legacy was in large part destroyed by post–World War II building development, but there are numerous vestiges of early Christian and medieval times. Some of the first and most significant early Christian places of worship were established here (S. Balbina, S. Prisca, S. Saba, S. Sabina), as well as monasteries and fortified settlements. Post-medieval architectural projects, such as the 18th-century compound of the Knights of Malta, by Giovanni Battista Piranesi, involved the modification and renovation of already existing buildings.

Casa dei Crescenzi

▦**6 D1.** The house of the Crescenzi, the most powerful Roman family from the 10th to the 12th century, was built between 1040 and 1065 to control the Tiber port that lay opposite. Like many of the fortresses built during the Middle Ages by the baronial class, the structure reutilized architectural elements from ancient monuments: the corbels with cherubs, the cornice, ceiling coffers with rosettes used as a window parapet. In addition to obvious practical and economic reasons, this recycling was dictated by a desire to "restore the ancient dignity of Rome," according to a long Latin inscription over the entrance arch. The building was used during the Middle Ages as the house of Pilate in the Easter Passion play along the Via Crucis, and the structure is also known by this name. ⊠ *Via Petroselli 54.*

Cimetero degli Inglesi
(English Cemetery)

▦**8 D1.** A source of fascination for many 19th-century Romantic artists, the Protestant or English cemetery is still extremely evocative. The cemetery was established in the 18th century for foreigners who were of other religious faiths and could not be buried in Catholic cemeteries. Set at the foot of the Pyramid of Gaius Cestius (the tomb of an eccentric 1st-century BC Roman, who wanted to emulate the pharaohs), it provides a solitary landscape of meadows, pines, and cypress trees that frames the tombs. Numerous famous figures are buried here, including poets John Keats and Percy Bysshe Shelley; painter Joseph Severn; and Antonio Gramsci, intellectual, co-founder of the Communist party in Italy,

aetheist, and one of the few Italians buried here. ⊠ *Via Caio Cestio.*

Complesso dell'Ordine dei Cavalieri di Malta
(Compound of the Order of Knights of Malta) ②

▦**5 F6.** The Order of the Knights of Malta grew out of the Order of St. John of Jerusalem. Established in the 11th century, the Knights of Malta were a charitable rather than military organization, although their holdings on Rhodes and Malta created an effective defense against the Turkish threat. The compound's current appearance is the result of a radical restoration, ordered in 1764 by Cardinal G.B. Rezzonico (grand master of the order and nephew of Clement XIII) and entrusted to the period's most well known engraver, Giovanni Battista Piranesi. This was Piranesi's only architectural project, and it is a masterpiece of Neoclassical urban design. Recurrent motifs from the artist's prints are translated into stone: walls punctuated by obelisks, niches and trophies of arms alluding to the order's history, and the heraldic symbols of the Rezzonico family. Similar motifs appear on the facade of the adjacent church, **S. Maria del Priorato**, which appears to be made of fragments of ancient marbles. A peek through the keyhole of the door at number 3 in the piazza offers an beautiful framed view of the gigantic dome of S. Pietro. ⊠ *Piazza Cavalieri di Malta 4.*

Isola Tiberina (Tiber Island) ①

▦**5 C5–C6.** Among the many legends that surround the island, the most famous refers to its boat-like shape, said to derive from the ship of Aesculapian, god of medicine, whom Romans invoked during a

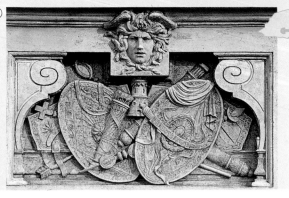

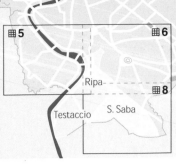

A shrine on the wall that encloses the Compound of the Order of the Knights of Malta, an exquisite Neoclassical project by Piranesi (1764–1766).

plague and to whom they dedicated a temple and hospital. From that time on the island was associated with healing. In 1584, the **Ospedale Fatebenefratelli** was built (and still stands in the piazza of the same name) by the Congregation of S. Giovanni di Dio. This group's members also were called "Fatebenefratelli" (literally "do good, brothers"), the phrase they would repeat when they asked for alms. The area was transformed into a leper asylum during the plague of 1656. The church of **S. Bartolomeo** (Piazza di S. Bartolomeo all'Isola) was built by the Holy Roman Emperor Otto II (10th century) on the ruins of the Temple of Aesculapian. The medieval well near the altar proba-bly served as the old hospital font, said to have had extraordinary ther-apeutic properties. Often damaged by frequent floodings of the Tiber, the church was rebuilt in 1113 by Pope Paschal II, who gave the build-ing one of the most harmonious Romanesque bell towers in Rome. The building was renovated in Baroque style in 1624. A porphyry basin beneath the high altar con-tains the remains of the apostle and martyr Bartholomew, who was famous for the miraculous healings he wrought during his work as an evangelist.

S. Alessio
5 F6. Dating from perhaps the 4th century and originally dedicated to St. Boniface, in the 10th century this church became a significant religious center for the Benedictines and a departure point for some of the most active evangelizers of the time, including St. Adalbert, bishop of Prague. Although totally renovat-ed in the 18th century, the church preserves some significant medieval structures, which for the most part date from the rebuilding under Pope Honorius III (1217). These are five bell towers; the mosaic entrance that reutilizes ancient marble from the imperial period; the two small columns in the apse, which come from the 13th-century choir; and the Romanesque crypt, the only one of its type in Rome, which contains the remains of St. Thomas of Canterbury. In the left nave, an ornate 18th-century chapel reveals vestiges of a staircase associated with the legend of St. Alexius. He was a young, wealthy 4th-century Roman who converted to Christianity and departed for the East, where he lived an ascetic life. Returning to Rome after 17 years, he worked as a slave in his father's house without being recognized, sleeping in a space beneath the staircase. The legend provided a wealth of material for music, poet-ry, and art during the Middle Ages and the Baroque period, when a great many chapels, altars, and staircases were dedicated to the saint. ⊠ *Piazza S. Alessio 23.*

S. Balbina
8 B3. According to tradition, St. Balbina, daughter of Quirinus, a Roman tribune, was killed with her father around the year 130 because they were both Christians. The church is first mentioned in a 6th-century document as Sanctae Balbinae, but its origins are older. Rebuilt many times, the church's current Romanesque appearance is the result of a radical restoration carried out in 1930. The high altar has a jasper urn containing the remains of the saint, her father, and St. Felicissimus. The sixth niche to the left has a fresco depicting the *Crucifixion of St. Peter* (12th centu-ry), perhaps connected to the leg-end that the chains of St. Peter were discovered by Balbina. A second legend relates how St. Balbina healed Pope Alexander I, who was also persecuted and imprisoned for his faith, by laying these same chains around his neck. For this reason Balbina is the patron saint of goiter patients. The most interesting work of art in the church is a mar-ble relief with a *Crucifixion* dating from the 15th century (the fourth niche on the right). ⊠ *Piazza S. Balbina 8.*

S. Cesareo de Appia
8 C5. Clement VIII, whose insignia are inscribed in the elegant gilded ceiling inside, rebuilt this church in the 16th century. It stands above a Roman house from the 2nd century AD, and a part of that build-ing's black and white mosaic floor with sea scenes is still visible. The column in front of the building, like many others in Rome, indicated that this was a hospice-hospital for medieval pilgrims. ⊠ *Via Porta S. Sebastiano.*

S. Eligio dei Ferrari
(St. Eligius of the Ironworkers)
6 C1. In 1453, Pope Nicholas V granted a small medieval church to the school of an assocation of iron artisans known as the Università dei Ferrari. The church was rebuilt and expanded in the following century, when it took on an exuberant Baroque appearance. St. Eligius was the patron saint of metal craftsmen, including goldsmiths, who left the university and the Confraternity of Ironworkers in 1509 and built their own church, S. Eligio degli Orefici. ⊠ *Via S. Giovanni Decollato 9.*

S. Giorgio in Velabro
6 D1. "In Velabro" comes from the ancient name for the swampy depression between the Campidoglio and the Palatine, which was subject to recurring floods of the Tiber. The building was erected in the 5th–6th centu- in a Greek neighborhood and w

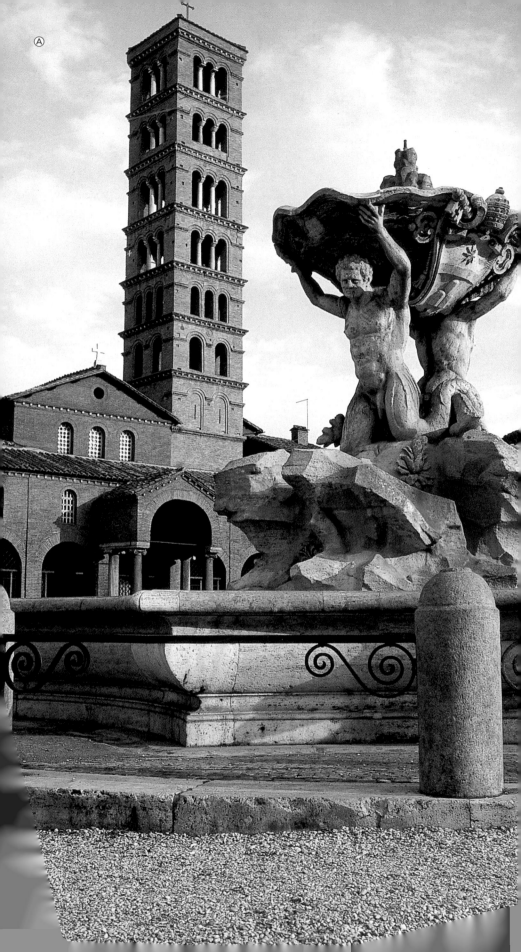

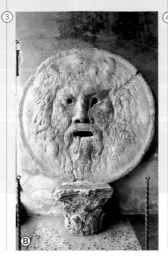

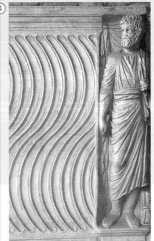

(A) The 18th-century Fontana del Tritone and, in the background, the facade and bell tower of S. Maria in Cosmedin ③.(B) The portico of the church contains the Bocca della Verità, a marble disk from the classical period, which is linked to a famous legend.

Detail of the decoration of a small, well-preserved sarcophagus in the 15th-century portico of S. Saba ④.

profoundly marked by Byzantine influences, which were also evident in other nearby churches (S. Anastasia, S. Maria in Cosmedin, S. Teodoro). The titular saint, St. George the Great, is a martyr from Cappadocia (a region in modern Turkey) who was venerated in the Middle Ages, particularly in the East, as a patron saint of soldiers and knights. A 20th-century restoration returned the church to its original Romanesque appearance, with a simple facade preceded by a portico and a basilica interior divided by recycled antique columns. ⊠ *Via del Velabro 19.*

S. Giovanni Decollato
(St. John Beheaded)
▦**6 D1.** The church was erected beginning in the late 15th century by the Florentine Archconfraternity of S. Giovanni Decollato, or the Misericordia, which was established to assist victims of capital punishment. In 1540, the confraternity obtained the privilege of yearly freeing one person sentenced to death. The church's interior is completely frescoed by Tuscan Mannerist artists, as is the lovely oratory, which is decorated with scenes from the life of St. John the Baptist. The adjacent porticoed cloister, inspired by the Florentine Renaissance, was a burial place for the condemned who were put to death. The compound houses an archive and a museum related to the confraternity's activities. ⊠ *Via S. Giovanni Decollato 22.*

S. Maria in Cosmedin ③
▦**6 D1.** The area in which the church stands, between the Velabrum and the Aventine, was inhabited by a populous Greek colony that was particularly important between the 7th and 9th centuries. Byzantium was politically supreme at that time, and there was an influx of refugees escaping to Rome from the iconoclast persecu-

tions in the Byzantine Empire. The church has its origins in a lay charitable organization from the 6th century and was founded above the ancient Ara Massima of Hercules. It was rebuilt many times over the centuries, until a 19th-century project restored the Romanesque forms from the 12th century, the period its greatest splendor. The name derives from the Greek "kosmein" (to embellish), referring to the church's considerable decorative scheme, much of which was executed by mosaic artists. The sacristy preserves a mosaic on a gold ground that depicts the *Epiphany* (8th century) and was removed from the ancient basilica of S. Pietro. The church has another popular attraction: the ancient drain-cover with the face of a river god, located beneath the portico. It is called the **Bocca della Verità** (Mouth of Truth), because, according to legend, the hand of a liar, placed in the mouth opening, would be bitten. ⊠ *Piazza Bocca della Verità 18.*

S. Omobono
▦**6 C1.** The 15th-century church of S. Salvatore in Portico (probably erected over a pagan edifice) was granted in 1575 to the Università dei Sarti, an association of tailors, who restored it and dedicated it to their patron saint, Homobonus of Cremona, a fabric merchant and miracle-worker. Near the church are the remains of a sacred area of exceptional archaeological importance, the two temples of Fortuna and Mater Matuta, discovered here in 1937. The temples were built by the Etruscan king Servius Tullius (579 BC–53 BC) and destroyed in the late 6th century when the republican regime was established, then

rebuilt in the 4th century BC. Subsequent excavations have uncovered ancient materials from the Bronze Age (14th–13th century BC). ⊠ *Vico Jugario*

S. Prisca
▦**8 B1-2.** Built between the 4th and 5th centuries, this church stands over a Roman residence that tradition identifies as the home of the young Prisca, daughter of Aquila and Priscilla, who offered hospitality to St. Peter and accompanied St. Paul on some of his missionary voyages. Prisca was baptized by Peter (the episode is depicted in the fine painting on the high altar). At the age of 13, she was condemned to be thrown to the lions and miraculously emerged unharmed, but was later decapitated. Numerous rebuilding projects have altered the early Christian appearance of the building, the most interesting part of which still stands underground. Archaeological excavations have revealed a sanctuary dedicated to the worship of the god Mithras and the Roman building that contained the original early Christian place of worship. ⊠ *Via S. Prisca 11.*

S. Saba ④
▦**8 C2.** In the 7th century this was the site of a monastery dedicated to St. Sabbas, a leading Eastern monastic figure (AD 439–AD 532). The Eastern monks were replaced in the 10th century by the Benedictines of Montecassino, who were succeeded in the 13th century by the Cluniac monks, who completely renovated the church, embellishing it with Roman marbles. Two centuries later the church was taken over by the Cistercians. The elegant entrance is by

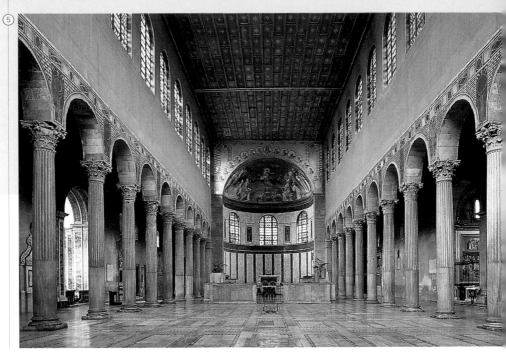

Giacomo, father of Cosma, whose name (cosmatesque) was taken for a famous dynasty of Roman marble-workers and mosaicists. The austere interior houses other works by these artists, most of which have been restored, including the floor, canopy, and episcopal throne. Above the latter is a dramatic 14th-century *Crucifixion*. ⊠*Piazza. G. L. Bernini 20.*

S. Sabina ⑤

▦**5 F6.** This church is an extraordinary example of a 5th-century Western Christian basilica, with original structure, furnishings, and decorations. It was founded in 425 by a priest, Peter of Illyria, during the papacy of Celestine I. Restored during the 8th and 9th centuries, it was granted by Honorius III to St. Dominic de Guzmán just after he approved the new Order of Dominicans (1216), to whom the church still belongs. Later additions during the Renaissance and Baroque eras were for the most part eliminated during the 20th century. The church contains precious elements that have been completely lost in other buildings, such as the magnificent colonnade in Greek marble, the schola cantorum (space for the choir), marble inlay of the side walls of the central nave, windows that make the interior so luminous, and the exceptional entrance with finely carved wooden doors. The doors depict *Scenes from the Old and New Testament*, which

illustrate correspondences between Moses (the Law) and Christ (the Gospel). The fine original mosaics are less well preserved; certain fragments remain from the interior of the facade, which still has a monumental inscription, in perfect gold letters against a blue background, that celebrates the donor, Peter of Illyria, and Pope Celestine I. The two female figures to the sides of the inscription personify the church of the pagans ("ecclesia ex gentibus") and the church of the Jews ("ecclesia ex circumcisione"). Adjacent to the church is a convent, founded by St. Dominic de Guzmán, where St. Thomas Aquinas taught. ⊠*Piazza Pietro d'Illiria 1.*

Ss. Nereo e Achilleo

▦**8 C4.** The establishment of this place of worship (4th century), originally called "titulus fasciolae," is connected to St. Peter, who, according to legend, while escaping from prison lost a bandage (fasciola) he had used to bind a wound caused by his chains. The church took its current name from the two martyrs, Nereus and Achilleus, who were killed by Diocletian in the 3rd century and buried in the Domitilla Catacombs. Their remains and those of St. Flavia Domitilla are buried beneath the high altar. In 814, Pope Leo III ordered some restoration work and embellished the church with mosaics, traces of which remain in the triumphal arch

(*The Transfiguration, The Annunciation, Madonna and Child*). The interior has 16th-century frescoes with scenes from the lives of the martyrs, a mosaic choir and episcopal throne, and a delicately ornamented marble candelabrum from the 15th century. ⊠*Viale delle Terme di Caracalla 28.*

Terme di Caracalla

▦**8 C3–C4.** The majestic ruins of the bath complex, opened by the emperor Caracalla in 217, were the most fascinating monument of the so-called Archaeological Walk, which was created between 1887 and 1914 to preserve and link within a single park the ancient remains between Piazza Venezia and the Appia Antica. This project was destroyed during the fascist regime by the transformation of the footpaths into traffic arteries. The gigantic bath complex included not only areas for bathing, but also gymnasiums, libraries, musical auditoriums, meeting rooms, gardens, and porticos. It was a place for both sports and cultural activity, and it offered Roman citizens an infinite variety of occasions for relaxation and amusement. Although well preserved, the Baths of Caracalla were originally much more magnificent, decorated with a profusion of statues, marbles, stuccowork, and mosaics. ⊠*Viale delle Terme di Caracalla 52.*

11

Esquilino, Castro Pretorio, Sallustiano, and Ludovisi

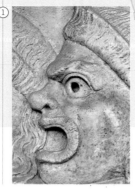

① An ancient roman bas-relief from the Museo Nazionale Romano, one of Italy's major museum of antiquity.

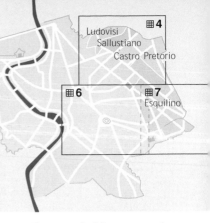

During the early imperial period, the Esquiline rione, which corresponded to the eastern part of the hill of the same name, had many public buildings, opulent villas, and a dense network of roads that are largely still in existence. During the 4th and 5th centuries, the villas were replaced by the basilicas of S. Croce in Gerusalemme and S. Maria Maggiore and some of the oldest Christian places of worship (S. Bibiana and S. Eusebio). Since the late 16th century, following Sixtus V's urban reorganization, the hill began to be repopulated with patrician villas. After 1870 these were demolished to make way for public buildings and the clerical class of the new state. The other three rioni developed in somewhat similar fashion, with a few notable examples of monumental structures from classical times (such as the Gardens of Sallust and the Barracks of the Praetorian Guard) and large 16th- to 18th-century patrician villas (including the magnificent Villa Ludovisi). Most of these were destroyed by late 19th-century development that created ministries, diplomatic buildings and missions, luxury hotels, and new street plans. After World War II, the area underwent further urban renewal, often of very high quality.

Anfiteatro Castrense

▦**7 E4.** This small amphitheater next to the basilica of S. Croce in Gerusalemme was part of the Sessorian Palace, an imperial building from the Severian period (3rd century AD), and owes its partial preservation to its inclusion in the Aurelian Walls. Next to the arch opened in the wall in modern times is the **Cappella di S. Maria del Buon Aiuto,** built by Sixtus IV in 1476 to house an image of the Virgin found on the site. The chapel is also known as S. Maria di Spazzolaria (*spazzola* means "brush" or "broom"), because of the alms that were gathered here, even with a broom. ✉*Piazza S. Croce in Gerusalemme 12.*

Arco di Sisto V

▦**7 A2 .** This is the only monument that officially bears the name of Pope Sixtus V, who worked tirelessly to transform the urban fabric of Rome (as well as the organization of the church). He built the Acquedotto Felice (the pope's name was Felice Peretti) and amid its arcades inserted one monumental arch with three barrel vaults of peperino and travertine, beneath which a road passed to the Baths of Diocletian. The aqueduct reutilized the water sources of an imperial aqueduct near Colonna and ended in the monumental Fountain of Moses in Piazza S. Bernardo. ✉*Piazzale Sisto V.*

Casino dell'Aurora

▦**4 B2.** Along with a large palazzo, now incorporated into the United States Embassy, the Casino dell'Aurora is the only surviving structure from the 17th-century Villa Ludovisi, once considered one of the most beautiful villaparks in the world. The villa was destroyed by postunification building speculation. The Casino is a 16th-century building, renovated by Cardinal Ludovisi in the mid-17th century on a cruciform plan, and altered again during the 19th-century. The building's name derives from the exceptional frescoes executed by Il Guercino in 1621. The depictions of *Aurora* in the vault and allegories of *Day* and *Night* in the side lunettes were decisive for the future of Baroque painting, anticipating by a decade the illusionism of Pietro da Cortona. ✉*Via Aurora.*

Collegium Russicum

▦**6 A6.** The college was established (1928–1929) by Pius XI, during a period of religious persecution in the Soviet Union, to provide the clergy with suitable training to reestablish relationships with the Russian world. Annexed to the college is the 14th-century church **S. Antonio Abate,** now presided over by Russian Catholics of Byzantine Slavic rite. A lovely Romanesque entrance still stands, and the church's 18th-century interior has been adapted to the needs of the Eastern rite. ✉*Via Carlo Alberto 2.*

Fontana del Mosè
(Fountain of Moses)
▦**4 D3.** Opposite the church of S. Maria della Vittoria, this famous monument was designed by Domenico Fontana for Sixtus V as a showpiece of the Acqua Felice, the ancient Claudian aqueduct restored by the pontiff. The water from the Alban Hills was carried to the city's highest elevations. Sculptures on the fountain evoke the voyage of the Jews in the desert under the guidance of Moses, whose statue stands in the central niche. ✉*Piazza S. Bernardo.*

Palazzo Massimo alle Terme, Museo Nazionale Romano ①
▦**4 E4.** Established in 1889 as the archaeological museum of Italy's

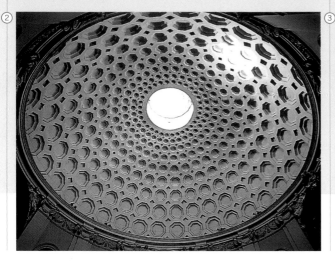

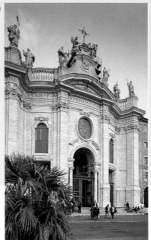

new capital city, this museum was first located in the complex made up of the Baths of Diocletian and the large cloister of S. Maria degli Angeli. The enormous quantity of materials, and the need to organize them more appropriately, made it necessary to find new exhibition spaces. The state acquired the Palazzo Massimo alle Terme and the Palazzo Altemps. A century after its birth, the Museo Nazionale Romano has been reorganized and modernized. Its collection of original documents illustrates the history and development of Rome in ancient times: art, public and private life, religion, economics, urban planning, and settlements outside the city. The museum's holdings are organized in four separate locations: Palazzo Altemps, Baths of Diocletian, Crypta Balbi, and Palazzo Massimo alle Terme. The latter was built in 1883–1887 by the Jesuit priest Massimiliano Massimo to house an educational institute on the grounds of the Pope Sixtus V's opulent Villa Peretti Montalto, which was built between 1576 and 1588 and later demolished to make way for the railway station. An enormous quantity of materials documents every aspect of Roman art, from the republican era to the time of Constantine. There are precious works of art from public buildings and the grand residences of the senatorial class, as well as original Greek sculptures imported to Rome in ancient times. ⊠*Largo di Villa Peretti 1,* ☎*06/489–03500.*

Porta Maggiore

⊞**7 C4.** The majestic architecture of this doorway through the Aurelian Walls, with two barrel vaults flanked by niches, was formed from the arcades of two aqueducts from the Roman period (1st century AD). Opposite the entrance is the **Tomb of Eurysace,** a Roman baker from the Augustinian period (30 BC), who built one of the most unusual funerary monuments in Rome. The cylindrical architectural elements simulate the containers in which he mixed bread dough, and the bas-relief frieze illustrates in detail the various phases of bread making. Facing the piazza is the entrance to the **basilica of Porta Maggiore,** a subterranean sanctuary from the 1st century AD. The basilica's walls are entirely decorated in stucco with mythological scenes, masks, and various decorative motifs. The interpretation of the images is uncertain, but they perhaps depict the liberation of the soul from the weight of the body and its metamorphosis into a different life. ⊠*Piazza di Porta Maggiore.*

S. Bernardo alle Terme ②

⊞**4 D3.** The church was built in 1598, in one of the corner circular halls of the Baths of Diocletian, by order of Caterina Nobili Sforza, niece of Julius III. It was dedicated to St. Bernard of Clairvaux, patron saint and founder of the Cistercians. The cylindrical construction is surmounted by a broad dome (72 feet in diameter) embellished with octagonal coffers that diminish in size toward the central opening, similar to that of the Pantheon. In 1647, a chapel in honor of St. Francis of Assisi was added. The various funerary monuments include one to the German painter Johann Friedrich Overbeck, founder of the Nazarene art movement, which had a certain success in Rome during the first half of the 19th century. ⊠*Piazza S. Bernardo.*

S. Bibiana

⊞**7 B2.** Pope Simplicius (AD 468–AD 483) had this church built in honor of Roman St. Bibiana, who was martyred a century before. According to tradition, the remains of 10,000 Christian martyrs lie in a cemetery on the site, but this has no basis in fact. The church was restored by Honorius III (1224), then given a Baroque renovation (1624–1626) by the young Gian Lorenzo Bernini, who began his career as an architect with this project. Bernini created the lovely statue of the saint for the high altar. A precious alabaster basin from the 4th century is said to contain the remains of the titular saint and her mother and sister, who also were martyrs. Near the entrance is the column to which Bibiana is said to have been tied before being whipped to death. Until the 18th century the dust from this column and the mint that grew on the saint's tomb were used as a remedy against epilepsy. ⊠*Via Giolitti 154.*

S. Croce in Gerusalemme ③

⊞**7 D4–E4.** The church was built on the site of the Sessorium (from the Latin *sedere,* "to stay"), the large imperial palace of Septimus Severus (3rd century), to which the Anfiteatro Castrense also belonged. (That amphitheater and the Coliseum are the only Roman amphitheaters still standing in Rome.) According to tradition the basilica was erected (AD 320) by Constantine to house the remains of the cross and other precious relics his mother, St. Helen, had brought back from Jerusalem. (The legend of the discovery of the true cross is illustrated in the late 15th-century fresco in the apse.) The

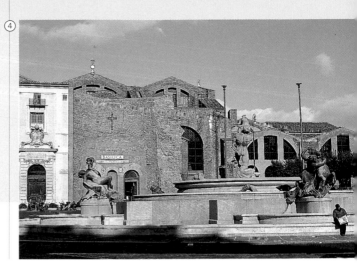

The vast dome of S. Bernardo alle Terme ② measures 72 feet in diameter. In the late 16th century, the church was created from one of the corner turrets of the ancient Baths of Diocletian.

Behind the 19th-century Fontana delle Naiadi is the facade of S. Maria degli Angeli ④, carved from the most monumental spaces of the central element of the great Baths of Diocletian.

church was modified many times during the Middle Ages (when the tall Romanesque bell tower was erected), and then completely transformed under Benedict XIV (1743), who added the delightful facade that functions as a backdrop for the Strada Felice (now Via S. Croce in Gerusalemme). The interior, dominated by 12 colossal antique columns, has elaborate stuccowork and a mosaic floor. The Chapel of St. Helen is decorated with a magnificent Renaissance reproduction of a 5th-century mosaic. The so-called "Calvary" staircase leads to the Chapel of Relics, which contains fragments of the cross, a nail, two thorns from Christ's crown, a piece of the sponge that was offered to him, a fragment of the scroll that hung on the cross, and one of the 30 coins of Judas. Earth from Calvary lies beneath the floor. The basilica is emblematic of a new mentality and a new era for Christianity. It is deliberately and clearly separate from the imperial building, from which it is independent and at the same time dominates. This relationship would have been unthinkable prior to the reign of Constantine, when early Christian meeting places were simply placed within a secular architectural context. ⊠ *Piazza S. Croce in Gerusalemme 12.*

S. Eusebio

▦**6 A6.** This is one of the oldest churches in Rome, and it is dedicated to the 4th-century Roman martyr who was a tireless opponent of Arianism. It seems that St. Eusebius of Bologna financed the construction (first mentioned in 474), and his remains lie beneath the altar. The facade is from the 18th century, and the interior preserves the Romanesque layout of the church rebuilt by Gregory IX (1238), with notable additions and embellishments from the 17th to

the 20th centuries. The Celestines, a Benedictine order founded in 1264 by the hermit St. Peter Celestine (the future Celestine V), had charge over the church and monastery for some time. Dispersed by the French Revolution, the order survived in Italy until 1807. The Celestines had the lovely carved wooden choir built (1600) behind the high altar. The former monastery, now a barracks, still has a harmonious 16th-century cloister. ⊠ *Piazza Vittorio Emanuele II 12/A .*

S. Isidoro

▦**4 C2.** Founded in 1622 by the Spanish Franciscans, this church is consecrated to St. Isidore (1070–1130), the patron saint of Madrid and of farm workers, who was canonized the same year the building was erected. In 1625, the building became a refuge for persecuted Irish Franciscans and is still the site of the Irish College. The church's most notable work is the Da Sylva Chapel, designed by Gian Lorenzo Bernini (1663). During the Napoleonic occupation, during which time the friars dispersed, the monastery became the home of the Nazarene painters, a group that revolved around the German artist Johann Friedrich Overbeck. Their name derived from the artists' "Nazarene-style," long hair and beards and from their communal and ascetic way of life. They proposed an anti-academic art, animated by strong religious sentiment and inspired by Christian medieval stories and legends. Their models were Giotto, Fra Angelico, and, most of all, Raphael and Dürer. ⊠ *Via degli Artisti 41.*

S. Maria degli Angeli ④

▦**4 D4.** In answer to the appeals of a Sicilian priest who had had a vision of angels in the Baths of Diocletian, Pius IV decided to construct a church dedicated to the angels and the Christian martyrs who, according to legend, had built the baths. Michelangelo was entrusted with the design of the basilica, which occupies the most monumental spaces in the center of the baths. The pope granted the complex to the Carthusians, who constructed a monastery (probably also according to a design by Michelangelo). Michelangelo was respectful of the classical ruins, and even with his modifications and later interventions by Luigi Vanvitelli (1750), the building has admirably preserved its antique appearance, which is characterized by eight gigantic monolithic columns and three broad cruciform vaults. The transept and presbytery walls have large altarpieces, many of which come from S. Pietro. One chapel, one statue, and various paintings commemorate St. Bruno of Cologne (1035–1101), founder of the Carthusians, who stayed in Rome for two years as an advisor to Urban II. The ascetic and extremely rigorous life of the order is evoked by the small, austere cells of the **Certosa** (monastery) **of S. Maria degli Angeli,** which presents a clear contrast to the majestic antique structures and opulent basilica. A central element of the monastery was the large cloister (completed in 1565), enclosed by a portico of some hundred travertine columns. ⊠ *Piazza della Repubblica.*

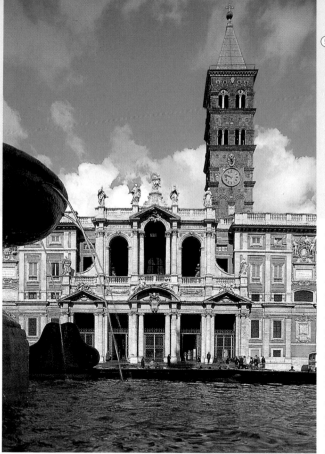

⑤ A large mid-18th-century portico, designed by Ferdinando Fuga, stands in front of the Baroque facade of the patriarchal basilica of S. Maria Maggiore. At the back of the basilica is a brick bell tower, the tallest in Rome, erected in 1377.

The Ecstasy of St. Teresa or, more correctly, *Teresa Transfixed by Love of God* (1646), the celebrated sculpture by Bernini, in S. Maria della Vittoria ⑦.

S. Maria della Concezione dei Cappuccini

⊞4 C2. The church was built in 1626 for the Capuchin cardinal Antonio Barberini, brother of Urban VIII, in a suburban area dominated by the noble Barberini family. It houses works by Guido Reni, Domenichino, Caravaggio, and Pietro da Cortona, but it is best known for its unusual **Capuchin Cemetery,** installed in the subterranean chapels. The chapels are furnished in a macabre style that was particularly popular in Spain, with the skulls and bones of 4,000 Capuchin friars (a similar cemetery is located in the church of S. Maria dell'Orazione e Morte, on the Via Giulia, ☞ 77). The skeletons were moved here from the old Capuchin monastery of S. Nicola de Portiis, now S. Croce e S. Bonaventura dei Lucchesi. ⊠ *Via Veneto 27.*

S. Maria Maggiore ⑤

⊞4 F4. The fourth of the patriarchal basilicas, this church was the centerpiece of Sixtus V's urban reconstruction (his Strada Felice led into the Piazza dell'Esquilino, behind the church). According to legend, the Madonna herself indi-cated to Pope Liberius (AD 352–AD 366) the site where he was to erect the church, with a miraculous snowfall on the peak of the Esquiline hill in August 356. For this reason, since the 11th century the church has also been known as S. Maria ad Nives, and every year, on the day of its founding, a high mass is celebrated, accompanied by a symbolic snowfall. In reality the basilica was erected by Sixtus III (AD 432–AD 440), immediately after the Council of Ephesus (431), which had proclaimed the dogma of Mary's virginity and maternity. The Marian cult, which is directly related to the birth of Jesus, expressed their beliefs in the mosaics of the triumphal arch and in relics from the Grotto of the Nativity in Bethlehem. The latter were brought to Rome in the 7th century and preserved in the oratory of the *presepio,* or crèche, beneath the Chapel of Sixtus V, which contains some nativity statues by Arnolfo di Cambio (1290). Despite innumerable interventions in later centuries (culminating in the 18th-century facade built by order of Benedict XIV), the grand layout of the original church is still visible, with three naves with 40 columns and magnificent mosaic decoration. Along the central nave, 36 panels illustrate *Scenes from the Old Testament,* which is styled in the Hellenistic-Roman tradition of continuous and realistic narration. The Byzantine-style mosaics of the triumphal arch illustrate episodes connected to Mary and the childhood of Christ and episodes that are not related in the Gospels and are therefore considered apocryphal. Above is an image inspired by the Apocalypse, with a bejeweled throne on which Christ will sit on Judgment Day. The apse mosaics, a masterpiece by Jacopo Torriti (1295), were created by order of Pope Nicholas IV. They depict *Scenes from the Life of the Virgin* and *The Coronation of Mary.* Two ornate side chapels are located in front of the high altar— the Sistine Chapel, conceived by Pope Sixtus V as his tomb and created by Domenico Fontana (1584–1587), and the Pauline Chapel, erected by Flaminio Ponzio for Pope Paul V Borghese (1611). The interior of the church is dominated not only by the mosaics, but also by the refined mosaic floor (12th century) and by the sumptuous coffered ceiling decorated with emblems of the client, Pope Alexander VI (1492–1503). It is said that the gilding was accomplished with the first gold brought from America. ⊠*Piazza S. Maria Maggiore.*

S. Maria della Vittoria ⑦

⊞4 C3. The Discalced Carmelites chose this site, where there was an earlier chapel dedicated to St. Paul, to erect a monastery and church. In 1608, Carlo Maderno was entrusted with the project, which was financed by Cardinal Scipione Borghese. Maderno reproduced the general design of his earlier S. Andrea della Valle, and the facade by Giovanni Battista Soria makes the structure appear to be a

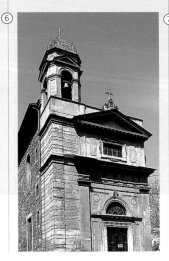

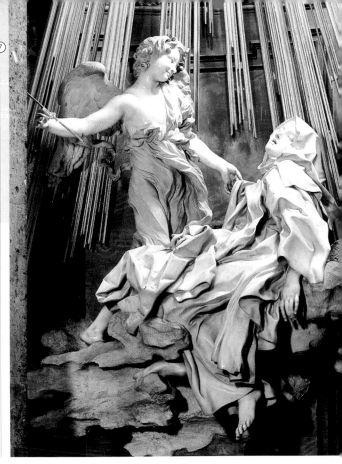

companion piece to the nearby church of S. Susanna. The church was reconsecrated to Mary after the victory of the Catholic imperial troops over the Lutherans near Prague, an event that was attributed to the prodigious influence of a painting of the Madonna and child carried Into battle by a Carmelite friar. It later assumed an ornate Baroque appearance, thanks in part to the intervention of Gian Lorenzo Bernini in the Cornaro Chapel (1646). The famous *Ecstasy of St. Teresa*, one of the high points of this sculptor's art, portrays an expression of mystical agitation that involves both spirit and flesh. The words with which the saint (1515–1582) described the ecstatic experience in her *Libro de su vida* found an extraordinary interpreter in Bernini, who was able to combine spiritual tension and sensuality, two inseparable qualities of 17th-century devotion. ⊠ *Via XX Settembre 17.*

Ss. Vito e Modesto ⑥
▦**6 A6.** In 1474 the church was rebuilt by Sixtus IV, on the site of an ancient place of worship. Changes made in subsequent centuries were eliminated for the most part by a 1973–1977 renovation that restored the 15th-century elements, such as the marble entrance and the two-mullioned Gothic-style windows of the facade. The interior houses two unusual altars in niches with Christ and the Virgin and, protected by a grate, the so-called "stone of iniquity." This was long believed to have been used for the martyrdom of many early Christians, but in reality it was a Roman funeral pillar. Next to the church is the **Arch of Gallienus**, with three barrel vaults,

an Augustinian reconstruction of a door in the Servian Wall (Porta Esquilina) that was dedicated to Emperor Gallienus and his wife in AD 262. ⊠ *Via Carlo Alberto 47.*

Terme di Diocleziano, Museo Nazionale Romano
▦**4 D4.** The largest bath complex in Rome (it could hold 3,000 people) was erected by Diocletian between AD 298 and AD 306. A colossal rectangular enclosure surrounded the central core, which had bath spaces and gymnasiums. The complex fell into ruins and, beginning in the 6th century, it was used to store grain and oil and for religious purposes. Under Pius IV (1561) a Carthusian monastery was installed; first Michelangelo (1561), then Luigi Vanvitelli (1749) contributed to the design and creation of the basilica of S. Maria degli Angeli. The best preserved structures in the ancient baths are those in the church: the two circular spaces in the corners of the enclosure (one has become S. Bernardo alle Terme) and the spaces adapted to house part of the collection of the Museo Nazionale Romano, namely the octagonal hall (planetarium) and the church

of S. Isidoro in Formis. The archaeological materials exhibited here are organized according to large-scale themes: the establishment and early development of the city, artistic development of the republican era, arts and social classes, the history of the Latin language, and writing. ⊠ *Via de Nicola 79,* ☎ *06/488–0530.*

12

Rome Outside the Walls

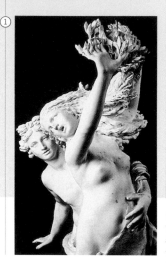

Bernini's *Apollo and Daphne* (1624), in the Galleria Borghese, depicts one of the metamorphosis described by the poet Ovid. Daphne, to escape Apollo's embrace, is transformed into a laurel plant.

The frescoes of the Catacombe di Priscilla ② are some of the oldest examples of sacred painting tied to Christianity. They depict scenes from the Old and New Testament and images of life of the early Christian community.

The Aurelian Walls (3rd century AD) marked the outer limits of the city from medieval times until the 19th century. In republican and imperial times, the suburban stretches of the great consular roads that radiated out from Rome were marked by an uninterrupted series of tombs and villas. In late antiquity the landscape began to change, with the creation of sanctuaries commemorating martyrs, basilicas, and Christian cemeteries, which immediately became popular pilgrimage sites. In subsequent centuries, while pagan monuments decayed into ruins, the most important of these Christian complexes became distinct villages. In the 9th century, devastating Saracen invasions made it necessary to move the martyrs' remains to protected locations within the city walls, condemning most of the early Christian sites to decline and abandonment. The Roman countryside was transformed into a deserted area, frequently described by Romantic writers and dominated by a few basilicas along devotional routes (S. Lorenzo, S. Paolo, and S. Sebastiano). Beginning in the late 16th century, some ornate suburban residences were built (such as the Villa Giulia and the Villa Albani). In the 20th century this formerly deserted area has become for the most part a sea of cement.

Abbazia delle Tre Fontane
(Abbey of the Three Fountains)
⊞ **1 E3.** This delightful complex on the Via Laurentina, surrounded by a eucalyptus grove, was built on the site of the apostle Paul's beheading. The name derives from the legend of three springs that gushed forth on the sites where Paul's head bounced, and where three churches were later built: **S. Paolo, Ss. Vincenzo e Anastasio,** and **S. Maria in Aracoeli.** Since 1868 the abbey has belonged to the Trappists, who then reclaimed the area, which was then malaria-infested and abandoned. In the 7th century a monastery for Greek monks was established near the first church dedicated to the apostle (5th–6th century). The head of the martyr St. Anastasius the Persian was brought here, then the body of St. Vincent of Saragossa, the Spanish martyr who resisted atrocious tortures. Innocent II gave the monastery to the Cistercians (1138), who rebuilt it (it was their second monastery in Italy, after Chiaravalle) according to the aesthetic principles dictated by their founder and patron saint, St. Bernard of Clairvaux. The last changes were made in 1599, on the eve of the 1600 Holy Year, when the churches of S. Maria in Aracoeli and S. Paolo were renovated. The former (1582) received its name (Aracoeli means "altar of heaven") from a vision St. Bernard had on the site, of a ladder on which the souls in purgatory were ascending. This is also the site where legend has it 10,203 legionnaires and their general, Zeno, martyred under Diocletian, are buried. The Romanesque **Ss. Vincenzo e Anastasio** chuch, rebuilt with the nearby monastery of **S. Bernardo**

(1221), preserves the austere monumentality of early Cistercian architecture. Seven altars contain the remains of both the titular martyrs and St. Zeno, as well as relics from the Holy Land. The monastery houses a fresco with a calendar of the months, a rare example of 14th-century secular painting. ⊠ *Via delle Acque Salvie.*

Catacombe di Domitilla
⊞ **1 D3.** The most well known monument along the Via Ardeatina, the Catacombs of Domitilla are one of the two largest early Christian burial sites in Rome (along with the Catacombs of St. Callixtus). Established in the 3rd century around some pagan underground tombs, the catacombs developed on three levels over the next two centuries. The name derives from the owner of the property, Flavia Domitilla, a relative of the emperor Domitian who was exiled because of her Christian beliefs. The most important martyrs buried here were Nereus and Achilleus, Roman soldiers who, after having persecuted Christians, converted and suffered martyrdom under Diocletian. Over their tomb, Pope Siricius (384–399) had a large basilica built, and that edifice contains a depiction of the martyrdom of Achilleus carved into a column. In the 16th century the martyrs' remains were moved inside the walls, along with those of Domitilla, to the church that bears their name. Petronilla (depicted in a 4th-century fresco), a martyr presumed to be the daughter of St. Peter, was also buried in these catacombs. Her remains were moved to the Vatican in 757 by Pope Paul I, to fulfill a promise to Pepin, king of the Franks. Petronilla later became the patron saint of France, and her tomb was the coronation site for the Carolingian sovereigns. ⊠ *Via Ardeatina 280.*

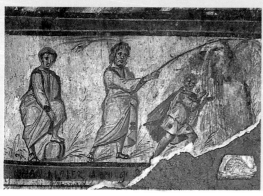

Catacombe Ebraiche di Villa Torlonia
(Jewish Catacombs of Villa Torlonia)

1 B4. In 1918 Jewish catacombs from the 3rd and 4th century were discovered in the park of the Villa Torlonia. They include two independent cemeteries, one of which has numerous inscriptions (mostly in Greek) with the names of the deceased. The other was probably more elaborate, judging from the presence of arched niches with paintings. ⊠ *Via Nomentana.*

Catacombe dei Ss. Marcellino e Pietro

1 C5. Located along the ancient Via Labicana (now the Via Casilina), these catacombs were built during the 3rd century next to a pagan cemetery. They contain the remains of a great many martyrs, including Marcellinus and Peter, who died during the persecutions of Diocletian (304). Constantine built a monumental sanctuary dedicated to the martyrs that included a large basilica and mausoleum, both circular in format. Constantine's mother, St. Helen, was buried here, although the site was almost certainly originally meant for the emperor himself. The catacombs have an incomparable pictorial legacy, with more than 85 spaces frescoed with both Christian and pagan scenes, all well preserved and of a high artistic level. In 827 a shocking event—the plundering of the bodies of the titular saints, ordered by Einhard, Charlemagne's minister and biographer—condemned the complex to decay and abandonment. ⊠ *Via Casilina 641.*

Catacombe di Priscilla ②

1 B3. The Christian cemetery takes its name from the Roman matron Priscilla, who, according to tradition, gave hospitality to the apostle Peter. It is one of the most important and popular pilgrimage sites, in part because of the presence of numerous papal tombs. Above the burial area, Pope Sylvester I (314–335) had a basilica built, which he then consecrated. Its present-day appearance is the result of a 1904–1907 renovation. The heart of the complex is the so-called *arenario*, originally a pozzolana quarry, which has always been considered one of the most ancient Roman catacomb sites (2nd–3rd century). It contains a great number of niches on which simple epitaphs of the deceased were painted in red. These are quite homogeneous, attesting to the egalitarian spirit that was typical of early Christianity, whereby social differences were ignored. One of the most important early Christian frescoes was discovered here, depicting a Madonna and child with a prophet. It dates from the years AD 230–AD 240, and is the oldest known image of the Virgin. ⊠ *Via Salaria 430.*

Catacombe di S. Callisto

1 D4. The oldest and most important cemetery along the Via Appia is named for Callistus. He was the deacon to whom Pope Zephyrnus entrusted the administration of the church's first official cemetery. The area includes the tombs of many martyrs and popes, including Sixtus II, a venerated pontiff who was killed with his deacons during the persecution of 258. Nine 3rd-century pontiffs; popes Caius, Eusebius, and Cornelius; and the martyrs Calocerus, Parthenius, and Caecilia (whose remains were moved here in 821) are buried here. As Christianity spread, the catacombs grew to monumental size, and it became necessary to create easily accessible pathways for pilgrims, through a system of galleries and stairways leading from one sanctuary to another. ⊠ *Via Appia Antica.*

Chiesa del Domine Quo Vadis

1 D3. Near the crossroads of the Via Appia and the Via Ardeatina is a little church, documented since the 9th century with the name S. Maria in Palmis. The current name, Domine Quo Vadis (Lord, where are you going?), refers to the well-known legend of the meeting between Christ and Peter, who was fleeing Rome to escape Nero's persecution. In answer to the apostle's question, Jesus replied, "I go to Rome to be crucified a second time," which led Peter to return to the city to face his martyrdom. The church's interior was renovated in the 17th century, and it houses a paving slab from the Via Appia, marked with footprints that the faithful have identified with those of Christ. ⊠ *Via Appia Antica 51.*

Galleria Borghese ①

1 B3. The Borghese Gallery is located within the gardens of the Villa Borghese on the Pincian Hill. It was built for Cardinal Scipione Caffarelli Borghese (1579–1633), nephew of Paul V, to house his art collection. Cardinal Borghese had extraordinary artistic instincts and was motivated by an insatiable passion for the most prized works, which pushed him to steal Raphael's *Deposition* from the Baglioni Chapel in Perugia and to imprison Domenichino, who had refused to sell him a painting. But the cardinal was also greatly admired for his patronage of exceptional talents, including Bernini, Caravaggio, Guido Reni, and Rubens. In keeping with the cardinal's wishes, the building was designed to be a "theater of the universe." Its primary function as a center for art and culture was merged with the contemplation of nature, and the immense grounds contained vineyards, orchards, an aviary, a zoo, and rare exotic plants. The importance of both patron and his villa went well beyond the

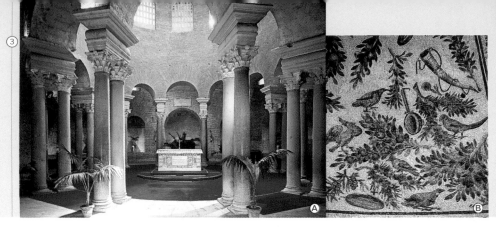

exceptional quality of his collection of ancient and modern art. "His" artists inaugurated a new style, the Roman Baroque, which would be imitated throughout Europe. The villa and park were renovated between 1770 and 1800 by Marcantonio Borghese, who gave the interiors a rich Neoclassical decorative scheme, with paintings and stuccowork by well known artists from Italy and abroad. Shortly thereafter his son Camillo (1775–1832), husband of Marie-Paulette Bonaparte, Napoléon's sister, was forced to sell the emperor 344 pieces from his archaeological collection. The artworks are now housed in the Louvre. The Borghese Gallery's art collection, which was expanded over the centuries, is one of the best private collections in the world. It includes Cardinal Scipione's beloved ancient marbles and sculptures and paintings by Italian and foreign artists from the 16th throught the 20th century. Raphael's dramatic *Deposition*, Correggio's sensuous *Danae*, Canova's scandalous *Paolina Borghese*, and works by Caravaggio and Bernini are only the most popular pieces in this treasure trove of masterpieces. ✉ *Piazzale Scipione Borghese 5,* ☎ *06/854–8577.*

Mausoleo di S. Costanza ③
⊞**1 B4.** This building is the burial site of Constantine's two daughters, Constantia (or Costanza) and Helena, neither of whom are saints. It is located near the large basilica of S. Agnese, where that saint is buried. The building was used as a baptistery, and it has been a church since 1254. The structure was thought to be a temple of Bacchus, because of the mosaics with harvest scenes, and it became a meeting place for artists in the 18th and 19th centuries. The solemn edifice on a central plan is covered with a dome resting on 12 pairs of granite

columns. The interior of the central space is a corridor with barrel vaults covered in elegant mosaics with floral, geometric, and figurative motifs. The spherical vault once contained mosaics illustrating scenes from the Old and New Testaments, but these have completely vanished. The building houses a cast of the large porphyry sarcophagus of Costantia, the original of which is in the Vatican Museums. ✉ *Via Nomentana 349.*

Moschea (Mosque)
⊞**1 A3.** This mosque and the adjacent Islamic cultural center were designed by Paolo Portoghesi and Vittorio Gigliotto (1984–1995). It is an eclectic building that combines rationalist and expressionist forms, reinterpreting the classical typology of the Islamic sanctuary according to the canons of postmodern architecture, of which Portoghesi is an active theoretician and practitioner. The large space is dominated by a series of piers and arches that support stepped domes. A museum and one of the largest Islamic libraries in Europe (40,000 volumes) are housed in the mosque complex. ✉ *Viale della Moschea,* ☎ *06/808–2167.*

Mura Aureliane (Aurelian Walls)
⊞**1 B2-B3-C2-C3-D3-C4.** Faced with a growing threat of barbarian invasion, the emperor Aurelian (270–275) realized the need to provide Rome with a new enclosing wall, and he commissioned one to follow the outline of the hills and encompass preexisting edifices (such as the Castrense Amphitheater and the Pyramid of Caius Cestius). The wall was later fortified, rebuilt, and furnished with a new course of crenellated turrets. One of the best preserved sections contains the Porta Latina and the Porta Appia (now the **Porta S. Sebastiano**), the most

monumental gateway in the entire complex. On the left pier are an image of the archangel Gabriel and a Latin inscription that recalls the 1327 victory of the Romans over the Angevins.

S. Agnese Fuori le Mura ④
⊞**1 B4.** Near the tomb of the young martyr Agnes (the same saint to whom the church in Piazza Navona is dedicated) is a basilica erected by Constantine, then rebuilt by Honorius I (625–638). The Constantinian basilica (334–357), like others of that time (S. Lorenzo, S. Sebastiano, and Ss. Marcellino e Pietro), had an unusual circular plan, with side naves around the semicircular apse. Now only a few impressive ruins of the apse and the adjacent mausoleum wall remain. The basilica Honorius built, which has undergone numerous renovations, contains a notable apse mosaic that depicts the saint with the attributes of her martyrdom: fire and the sword. On the right is an image of a phoenix, symbol of immortality. The canopy above the high altar dates from a restoration from the time of Paul V (1614). It includes a statue of the saint by Nicolas Cordier (1605), who added a gilded bronze head, clothing, and hands to an antique alabaster torso. The nearby **Cimitero Maggiore Catacombs** (3rd–4th century) contain the remains of St. Emerentiana, thought to be the foster-sister of St. Agnes. The catacombs also have numerous paintings with biblical scenes and chairs carved into the tufa stone, perhaps used for funeral banquets. ✉ *Via Nomentana 349.*

S. Andrea
⊞**1 B3.** Julius III ordered this church built in memory of his escape from prison during the sack of Rome in 1527. The design by Vignola (it was renovated in the 19th century) is cubic in form, with

(A) The tomb of S. Costantia ③, erected in the late 4th century.
(B) The interior, which is still tied to the style of Roman architecture, is embellished with mosaics of rare beauty, with fanciful naturalistic decorative schemes.

The interior of S. Agnese Fuori le Mura ④, with three naves divided by columns with beautiful Corinthian capitals. The apse contains a splendid Byzantine mosaic that depicts St. Agnes with popes Symmachus and Honorius.

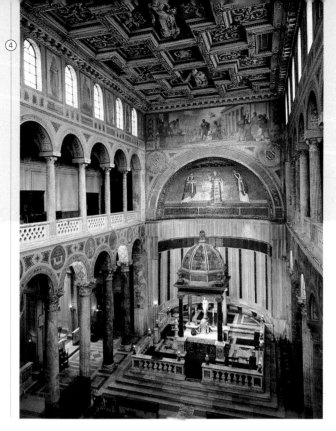

an entrance with tympanum and a small elliptical dome, a new element in this architect's work. ✉ *Viale Tiziano.*

S. Lazzaro
▦**1 B2.** This Romanesque church, which takes its name from the surrounding district, stands at the foot of Monte Mario, below the Via Trionfale. It was built shortly after the year 1000 and originally was known as S. Maria Maddalena, which was also the name of a hospice for pilgrims. Via Trionfale was one of the roads traveled by pilgrims arriving from the north. After an asylum for lepers was established, the church was dedicated to Lazarus, the patron saint of lepers. The original Romanesque interior of the church is preserved, with three naves with recycled columns. A chapel is dedicated to St. Mary Magdalen, patron of vinedressers, who worked in the vicinity. ✉ *Via Trionfale.*

S. Lorenzo Fuori le Mura
▦**1 C4.** In AD 303, Constantine honored venerated Roman martyr St. Laurence of Rome by building a large basilica near the saint's tomb in the Cemetery of Cyriaca, on the Via Tiburtina. The basilica was flanked by the church of Pope Pelagius II (579–590), built directly over that martyr's tomb, which also contained the remains of the early martyr St. Stephen, brought from Byzantium. In subsequent centuries, while the Constantine basilica fell into ruin, the new church became the center of a fortified village, Laurentiopoli, which included two monasteries, churches, libraries, baths, and all the welfare structures necessary for aiding the poor and pilgrims. Pope Honorius III (1216–1227) is responsible for the present appearance of the basilica, which incorporated the Pelagian church into its presbytery. A tragic bombing in 1943 destroyed

the portico, the facade, and much of the central nave, which were rebuilt with their original stones. The floor and the two pulpits of the central nave are precious examples of mosaic work from the time of Honorius. At the end of the nave is the dramatic presbytery, delimited by imposing columns that were taken from the underlying Pelagian basilica and which support an arched women's gallery. The episcopal throne (1254) and canopy (1148) are a fine examples of Romanesque marble work. The interior face of the triumphal arch contains a mosaic showing Christ enthroned between saints that comes from the church of Pelagius II. The cloister (late 12th century) is one of the few vestiges of medieval Laurentiopoli. ✉ *Piazzale del Verano.*

S. Pancrazio
▦**1 B2.** The basilica rises along the Via Aurelia, the ancient consular road that linked Rome to Etruria, Liguria, and Provence. It was also one of the principal arteries that passed through the Trastevere. The road began at the gateway of the same name, which in medieval times became Porta S. Pancrazio, in honor of the area's most venerated martyr. According to hagiographic tradition, Pancras came from

Phrygia (Asia Minor) and died at age 15 in Rome during Diocletian's persecution (ca. 304). The young saint began to be venerated immediately after his death, particularly in his capacity as a protector of those accused of perjury. A cemetery grew up in the area around his tomb, and a small oratory later was transformed into a basilica by Pope Symmachus (498–514), who also ordered the construction of a hospice for pilgrims. The present basilica, built under Honorius I (625–638), was reconstructed in the 12th and again in the 17th century. ✉ *Piazza S. Pancrazio 5/D.*

S. Paolo Fuori le Mura ⑤
▦**1 D3.** The basilica dedicated to the apostle Paul rises above his tomb, a short distance from the site of his martyrdom (Abbey of the Three Fountains). In the Middle Ages this basilica, along with the Vatican, was the principal destination for pilgrims traveling to Rome. The basilica remained the largest in Rome until the construction of the new S. Pietro. Its history is an uninterrupted sequence of restorations, repairing damage from numerous earthquakes and fires, until the fire of 1823, which almost destroyed the original medieval structure. It was entirely rebuilt, following the ancient plan, and consecrated by

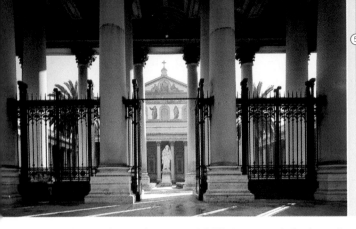

Pius IX in 1854. Constantine was responsible for the construction of the first, modest basilica. But popular veneration for St. Paul and his primary role in the conversion of the educated pagan classes resulted in a new, grander structure (375–423), the size of the present-day church. In the 8th century, a Benedictine monastery was added (this is the only of the four patriarchal basilicas still presided over by monks). Faced with the threat of Saracen invasions, John VIII (872–882) transformed the complex into a fortified citadel, which took the name of Giovannopoli, in honor of its founder. The bronze doors of the Porta Santa were made in Constantinople (1070) specifically for this building. Above the crypt, the high altar containing the tomb of the apostle is surmounted by an elegant Gothic canopy by Arnolfo di Cambio (1285), which miraculously survived the fire, as did the mosaics in the triumphal arch (5th century). The apse mosaics, executed for Honorius III by Venetian masters (ca. 1220), were heavily restored in the 19th century. The marble Easter candelabrum, nearly 20 feet tall, is decorated with scenes from the Passion and Resurrection. A masterpiece of 13th-century art, it was created by Pietro Vassalletto, who also designed the cloister, which, with its harmonious structure and decorative refinement, is one of the most beautiful in Rome. ✉ *Via Ostiense 186.*

S. Sebastiano

▦**1 D4.** This church stands in an area of the Via Appia called "ad catacumbas," from the Greek "katà kymbas," that is "near the hollow," perhaps referring to the pozzolana quarries that had contained first a pagan, then a Christian cemetery. The word catacombs was then extended to all the underground Christian burial places. This tomb area was well known throughout the Middle Ages, not only for the tomb of St. Sebastian, but also because of the tradition, perhaps legendary, that the remains of Sts. Peter and Paul were temporarily interred here. The first basilica, built by Constantine, was called Basilica Apostolorum, and it wasn't until the 9th century that it was consecrated to St. Sebastian, the Roman soldier shot to death by arrows during the persecution of Diocletian (298). The circular basilica that Constantine erected was rebuilt by order of Cardinal Scipione Borghese (1608). Above the tomb of St. Sebastian, the cardinal erected a new chapel, which contains a statue of the martyr made from a drawing by Gian Lorenzo Bernini. The Chapel of Relics contains what tradition holds is one of the arrows that pierced the saint and the column of his martyrdom. The cultural centerpiece of the catacombs is a porticoed courtyard where rites and funeral banquets in honor of Peter and Paul were held. The walls are covered with more than 600 examples Latin and Greek graffiti from the 3rd and 4th centuries, with invocations to the two apostles. The **Via delle Sette Chiese** ends nearby; this street, which leads out from S. Paolo Fuori le Mura, takes its name from the devotional route established by St. Philip Neri, which included visits to the four patriarchal basilicas and S. Lorenzo Fuori le Mura, S. Croce in Gerusalemme, and S. Sebastiano. ✉ *Via Appia Antica 136.*

S. Urbano

▦**1 D4.** This church, built in the 10th century, transformed an ancient Roman temple, probably constructed by Herodes Atticus (2nd century AD). A cultivated and wealthy Athenian and friend of the emperors Hadrian and Antoninus Pius, he had extensive landholdings in this area. The pagan building had a portico with four columns and brick walls. A 1634 addition result-ed in the exterior walls between the columns and various interior restorations. Very little is known about the life and works of St. Urban. He was pope from 222 to 230 and, according to tradtion, was buried either in the Catacombs of St. Calixtus or in the Catacombs of Pretestato, near the church. ✉ *Vicolo S. Urbano*

Santuario della Madonna del Divino Amore

▦**1 E5.** This sanctuary was constructed in 1744 to house an image of the Madonna, considered miraculous, that had been removed from a tower of the nearby Castel di Leva. It immediately became a popular destination for pilgrims from the Roman countryside and the Castelli Romani. After the Allied troops disembarked in Anzio in 1944, the image was carried to safety in Rome, where Pius XII proclaimed it the protector of the city. ✉ *Via Ardeatina, Km 12.*

Via Appia ⑥

▦**1 D3-D4-E4.** The Appian Way was laid out in 312 BC by Appius Claudius Cieco, the Roman censor from whom the road takes its name. This famous road played a decisive role in the economic development of Rome, because it linked the city to southern Italy and thus to the rich trade from the eastern Mediterranean. Its initial segment traverses one of the most fascinating landscapes around the capital city, perhaps the only one that can evoke an image of the ancient outskirts of Rome, with its luxurious villas (which belonged to the Quintili, the Gordiani, and the Massenzio families) and tombs (the most famous and best preserved is that of Cecilia Metella). The road's reputation as a burial site continued with the rise of Christianity, when the first Christian cemeteries, S. Sebastiano and S. Callisto, emerged along its route.

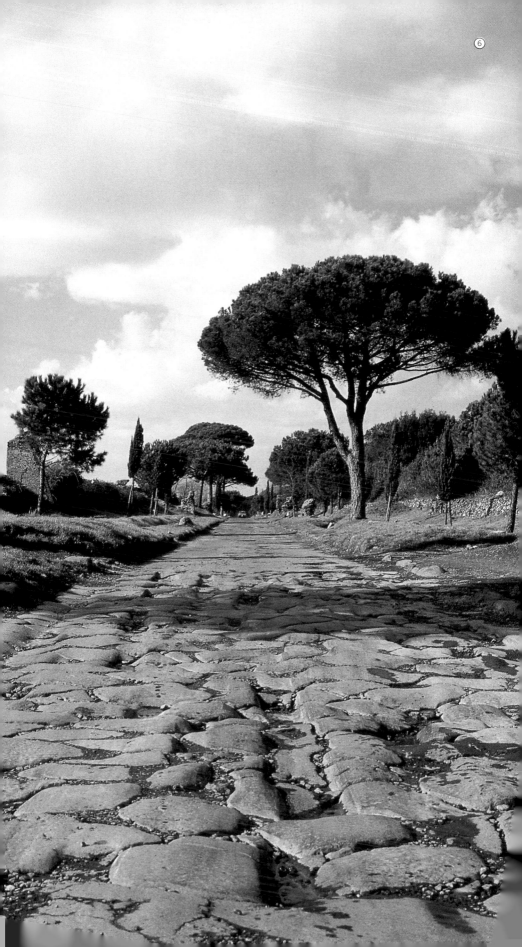

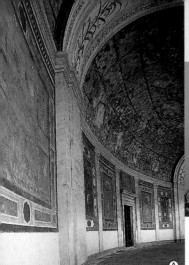

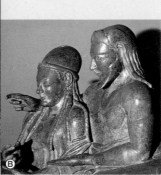

⑦ The Villa Giulia was the result of a mid-16th-century competition among the talented architects Vasari, Ammannati, and Vignola. It is embellished with splendid decorations, such as the frescoes in its ambulatory. Its interior houses the Museo Nazionale Etrusco and contains pieces that have come from throughout Lazio (the exceptional *Sarcophagus of the Bride and Bridegroom* was found in Cerveteri).

Opposite:
The church of S. Francesca Romana amid the columns of the Forum.

Via Appia Pignatelli

⌗1 D4-E4. This road was completed in the 17th century as a link between the Via Appia Antica and the Via Appia Nuova. It is the site of the **Catacombs of Pretestato** (Pretestato's identity is unknown), which were developed within a pagan cemetery. The latter area was very likely set aside for members of the aristocracy, judging from the luxurious sarcophagi discovered here and the presence of an exceptionally large gallery, the so-called "spelunca magna" (large cave). According to tradition this is the burial site of Januarius (killed under Marcus Aurelius), Urban I, and the deacons Felicissimus and Agapitus, who were beheaded with Sixtus II in 258. Some burial chambers, particularly that of St. Januarius, have fine pictorial decorations. The **Jewish Catacombs of Vigna Randanini**, also on this road, are, along with the Villa Torlonia burial ground, the only Jewish cemeteries still in use in the city.

Via Ardeatina

⌗1 D3-D4-E4. The Via Ardeatina, the ancient artery that connected Rome to Ardea, emerges from the Aurelian Wall through the Porta Ardeatina and for quite some distance runs almost parallel to the Via Appia. The most famous and well preserved of its monuments are the **Catacombs of Domitilla** (Via Ardeatina 280), the most extensive in Rome. In 1991 the ruins of a circular basilica were discovered near the church of Domine Quo Vadis. Scholars have hypothesized that this may be the church built by Pope Mark in 336. Sources and old itineraries mention many other Christian structures along the

Via Ardeatina, including the funerary basilicas of Pope Damasus I (366–384); the martyrs Mark, Marcellian, and St. Soter; and the sanctuary of the so-called "Greek Martyrs." Most of these can no longer be identified.

Via Salaria

⌗1 B3-A3. Perhaps the most ancient of the roads that led out from Rome, the Via Salaria takes its name from the exportation of salt from Rome to the hinterlands. Exiting from the Aurelian Walls, the road forked into the Salaria Vecchia, which soon become insignificant, and the Salaria Nuova, which roughly corresponded to the present road. Along the first section are various devotional stops mentioned in medieval itineraries: the **Catacombs of Bassilla**; the underground basilica of the martyr St. Hermes, built by Damasus in the 4th century and then replaced by a small oratory that housed a fresco with the oldest known image of St. Benedict; the **Catacombs of S. Panfilo** (Via Paisiello 24b), on the walls of which are numerous examples of graffiti by pilgrims. On the Salaria Nuova, in addition to the Catacombs of Priscilla, pilgrims visited the **Catacombs of S. Felicita** (Via Simeto 2), who, according to tradition, was the mother of seven sons martyred together because of their faith. She is the patron saint of women and mothers, and her blessing is invoked for the bendiction of children and the birth of sons. The small underground basilica contains an interesting 7th-century fresco. Farther along is the so-called **Cemetery of the Giordani** (at the corner of the Via Taro), known for the fine painting cycle with scenes from the Old and New Testaments (3rd–4th century).

Villa Albani Torlonia

⌗1 B3. During the Renaissance, palazzi were decorated with antique sculptures, but in the two subsequent centuries many buildings were erected specifically to house immense collections, such as the Villa Borghese in the 17th century and the Villa Albani in the 18th century. Cardinal Alessandro Albani, nephew of Pope Clement XI and the unrivaled collector in Rome during that period, built a grand museum-villa on the Via Salaria (1747–1767), where obelisks, sarcophagi, statues, and busts of emperors filled the rooms and dotted the park. Here Winckelmann, the cardinal's librarian, conducted his research, which became the basis of modern archaeological and art history. Much of the collection was moved to Paris by Napoléon, but in the subsequent century the Torlonia family restored the villa's splendor, filling it with works of exceptional value. ✉ *Via Salaria 92,* ☎ *06/686–1044*

Villa Giulia ⑦

⌗1 B3. The suburban villa (1551–1555) of Pope Julius III is a compendium of Mannerist architecture. Its many wings spread over terraces on different levels, with a juxtaposition of rectilinear and curvilinear elements, a dramatic succession of spaces along a longitudinal axis, and a close relationship between external and internal spaces. The theatrical loggia-enclosed grotto is the work of Ammannati and Vasari, and the severe, monumental facade is by Vignola. The building houses the **National Etruscan Museum,** which has a vast collection of sculptures, gold work, ceramics, bronzes, and other archaeological remains from Etruscan culture. ✉ *Piazzale di Villa Giulia 9,* ☎ *06/320–1951.*

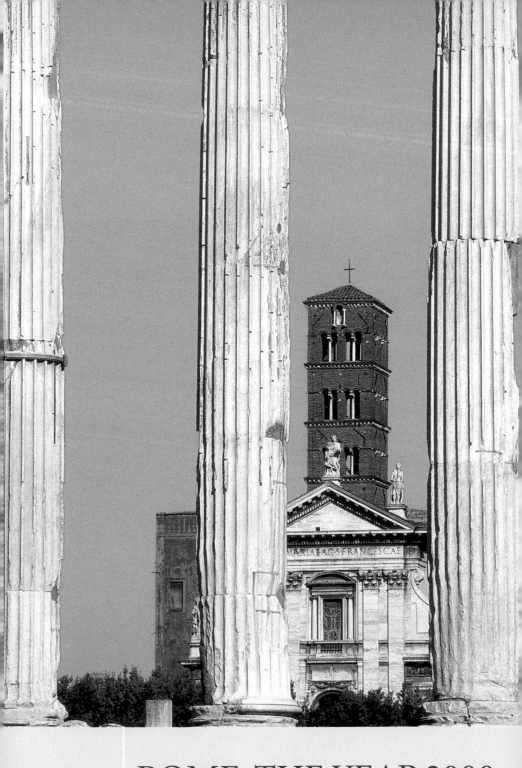

AGENZIA ROMANA
PER LA PREPARAZIONE
DEL GIUBILEO

ROME, THE YEAR 2000, AND THE CHRISTIAN JUBILEE

Rome, the year 2000 and the Christian Jubilee

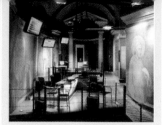

The Rome Agency for Jubilee Preparations welcomes all visitors, tourists, and pilgrims to Rome to explore the city, to see its artistic treasures, and to participate in the celebration of the Jubilee and the passage to the year 2000.

This section offers visitors information on the projects that have been prepared for the year 2000, the calendar of major cultural events, and the official calendar of religious events prepared by the Holy See. An overview of the main Jubilee destinations and itineraries is also provided.

In addition to religious celebrations, a wide variety of cultural events will take place during the year 2000. Major art exhibitions and a rich program of theatrical and musical events will celebrate Rome's unparalleled artistic tradition from antiquity to today. The playbill for the year 2000 has something to offer the widest of audiences.

To prepare for this historic event, Rome and the Lazio Region have undertaken a major organizational effort. With funds provided by the Italian State, all the government departments involved have built new infrastructure, restored cultural heritage sites, and organized reception services. The private sector has also made a significant contribution to these preparations.

The Agency has a special role in the organization of events in the year 2000, including planning services, event management, and promoting cultural activities. The services that affect pilgrims and visitors most directly are the Jubilee volunteer activities and information services.

VOLUNTEER SERVICES
The Center for Jubilee Volunteers for Reception Activities, which is organized by the Central Committee of the Great Jubilee and the Rome Agency for Jubilee Preparations, is charged with recruiting, training, and organizing volunteers.

More than 50,000 volunteers have been recruited for the year 2000 to assist and inform pilgrims along the Jubilee itineraries and during celebrations, aid travelers with disabilities and children at places of worship, and monitor cultural heritage sites and parks.

The Center's office is open to all those who would like to help with reception activities and is located in Rome in Largo Santa Lucia Filippini 20, phone 06/678-9695.

INFORMATION
The Information Centers organized by the Agency offer computers and audiovisual rooms to provide information on reception services, the calendar of religious celebrations, and other events connected with the Jubilee year and the history and culture of the Jubilee.

The Centers are located at:

☞ the Museo del Risorgimento on Via di San Pietro in Carcere;
☞ the Auditorium on Via della Conciliazione;
☞ the Ala Mazzoniana of Termini railway station on Via Giolitti.

Additional information centers have been set up at train stations, airports, and the patriarchal basilicas in Rome; the main access routes into Rome; and at various sites around Lazio.

The Agency's Web site (www.romagiubileo.it) provides constantly updated information on services, cultural activities, special events, and other initiatives for the Jubilee and the start of the new millennium.

THE PILGRIMAGE TO ROME IN THE YEAR 2000
The Jubilees, or Holy Years, are normally called every 25 years. The great Jubilee of the year 2000 is the 26th ordinary Jubilee called in the past 700 years, although numerous "extraordinary" Jubilees have been decreed on special occasions outside the normal calendar. During a Jubilee year it is possible to obtain an indulgence (cancellation of punishments imposed for sins), which is why the year is known as a Year of Pardon. Over the years, the concept of forgiveness has been supplemented by many other spiritual and moral themes: conversion, reconciliation, solidarity, justice and service to others.

The Holy Year 2000 is the first to be celebrated simultaneously in Rome, Jerusalem, and all the churches of the world, making it a truly universal Jubilee.

In promoting the spiritual aspects of the event, Pope John Paul II set out the characteristics of the Jubilee pilgrimage to Rome in the *Bull of Indiction of the Great Jubilee of the Year 2000*:

"make a pious pilgrimage to one of the Patriarchal Basilicas, namely, the Basilica di S. Pietro in the Vatican, the Archbasilica of the Most Holy Savior at the Lateran (S. Giovanni in Laterano), the Basilica di S. Maria Maggiore and the Basilica di S. Paolo on the Ostian Way, and there take part devoutly in Holy Mass or another liturgical celebration; ... visit, as a group or individually, one of the four Patriarchal Basilicas and there spend some time in Eucharistic adoration and pious mediations, ending with the 'Our Father,' the profession of faith in any approved form, and prayer to the Blessed Virgin Mary. To the four Patriarchal Basilicas are added, on this special occasion of the Great Jubilee, the following further places, under the same conditions: the Basilica di S. Croce in Gerusalemme, the Basilica di S. Lorenzo in Campo Verano, the Santuario della Madonna del Divino Amore, and the Christian Catacombs."

The Main Jubilee Destinations

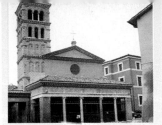

The main Jubilee destinations and itineraries have been defined by the agency in coordination with the Central Committee of the Great Jubilee of the Year 2000.

Numbers listed with each site refer to the map on pages 138–139.

PATRIARCHAL BASILICAS
Historically these are the main destinations of Jubilee pilgrimages. The majority of pilgrims will be visiting these sites during the great Jubilee of the year 2000.

1   S. Pietro
2   S. Paolo Fuori le Mura
3   S. Giovanni in Laterano
4   S. Maria Maggiore

WAY STATIONS
These comprise the churches near the patriarchal basilicas. They will serve as places for meditation, prayer, and preparation for the visit to the patriarchal basilica.

5   S. Lorenzo in Piscibus
6   S. Maria del Rosario in Prati
7   S. Maria in Traspontina
8   S. Monica
9   S. Spirito in Sassia
10 Abbazia delle Tre Fontane
11 Battistero Lateranense
12 S. Antonio da Padova a Via Merulana
13 S. Clemente al Laterano
14 S. Croce in Gerusalemme
15 S. Lorenzo in Palatio ad Sancta Sanctorum (Scala Santa)
16 SS. Quattro Coronati al Laterano
17 S. Prassede all'Esquilino
18 S. Pudenziana al Viminale
19 S. Antonio Abate all'Esquilino

CATACOMBS
The catacombs are sacred sites that date from the very origins of Christianity. In addition to their spiritual significance as burial sites of the martyrs and the first Christians, they are also one of the most important examples of subterranean architecture.

The main catacombs are:
20 S. Callisto

21 S. Sebastiano
22 Domitilla
23 Priscilla
24 S. Agnese
25 S. Pietro e Marcellino

PALEOCHRISTIAN BASILICAS
These basilicas are the first appearance of the church in public life, testifying to the growth and development of Christianity.

26 S. Agnese Fuori le Mura
27 S. Anastasia al Palatino
28 S. Balbina all'Aventino
29 S. Cecilia in Trastevere
30 S. Giovanni a Porta Latina
31 S. Lorenzo Fuori le Mura
32 S. Lorenzo in Damaso
33 S. Lorenzo in Lucina
34 S. Maria in Cosmedin
35 S. Maria in Domnica
36 S. Maria in Trastevere
37 S. Sabina all'Aventino

OTHER CHURCHES OR BASILICAS
Other destinations connected with the tradition of the Jubilee pilgrimage.

38 S. Agnese in Agone
39 S. Agostino in Campo Marzio
40 S. Andrea della Valle
41 S. Bartolomeo all'Isola
42 S. Crisogono
43 S. Giorgio in Velabro
44 S. Giovanni Battista dei Fiorentini
45 S. Ignazio di Loyola in Campo Marzio
46 S. Maria Ad Martyres (Pantheon)
47 S. Maria degli Angeli e dei Martiri
48 S. Maria del Popolo
49 S. Maria della Vittoria
50 S. Maria in Vallicella
51 S. Maria Sopra Minerva
52 S. Pietro in Montorio
53 S. Pietro in Vincoli a Colle Oppio
54 S. Stefano Rotondo al Celio
55 SS. XII Apostoli
56 SS. Cosma e Damiano in via Sacra

57 Ss. Giovanni e Paolo al Celio
58 SS. Nome di Gesù all'Argentina

NATIONAL CHURCHES
Traditional destinations where foreign pilgrims can participate in services given in their native language and receive spiritual, theological, and practical guidance.

59 **Argentina**—S. Maria Addolorata a Piazza B. Aires
60 **Armenia**—S. Nicola da Tolentino agli Orti Sallustiani
61 **Belgium**—S. Giuliano dei Fiamminghi
62 **Canada**—Nostra Signora del SS. Sacramento and SS. Martiri Canadesi
63 **Croatia**—S. Girolamo dei Croati a Ripetta
64 **Ethiopia**—S. Tommaso in Parione
65 **France**—S. Luigi dei Francesi in Campo Marzio
66 **Germany**—S. Maria dell'Anima
67 **Great Britain**—S. Silvestro in Capite
68 **Greece**—S. Atanasio
69 **Ireland**—S. Isidoro a Capo le Case
70 **Ireland**—S. Patrizio a Villa Ludovisi
71 **Lebanon**—S. Giovanni Marone
72 **Lithuania**—S. Casimiro a Via Appia Nuova
73 **Mexico and Latin America**—Nostra Signora di Guadalupe and S. Filippo Martire in Via Aurelia
74 **Poland**—S. Stanislao alle Botteghe Oscure
75 **Portugal**—S. Antonio in Campo Marzio
76 **Rumania**—S. Salvatore alle Coppelle
77 **Slovenia**—Collegio Sloveno
78 **Spain**—S. Maria in Monserrato degli Spagnoli
79 **Sweden**—S. Brigida a Campo de' Fiori
80 **Syria**—S. Maria in Campo Marzio
81 **Ukraine**—S. Giosafat al Gianicolo
82 **United States**—S. Susanna alle Terme di Diocleziano

OTHER PLACES OF DEVOTION
Sites that will host religious celebrations during the Jubilee.

83 Santuario del Divino Amore
84 Colosseo

The Main Jubilee Itineraries

The Jubilee itineraries indicated here are the oldest such routes and those that, in conformity with the desire of the popes to create a "holy city," are part of the devotional aspects of the Jubilee. Their total length is about 26 miles, and secondary itineraries add a further 15 miles, for a total of about 41 miles..

(*Use the list below as a key for the itineraries shown on the map)

S. Pietro–S. Paolo Fuori le Mura. Medieval devotional itinerary

S. Pietro–S. Maria del Popolo. Medieval devotional itinerary

S. Giovanni in Laterano–S. Maria Maggiore–S. Maria del Popolo. 16th-century devotional itinerary

S. Giovanni in Laterano– Colosseo– S. Maria del Popolo. 16th-century devotional itinerary

S. Pietro–S. Sebastiano Fuori le Mura. Devotional itinerary of the sites of the apostles

S. Pietro–S. Maria Maggiore. 16th–century devotional itinerary (in part)

S. Sebastiano Fuori le Mura–Santuario del Divino Amore. Modern devotional itinerary

S. Paolo Fuori le Mura–Abbazia delle Tre Fontane. Devotional itinerary at the site of St. Paul's martyrdom

The Tour of the Seven Churches was begun by St. Philip Neri around the middle of the 16th century. It included S. Pietro, S. Paolo Fuori le Mura, S. Sebastiano Fuori le Mura, S. Giovanni in Laterano, S. Croce in Gerusalemme, S. Lorenzo Fuori le Mura, and S. Maria Maggiore.

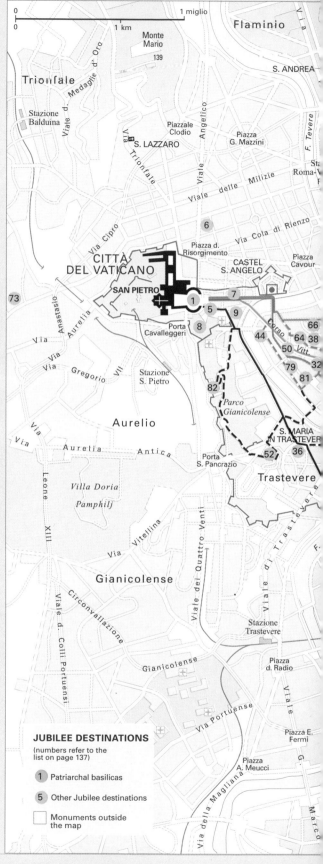

JUBILEE DESTINATIONS
(numbers refer to the list on page 137)

1 Patriarchal basilicas

5 Other Jubilee destinations

☐ Monuments outside the map

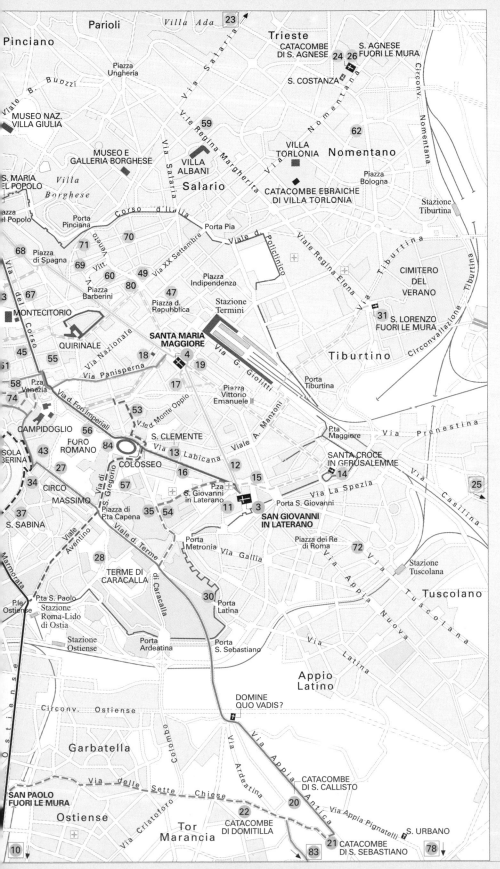

Calendar of the Holy Year 2000

This is the official calendar of religious celebrations prepared by the Holy See. The Central Committee of the Great Jubilee of the Year 2000 graciously authorized the publication of the calendar here. Updates will be publicized on the Central Committee's official Web site (www.jubil2000.org).

December 1999[1]

24 Friday
Solemnity of the Birth of the Lord
Basilica di S. Pietro
Opening of the Holy Door
Mass at Midnight

25 Saturday
Solemnity of the Birth of the Lord
Basilica di S. Giovanni in Laterano and S. Maria Maggiore
Opening of the Holy Door
Mass during the day
Basilica di S. Pietro
Urbi et Orbi Blessing
Holy Land
Opening of the Jubilee
Local Churches
Opening of the Jubilee

31 Friday
Basilica di S. Pietro
Prayer vigil for the passage to the year 2000

January 2000

1 Saturday
Solemnity of Mary, Mother of God
Basilica di S. Pietro
Holy Mass
World Day of Peace

2 Sunday
Second Sunday after Christmas
Basilica di S. Pietro
Day for Children

6 Thursday
Solemnity of the Epiphany of the Lord
Basilica di S. Pietro
Holy Mass
Episcopal Ordinations

9 Sunday
Feast of the Baptism of the Lord
Holy Mass
Celebration of the sacrament of Baptism for children

18 Tuesday
Beginning of the Week of Prayer for Christian Unity[2]
Basilica di S. Paolo Fuori le Mura
Opening of the Holy Door
Ecumenical celebration

25 Tuesday
Feast of the Conversion of St. Paul
Basilica di S. Paolo Fuori le Mura
Ecumenical celebration for the conclusion of the Week of Prayer for Christian Unity

28 Friday
Memorial of St. Ephrem
Basilica di S. Cecilia in Trastevere
Divine Liturgy in the East Syrian Rite (Malabarese)

February 2000

2 Wednesday
Feast of the Presentation of the Lord
Basilica di S. Pietro
Liturgy of light and Holy Mass
Jubilee of Consecrated Life

9 Wednesday
Memorial of St. Maron
Basilica di S. Maria Maggiore
Divine Liturgy in the Syro-Antiochene Rite (Maronite)

11 Friday
Memorial of Our Lady of Lourdes
Basilica di S. Pietro
Holy Mass
Celebration of the Sacrament of the Anointing of the Sick
Jubilee of the sick and health-care workers

18 Friday
Memorial of Blessed John (Beato Angelico)
Basilica di S. Pietro
Jubilee of artists

20 Sunday
Jubilee of permanent deacons

22 Tuesday
Solemnity of the Chair of St. Peter Apostle
Basilica di S. Pietro
Holy Mass
Jubilee of the Roman Curia

25 Friday–27 Sunday
Study convention on the implementation of the Second Vatican Ecumenical Council

March 2000

5 Sunday
Ninth Sunday in Ordinary Time
Basilica di S. Pietro
Beatification of Martyrs

8 Wednesday
Ash Wednesday
Penitential procession from the *Basilica di S. Sabina to the Circus Maximus*
Holy Mass and imposition of ashes
Request for pardon[3]

9 Thursday
Basilica di S. Paolo Fuori le Mura
Eucharistic Adoration

10 Friday
Basilica di S. Giovanni in Laterano
Way of the Cross and penitential celebration

11 Saturday
Basilica di S. Maria Maggiore
Recitation of the Rosary

12 Sunday
First Sunday of Lent[4]
Basilica di S. Giovanni in Laterano
Rite of Election and the enrolment of the names of the catechumens

16 Thursday
Basilica di S. Paolo Fuori le Mura
Eucharistic Adoration

17 Friday
Basilica di S. Giovanni in Laterano
Way of the Cross and penitential celebration

18 Saturday
Basilica di S. Maria Maggiore
Recitation of the Rosary

19 Sunday
Second Sunday of Lent
Basilica di S. Maria degli Angeli
East Syrian Rite (Malabarese)
Basilica di S. Giovanni in Laterano
First scrutiny of catechumens

20 Monday
Solemnity of S. Joseph, husband of the Blessed Virgin Mary
Jubilee of craftsmen

23 Thursday
Basilica di S. Paolo Fuori le Mura
Eucharistic Adoration

24 Friday
Basilica di S. Giovanni in Laterano
Way of the Cross and penitential celebration

25 Saturday
Solemnity of the Annunciation of the Lord
Nazareth Basilica of the Annunciation
Liturgical celebration linked with the Basilica di S. Maria Maggiore and the world's major Marian shrines to underscore the dignity of women in the light of Mary's mission (*Mulieris dignitatem*)

26 Sunday
Third Sunday of Lent
Basilica di S. Giovanni in Laterano
Second scrutiny of catechumens

30 Thursday
Basilica di S. Paolo Fuori le Mura
Eucharistic Adoration

31 Friday
Basilica di S. Giovanni in Laterano
Way of the Cross and penitential celebration

April 2000

1 Saturday
Basilica di S. Maria Maggiore
Recitation of the Rosary

2 Sunday
Fourth Sunday of Lent
Basilica di S. Giovanni in Laterano
Third scrutiny of catechumens

6 Thursday
Basilica di S. Paolo Fuori le Mura
Eucharistic Adoration

7 Friday
Basilica di S. Giovanni in Laterano
Way of the Cross and penitential celebration

8 Saturday
Basilica di S. Maria Maggiore
Recitation of the Rosary

9 Sunday
Fifth Sunday of Lent
Basilica di S. Pietro
Beatification of Confessors
Basilica di S. Giovanni in Laterano
Rite of giving the Creed and the Lord's Prayer to the catechumens

13 Thursday
Basilica di S. Paolo Fuori le Mura
Eucharistic Adoration

14 Friday
Basilica di S. Giovanni in Laterano
Way of the Cross and penitential celebration

15 Saturday
Basilica of S. Maria Maggiore
Recitation of the Rosary

Holy Week

16 Sunday
Palm Sunday of the Lord's Passion
Piazza S. Pietro
Commemoration of the Lord's entry into Jerusalem and Holy Mass

18 Tuesday
Tuesday of Holy Week
In the Major Basilicas
Communal celebration of the sacrament of Penance with individual absolution

20 Thursday
Holy Thursday
Basilica di S. Pietro
Chrism Mass
Basilica of St. John Lateran
Mass of the Lord's Supper

21 Friday
Good Friday
Basilica di S. Pietro
Celebration of the Lord's Passion
Colosseum
Solemn Way of the Cross

23 Sunday
Easter Sunday—the Resurrection of the Lord
Basilica di S. Pietro
Easter Vigil of the Holy Night: Service of Light, Liturgy of the Word, Baptismal Liturgy (Celebration of the Rite of Christian Initiation of Adults), Eucharistic Liturgy
Mass during the Day
Urbi et Orbi Blessing

30 Sunday
Second Sunday of Easter
Basilica di S. Pancrazio
Mass for newly baptized adults

May 2000

1 Monday
Memorial of St. Joseph the Worker
Holy Mass
Jubilee of workers

6 Saturday
Basilica di S. Maria Maggiore
Recitation of the Rosary

7 Sunday
Third Sunday of Easter
Colosseo
Ecumenical service for the "new martyrs"

13 Saturday
Basilica di S. Maria Maggiore
Recitation of the Rosary
Piazza S. Pietro

14 Sunday
Fourth Sunday of Easter
Basilica di S. Pietro
Holy Mass
Priestly Ordinations
World Day of Prayer for Vocations

18 Thursday
80th Birthday of the Holy Father
Piazza S. Pietro
Holy Mass
Jubilee of clergy

20 Saturday
Basilica di S. Maria Maggiore
Recitation of the Rosary

25 Thursday
Jubilee of scientists

26 Friday
Basilica di S. Maria degli Angeli
Divine Liturgy in the Alexandrian-Ethiopian Rite
(Feast of Mary Covenant of Mercy)

27 Saturday
Basilica di S. Maria Maggiore
Recitation of the Rosary

28 Sunday
Sixth Sunday of Easter
Holy Mass
Jubilee of the Diocese of Rome

31 Wednesday
Vigil of the Solemnity of the Ascension of the Lord
Basilica di S. Pietro
First Vespers of the Solemnity

June 2000

1 Thursday
Solemnity of the Ascension of the Lord
Basilica di S. Pietro
Holy Mass

2 Friday
Jubilee of migrants and itinerants

4 Sunday
Seventh Sunday of Easter
Holy Mass
Day of Social Communications
Jubilee of journalists

10 Saturday
Vigil of the Solemnity of Pentecost
Piazza S. Pietro
Solemn Vigil of Pentecost

11 Sunday
Solemnity of Pentecost
Basilica di S. Pietro
Day of Prayer for collaboration
among the different religions[5]

18 Sunday
Solemnity of the Holy Trinity
Basilica di S. Giovanni in Laterano
Celebration of the opening of the
International Eucharistic Congress

22 Thursday
Solemnity of the Body and Blood
of Christ
Basilica di S. Giovanni in Laterano
Eucharistic procession

25 Sunday
Closing of the International
Eucharistic Congress

29 Thursday
Solemnity of the Apostles Peter
and Paul
Basilica di S. Pietro
Holy Mass and imposition of the
pallium on Metropolitan
Archbishops

July 2000

2 Sunday
13th Sunday in Ordinary Time
Station Mass of the Jubilee

9 Sunday
14th Sunday in Ordinary Time
Jubilee celebration in the prisons

16 Sunday
15th Sunday in Ordinary Time
Station Mass of the Jubilee

23 Sunday
16th Sunday in Ordinary Time
Station Mass of the Jubilee

30 Sunday
17th Sunday in Ordinary Time
Station Mass of the Jubilee

August 2000

5 Saturday
Vigil of the Feast of the
Transfiguration of the Lord
Basilica di S. Maria Maggiore
Prayer vigil[6]

6 Sunday
Feast of the Transfiguration
of the Lord

Basilica di S. Paolo Fuori le Mura
Second Vespers of the Feast

14 Monday
Vigil of the Solemnity of the
Assumption of the Blessed Virgin
Mary
Basilica di S. Maria Maggiore
Incense Rite of the Coptic Liturgy

15 Tuesday
Solemnity of the Assumption of
the Blessed Virgin Mary
Opening of the 15th World Youth
Day

19 Saturday–20 Sunday
20th Sunday in Ordinary Time
Prayer Vigil and Holy Mass
Conclusion of the 15th World
Youth Day
Jubilee of youth

27 Sunday
21st Sunday in Ordinary Time
Station Mass of the Jubilee

September 2000

3 Sunday
22nd Sunday in Ordinary Time
Basilica di S. Pietro
Beatification of Confessors

8 Friday
Feast of the Birth of the Blessed
Virgin Mary
Solemn Celebration to recall the
birth of the Mother of the Lord in
relation to the birth of our Savior
Jesus Christ

10 Sunday
23rd Sunday in Ordinary Time
Basilica di S. Pietro
Holy Mass
Jubilee of university teachers

14 Thursday
Feast of the Exaltation of the Holy
Cross
From the *Basilica di Santa Croce in
Gerusalemme* to the *Basilica di
S. Giovanni in Laterano*
Stational Procession
Basilica di S. Giovanni in Laterano
Vespers in the Armenian Rite and
the Rite of Antasdan

15 Friday
Opening of the International
Marian-Mariological Congress
Jubilee of Pontifical Representatives

17 Sunday
24th Sunday in Ordinary Time
Jubilee of senior citizens

24 Sunday
25th Sunday in Ordinary Time

Holy Mass
Conclusion of the International
Marian-Mariological Congress

October 2000

1 Sunday
26th Sunday in Ordinary Time
Piazza S. Pietro
Canonization

3 Tuesday
Day for Jewish-Christian Dialogue

7 Saturday
Memorial of Our Lady of the
Rosary
Recitation of the Rosary and
torchlight procession

8 Sunday
27th Sunday in Ordinary Time
Basilica di S. Pietro
Holy Mass
Jubilee of Bishops on the occasion
of the 10th Ordinary General
Assembly of the Synod of Bishops
Act of dedicating the new
millennium to the protection of
Mary

14 Saturday–15 Sunday
Third Worldwide Meeting of the
Holy Father with Families

15 Sunday
28th Sunday in Ordinary Time
Piazza S. Pietro
Holy Mass
Celebration of the Sacrament
of Matrimony
Jubilee of families

20 Friday–22 Sunday
International Missionary-
Missiological Congress

21 Saturday
Basilica di S. Maria Maggiore
Celebration of the Rosary

22 Sunday
29th Sunday in Ordinary Time
Basilica di S. Pietro
Holy Mass
World Mission Day

28 Saturday
Basilica di S. Maria Maggiore
Recitation of the Rosary

29 Sunday
30th Sunday in Ordinary Time
Olympic Stadium
Holy Mass
Jubilee of athletes

31 Tuesday
Vigil of the Solemnity of All Saints
Basilica di S. Pietro
First Vespers of the Solemnity

November 2000

1 Wednesday
Solemnity of All Saints
Basilica di S. Pietro
Holy Mass

2 Thursday
Commemoration of All the
Faithful Departed

4 Saturday
Celebration in the Ambrosian Rite

5 Sunday
31st Sunday in Ordinary Time
Holy Mass
Jubilee of those involved in public
life

12 Sunday
32nd Sunday in Ordinary Time
Holy Mass
Day of thanks for the gifts of
creation
Jubilee of the agricultural world

19 Sunday
33rd Sunday in Ordinary Time
Basilica di S. Pietro
Holy Mass
Jubilee of the military and the
police

21 Tuesday
Feast of the Presentation of the
Blessed Virgin Mary
Basilica di S. Maria in Trastevere
Divine Liturgy in the Syro-
Antiochene Rite (Syrian and
Malankarese)

24 Friday
Opening of the World Congress
for the Apostolate of the Laity

26 Sunday
Solemnity of Christ the King
Basilica di S. Pietro
Holy Mass
Conclusion of the World Congress
for the Apostolate of the Laity

December 2000 [7]

2 Saturday
Vigil of the First Sunday of Advent
Basilica di S. Pietro
First Vespers of Sunday

3 Sunday
First Sunday of Advent
Basilica di S. Paolo Fuori le Mura
Holy Mass
Basilica di S. Pietro
Holy Mass
Jubilee of the disabled

8 Friday
Solemnity of the Immaculate
Conception of the Blessed Virgin
Mary
Basilica di S. Maria Maggiore
Akathistos Hymn

10 Sunday
Second Sunday of Advent
Basilica di S. Giovanni in Laterano
Holy Mass

16 Saturday
Basilica di S. Maria Maggiore
Celebration in the Mozarabic Rite

17 Sunday
Third Sunday of Advent
Basilica di S. Paolo Fuori le Mura
Holy Mass
Jubilee of the entertainment world

24 Sunday
Solemnity of the Birth of Our Lord
Basilica di S. Pietro
Midnight Mass

25 Monday
Solemnity of the Birth of Our Lord
Basilica di S. Pietro
Mass during the day
"Urbi et Orbi" Blessing

31 Sunday
Basilica di S. Pietro
Prayer Vigil for the passage to the
new millennium [8]

January 2001

1 Monday
Solemnity of Mary Mother of God
Basilica di S. Pietro
Holy Mass
World Day of Peace

5 Friday
Vigil of the Solemnity of the
Epiphany of the Lord
*Basilica di S. Giovanni in Laterano,
S. Maria Maggiore, and S. Paolo
Fuori le Mura*
Holy Mass
Closing of the Holy Door [9]
Holy Land
Closing of the Jubilee
Local Churches
Closing of the Jubilee

6 Saturday
Solemnity of the Epiphany of
the Lord
Basilica di S. Pietro
Closing of the Holy Door

NOTES

*(1) Material will also be prepared for
the local churches for the season of
Advent, for the ceremony of opening of
the Holy Door, and for the prayer vigil
for the passage to the year 2000.*

*(2) During the week ecumenical cele-
brations will take place in the basilicas
and churches of Rome, presided over
by representatives of the Christian
denominations. Material will also be
prepared for the local churches.*

*(3) The church "cannot cross the
threshold of the new millennium without encouraging her children to purify
themselves through repentance of past
errors and instances of infidelity,
inconsistency, and slowness to act"
(Tertio millennio adveniente, n. 33;
cf. also ibid., nn. 34–36).*

*(4) For the season of Lent, material
will also be prepared for the local
churches.*

*(5) Material will also be prepared for
the local churches.*

*(6) In response to the request of the
Patriarch of Constantinople,
Bartholomew I.*

*(7) Material will be prepared for the
local churches for the season of Advent.*

*(8) Material will also be prepared for
the local churches.*

*(9) Material will also be prepared for
the local churches for the closure of the
Holy Door.*

Rome Above and Below

New excavations, museums, and architecture for the city in the year 2000

"For 364 days of the year you can be completely detached from Rome as a city, live there without seeing it or, worse, suffer through it. But then, wrapped up in your troubles in the back of a taxi stopped at a traffic light, a familiar street suddenly appears in a play of color and light that you had never seen before ... and you feel that a magical connection has been formed, a feeling of peace that melts away your tension ... it gives you another sense of time, of life, of yourself." Thus Federico Fellini described the moments in which the "ancient charm" of the city would strike him and touch his heart. So many Romans and foreigners, pilgrims, artists, and harried tourists have felt the same sensation, one that you never forget once you have experienced it.

This is a special season for that "ancient charm." Above all, the city is preparing itself to host the extraordinary human and religious event of the Jubilee, an occasion through which an ancient and deep spirit will transmit a strengthened sense of its universality. An event that will introduce millions of pilgrims and visitors to the splendor of the Rome of the great basilicas, while the more curious will be able to rediscover the multitude of less-evident traces of a religious history, details that will sharpen their memories of the event and enhance the emotion of the experience.

The Forums, the Coliseum, the Oppian Hill *History Uncovered*

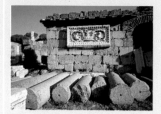

The excavations at the Imperial Forums are the most extensive ongoing archaeological works in the world. Following the recent excavations at the Forum of Nerva, in the next few years some 37,660 square feet of the Forum of Caesar, 59,180 square feet of the Forum of Peace, and 64,560 square feet of the Forum of Trajan will be brought into the light of day. The last is perhaps the most majestic, built on the orders of the emperor after his conquest of the Dacians and inaugurated in AD 112. The recovery effort will create a giant open-air museum stretching from the Coliseum to the Capitoline Hill and the Markets of Trajan, where a Museo dei Fori will be established, devoted principally to Roman architecture from the imperial period. The entire area is accessible along the Via Sacra itinerary, which runs past the Temple of Vesta and the Roman Curia.

The Coliseum is also due to receive an upgrade for the Jubilee: an internal elevator will facilitate access, and the arcades, tunnels, and the floor of the Coliseum arena will be open. By the year 2002 the entire monument will be accessible to the public, from the underground chambers (which will host museum exhibits) to the balcony of the attic.

Across the road from the Coliseum, the Oppian Hill area is an inexhaustible source of new discoveries: Nero's Domus Aurea, a vast residence with more than 500 rooms, was built over by Trajan and is undergoing a complex restoration. During recent excavations, the "fresco of the painted city" was discovered under the Trajan library, depicting a fascinating turreted city. The work's subject and size (about 110 square feet) make it one of the most important archaeological discoveries in years.

The Great Capitoline Hill *A Hill Regained*

The Great Capitoline Hill project promoted by the city government is restoring the Capitoline Hill to its ancient central role. Once completed, the hill will be the focal point for a "city of archaeology and art," and it will stretch from the Circus of Flaminius and the Theater of Marcellus to the Imperial Forums and the Parco della Via Appia. Following the restoration of the palazzi designed by Michelangelo, the entire museum complex, comprising the Tabularium, the Palazzo Senatorio, and the Casina dei Pierleoni, will be refurbished. The Pinacoteca Capitolina will also be restored and improved. The entire hill will be enclosed, turning it into an oasis in the center of the modern city and a wonderful cultural attraction with breathtaking views.

In the year 2000 the exhibition area will be supplemented with a new space designed by architect Carlo Aymonino, to be constructed in the Giardino Romano of the Palazzo dei Conservatori and the adjacent Giardino Caffarelli. The hall, covered by a 17-foot transparent roof, will be the final home of the original statue of Marcus Aurelius. A glass wall will open to the garden and another wall will serve as a background to the decorations of the pediment of the Temple of Apollo Sosiano. To its right will be placed the reconstruction of the cella of the temple, recovered thanks to the intelligent use of existing remains.

Crypta Balbi, built on the ancient theater erected in 13 BC by Lucius Cornelius Balbus and not far from the Capitoline Hill (between Via Caetani and Via delle Botteghe Oscure), will also be restored. It is one of the few examples of archaeological excavations of a medieval site in Rome. The restored spaces will house an exhibit on the history of the site and of medieval Rome between the 5th and 9th centuries.

Via Appia, Via Latina
The Southern Reaches

The area to the south of the Coliseum extends all the way to the slopes of the Colli Romani and is home to one of the world's largest archaeological sites. This is a countryside unique in its extraordinary balance of history and environment. The leading minds of the city fought a long and courageous battle to defend the area, and now we are seeing the fruits of their efforts.

For the year 2000 the Appia Antica will finally be healed of the terrible wound inflicted by the construction of Rome's Ring Road during the 1950s and 1970s. Two 14,000-foot tunnels will banish the cars that divide the queen of Roman roads, and the area will be replanted and repaved. It will form the largest pedestrian area in Europe, extending from the Circus of Maxentius to the Mausoleo di Cecilia Metella in a continuous itinerary alternating between countryside and ancient, often monumental, ruins. The restoration will bring the Parco della Caffarella together with the Appia Antica as its axis, creating a single space of unmatched archaeological and naturalistic value, with a total area of more than 49,400 acres punctuated by Roman tombs, catacombs, aqueducts, and sacred sites against the background of the Roman hinterland.

The archaeological oasis will include the Parco delle Tombe di Via Latina, a vast necropolis with perfectly preserved frescoes and stuccowork. The park comprises the tombs of the Barberini, the Pancrazi, and the Valeri, along with related structures (tabernae, terrace with nymph, fountain) and the paleochristian church dedicated to St. Stephen. The Sepolcreto degli Scipioni will also be reopened, and the Museo delle Mura Aureliane at Porta San Sebastiano will be refurbished. An upgrade is also in store for the famous Villa of the Quintili, the extraordinary residence of the two consuls (and brothers) that has furnished statuary to museums around the world. The spectacular terraced structure of the complex offers a view of the surrounding countryside. Recent excavations have uncovered marvelously preserved thermal baths.

S. Pietro
A "Factory" at Work

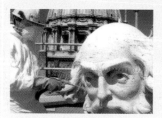

A delicate, scientific cleaning job has been performed at S. Pietro to restore the original brilliant splendor of the Maderno facade and the statues of the attic level. The job began with careful preliminary studies and has been carried out with sophisticated techniques. Execution of the works has been supervised by the Fabbrica di San Pietro (the "factory" of St. Peter's), whose plans for restoring the massive wall called for cleaning the travertine, followed by stuccoing and replacement of missing pieces and a final surface treatment.

The surface is enormous: some 753,200 square feet. After a long study, a low-pressure (no more than 0.4 atm) water-based cleaning technique, using a stream of water mixed with travertine powder (a soft abrasive), was adopted. The subsequent stuccoing has been particularly challenging, because some stuccowork had to be replaced completely, and other areas had to be repaired. Particularly difficult was stuccowork done in 1985-1986 that had turned gray and cracked into a dense network of lines across the surface, problems that were revealed in a complex photogrammetric analysis by ENI.

The Fabbrica has also been at work in the atrium of the basilica to restore the stuccowork and in the Vatican necropolis in the area around St. Peter's Tomb under the altar of the Confessione and the great baldacchino of Bernini: a place of unequaled emotion and faith.

Palazzo Braschi
The Past Finds a Home

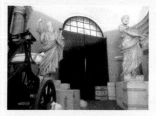

The year 2000 will see the return of Rome's museum. After being closed to the public for 10 years, the Museo di Roma will finally reopen, with its varied collection of iconography, ceramics, sculptures, medieval lapidary, and furnishings, all housed in one of the last great palazzi in the city center, Palazzo Braschi. The Braschi family and Pope Pius VI spared no expense in its construction towards the end of the 18th century, and they are the subject of an exhibition that is temporarily interrupting the restoration works.

The restoration of the palazzo, which in addition to the Museo di Roma also houses the Gabinetto delle Stampe and the Archivio Fotografico Comunale, will be carried out in two stages. The first stage will conclude with the inauguration of the exhibition, while the inventory and reorganization of the vast collection of material will continue. A permanent exhibit on the pomp and circumstance of city life between the 16th and 19th centuries will be created. Temporary exhibits on a range of themes will gradually bring the entire collection to the public eye.

The building's location—between Piazza Navona, where the traditional entry door will be reopened, Piazza di San Pantaleo, and Piazza Pasquino—makes it an ideal place for a museum visit to the city. The addition of a multimedia system for consulting documents and works will raise the museum to the international standards represented by the Musée Carnavalet in Paris and the Victoria & Albert Museum in London.

The Great Museums
The Ancient Goes to Court

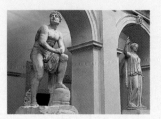

The Scuderie Papali
Exhibitions in the Stables

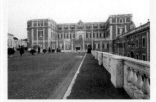

Villa Borghese
Museum Park

The Museo Nazionale Romano opened several new buildings—the Renaissance-era Palazzo Altemps, which holds the statuary of the great collections of the nobility, and the Museo di Palazzo Massimo, which offers a view of the Imperial Age through statues, mosaics, and above all the extraordinary frescoes from the villas of the emperors—that completed its integrated system, but the comprehensive refurbishing was capped by the definitive relocation of museum headquarters at the Baths of Diocletian, which had been the original nucleus since 1889. The new epigraphical section in the former masterpiece hall has been completed, and the public will be readmitted to the section on the pre- and protohistory of Rome. The large chapel by Michelangelo will be reopened after meticulous restoration work.

The Galleria Nazionale d'Arte Antica will be housed in more appropriate quarters after the full recovery of Palazzo Barberini, a masterpiece of Roman Baroque architecture constructed by Pope Urban VIII. The extensive restoration involved the facade, the furnishings, the gallery spaces, and the Princess Carolina Apartments. Other rooms are now being restored and will be used for international exhibitions. A modern reception center will direct visitors to all museums, which hold works dating from the Renaissance through the 18th century.

Beloved by Romans and one of the most popular destinations among tourists—thanks in part to its strategic location—Castel Sant' Angelo, with its roughly 2000 years of history, is already a museum. For the Jubilee, its numerous collections will be reorganized and a visitor orientation and assistance service will be created to make visits easier and more enjoyable.

Built between 1722 and 1732, the Scuderie Papali (Papal Stables), together with the Palazzo del Quirinale and the Palazzo della Consulta, mark the broad space of Piazza del Quirinale, an example of the perfect melding of buildings of different eras and styles into an integrated whole.

As part of the major events planned for the year 2000, the Presidency of the Italian Republic has granted the City of Rome the use of the Scuderie for cultural activities related to the Jubilee celebrations. The city has in turn entrusted management of the space to the Rome Agency for Jubilee Preparations, which plans to use it as a center for temporary exhibitions. To ensure the complete accessibility of the building, the Soprintendenza per i Beni Ambientali e Architettonici (the Department of the Preservation of Architectural and Environmental Landmarks) has begun restoration and restructuring works designed by architect Gae Aulenti.

The Scuderie abut the wall enclosing the Colonna garden and are built on the site of the Roman Temple of Serapis. The original design for the complex was prepared by Roman architect Alessandro Specchi (1668–1729), on a commission from Pope Innocent XIII. Clement XII completed the work, assigning the job to Florentine architect Ferdinando Fuga (1699–1781), who was also responsible for the Palazzo della Consulta. The building kept its original function until 1938, when it was turned into a garage. The restoration will recover a building with an excellent location, making available more than 32,280 square feet of exhibition space of unparalleled value to the city.

Cardinal Scipione Borghese transformed 200 acres of former vineyard outside the city walls into a villa, which is today experiencing a renaissance. The plan for the comprehensive restoration and reorganization of Villa Borghese and its many treasures is already producing results. The public will for the first time be able to visit the Casino del Graziano, a delightful 16th-century villino previously used as a storehouse, with frescoes by students of Domenichino and Reni. But this is only one part of the project, which is also slated to restore the villa's entire treasure of green spaces, monuments, sculptures, fountains, and decorative niches.

The rebirth is completed by the recent reopening of the Galleria Borghese in the heart of the villa, after years of restoration work that has returned the splendors of the collection to the admiring gaze of the public. This extraordinary mixture of park, nature, and art in the center of the city is joined by two more major attractions: the Galleria Nazionale d'Arte Moderna e Contemporanea and the Museo Nazionale Etrusco in Villa Giulia.

At Villa Giulia, the museum's permanent collection is being expanded in the splendid Renaissance building commissioned by Pope Julius III, with a new wing devoted to the pre-Italic civilization of the Falisci. Work is also under way on a radical refurbishment involving the expansion of exhibition space in nearby Villa Poniatowski, which can be visited by way of a connecting passage running alongside the park of Villa Strohl-Fern.

Near Villa Borghese is the Hendrik Christian Andersen Museum, the home, museum, and studio of the American sculptor and painter born in Bergen, Norway, in 1872. Andersen lived in Rome from 1896 until his death in 1940. The neo-Renaissance building, erected in the 1920s, is being restored and contains the artist's sculptures, paintings, and drawings for his utopian design for a "Global City."

New Spaces
Art with a Diesel Engine

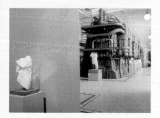

The Centrale Montemartini is home to some of the masterpieces of the Capitoline Museums, including the sculptures. Their stay at the former electric plant, inaugurated by King Vittorio Emanuele III in 1912, was supposed to have been temporary, but the juxtaposition of ancient statuary and industrial archaeology was an immediate hit with the public.

The Galleria Comunale d'Arte Moderna has found its own home in another monument of old industrial Rome, on the premises of the former Birreria Peroni, which was designed in a Liberty-inspired style by architect Giovannoni between 1902 and 1922. The large complex covers more than 172,160 square feet. Not only will the site have temporary and permanent exhibits, it will also become a fully operational center for cultural production for the visual arts, similar to other such initiatives around the world. The permanent collection of works by the masters of Italian contemporary art at Villa Glori, the city's first open-air art park, will be expanded.

Finally, the 387,360 square feet of the former Montello barracks, a short distance from the Città della Musica, will be the site of the new Centro per le Arti Contemporanee, based on the design by architect Zaha Hadid, winner of the international competition. The center, which will be a full-fledged community for the promotion of today's languages of expression, will house contemporary art dating from 1960 on. It will also host temporary exhibits and will have sections devoted to architecture, multimedia, and the visual arts.

New Architecture

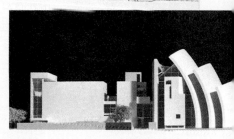

RICHARD MEIER

Richard Meier, the Pritzker Prize winner in 1984, is the creative force behind the design of the church at Tor Tre Teste, one of the works symbolizing the Jubilee of the year 2000.

The design, shown in the model at right embodies the theme of welcome and dialogue. Three large shells close one of the sides.

Meier is also responsible for the refurbishment of the Ara Pacis of Augustus, the altar celebrating the triumph of the Pax Romana. The glassed-in structure dating from 1939 will be removed and replaced by a museum that will give the monument the visibility and accessibility it deserves. In the drawing above, the view from the east.

RENZO PIANO

For Rome, the creation of the Città della Musica in the Flaminio quarter of the city marks the end of a 60-year gap, from the demolition of the old concert hall at the Mausoleo di Augusto. The three separate halls of the new complex were conceived by Renzo Piano as three enormous beetles. At left, a model of the complex and, below, a sectional view of one of the halls.

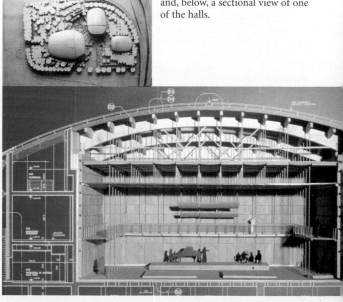

The Jubilee and Culture

A program of some of the events planned for the year 2000 in Rome. The complete and updated program of the cultural events is available at the Agency's Web site (www.romagiubileo.it).

Exhibitions

Pilgrims and Jubilees in the Middle Ages: Medieval Pilgrimages to St. Peter's Tomb (350–1350)
October 1999–February 2000
The pilgrimage seen as a journey of faith and an encounter between different peoples and cultures.
Museo Nazionale di Palazzo Venezia (the Saloni Monumentali and the Barbo Apartment)
⊠ *Via del Plebiscito 118*
☎ *06/841–2312*

Francesco Borromini Architect 1599–1667: Structure and Metamorphosis
December 1999–February 2000
The complete work of Francesco Borromini: drawings (those preserved at the Albertina and never before exhibited), casts, relief models, medals, portraits, a scientific seminar, an international conference, guided tours and Borromini itineraries.
Palazzo delle Esposizioni
⊠ *Via Nazionale 194*
☎ *06/474–5903*

Impressionists and the Avant-garde
December 1999–June 2000
Masterpieces of Impressionist and Post-Impressionist painting from the Hermitage Museum in St. Petersburg. The exhibit presents some 100 paintings by 25 great artists from between 1870 and 1920, tracing the development of art over the period from Monet to Léger.
Scuderie Papali
⊠ *Via XXIV Maggio 16*
☎ *06/678–6648.*

Roma: Universalitas Imperii
Throughout the Jubilee year.

The dislocation of the various ethnic groups that were absorbed into Roman society is conveyed through itineraries designed around monuments, archaeological sites, and subterranean areas, many of which are little known to the general public.
Circuito dei Musei Archeologici Romani (Roman archeological museums).

Villa Medici, the Dream of a Cardinal
November 1999–March 2000
Following the restoration of Villa Medici, the French Academy will present the most important works from the collection of Cardinal Ferdinando de' Medici, one of the greatest art patrons and collectors of the 16th century.
Villa Medici
⊠ *Viale Trinità dei Monti 1/A*
☎ *06/676–11*

Cassiano dal Pozzo (1588–1657): Artistic Culture and Scientific Experimentation in the Rome of the Barberinis
December 1999–February 2000
Palazzo Barberini (Cardinal Francesco Library)
⊠ *Via delle Quattro Fontane 13*
☎ *06/482–4184*

Roy Lichtenstein
December 1999–April 2000
Works and sketches by the great U.S. artist, recently deceased. With the contribution of the Estate of Roy Lichtenstein.
Chiostro del Bramante
⊠ *Via Arco della Pace 5*
☎ *06/688–09035*

Islamic Art in Lazio
December 1999–March 2000
An exhibition divided in two sections: sacred vestments and Oriental fabrics: a meeting of Christianity and the Islamic world; and elements of Oriental art in Christian iconography.
Palazzo Brancaccio, Museo Nazionale d'Arte Orientale
⊠ *Via Merulana 248*
☎ *06/487–4415*

Capogrossi: The Centenary of His Birth
January 2000
Sixty paintings by the Roman artist born in 1900.
Galleria Nazionale d'Arte Moderna
⊠ *Viale delle Belle Arti 131*
☎ *06/322–981*

The Braschi Family and Palazzo Braschi
January–March 2000
To celebrate the restoration and reorganization of the museum, an exhibition will pay homage to the Braschi family, reconstructing its history and its role in politics and commissioning artwork in the last decade of the 18th century.
Palazzo Braschi
⊠ *Piazza di San Pantaleo 10*
☎ *06/688–02713*

Goya
February–April 2000
Palazzo Barberini (the salone Pietro da Cortona)
⊠ *Via delle Quattro Fontane 13*
☎ *06/481–4591*

Yemen: The Queen of Sheba
March 2000
Palazzo Ruspoli
⊠ *Via del Corso 418*
☎ *06/687–4704*

Modern and Ancient Rome in the 17th Century as Seen by a Contemporary: Giovan Pietro Bellori
March–June 2000
An overview of the figurative arts in 17th-century Rome described by a unique contemporary observer: Giovan Pietro Bellori, archaeologist, historiographer, and driving force behind major artistic events and important archaeological discoveries. In connection with a related exhibition in Bologna.
Palazzo delle Esposizioni
⊠ *Via Nazionale 194*
☎ *06/474–5903*

The Year 1300: The First Jubilee. Boniface VIII and His Times
March–July 2000
Artworks produced in Rome at the end of the 13th century by Giotto, Arnolfo, Cavallini, Torriti. Exhibitions, seminars, music, theater, itineraries, and art, with links to satellite exhibits and events.
Museo Nazionale di Palazzo Venezia (the saloni monumentali and the Barbo Apartment)
⊠ *Via del Plebiscito 118*
☎ *06/841–2312*

Meetings: Contacts and Exchanges Between Cultures
March–December 2000
Everyday objects as evidence of the vital circulation of cultural

experience.

Museo Preistorico e Etnografico
Luigi Pigorini
✉ *Piazza Marconi 14*
☎ *06/549–52238*

Roman Fraternitas
September–December 2000
Museo Nazionale di Palazzo
Venezia (the Saloni Monumentali
and the Barbo Apartment)
✉ *Via del Plebiscito 118*
☎ *06/841–2312*

The Road and the Holy City: Music and Art in Interreligious Dialogue
Throughout the Jubilee year.
Exhibitions, musical events and an
international conference at dates
throughout the Jubilee year on the
theme "Pilgrimage and the Holy
City" viewed in the light of the five
major religions: Christianity,
Judaism, Islam, Hinduism and
Buddhism.
S. Andrea al Quirinale and the
Pontifical Gregorian University

Arts and Music
April 2000
A critical assessment of the
relationship between two
disciplines that have been closely
linked throughout the 20th
century: music and the figurative
arts. The exhibition will be housed
in the new premises of the Galleria
Comunale d'Arte Moderna e
Contemporanea (Municipal
Gallery of Modern and
Contemporary Art).
Ex stabilimento Birra Peroni
(the former Peroni Brewery)
✉ *Via Cagliari 29*
☎ *06/474–2848*

Christiana Loca
April 2000
The conclusion of a series of
conferences that began in 1998 and
will continue in 1999. An exhibit
on ancient Christianity: the
integration of Christianity within
the city with objects, relief models,
and charts.
The vaults of the Basilica di
S. Maria Maggiore

Paris Expo 1900: The Universal Exposition of 1900 in Paris
May–July 2000
Paintings, posters, prints,
photographs, illustrated books,
magazines, souvenir objects,
postcards, and official programs
from the spectacular Exposition of
the Belle Epoque.

Area Domus
✉ *Via del Pozzetto 124*
☎ *06/442–37261*

Views of Rome
May 2000
Calcografia
✉ *Via della Stamperia 6*
☎ *06/699–801*

City, Garden, Memory
May–August 2000
A series of exhibitions inaugurated
in 1998 and devoted to
contemporary art. The works of
the leading artistic figures weave a
dialogue with the ancient against
the background of Villa Medici
and its gardens.
Villa Medici
✉ *Viale Trinità dei Monti 1/A*
☎ *06/676–11*

"Exodus": Photographs by Sebastião Salgado
June–September 2000
The photographs, presented in
Rome in their world premiere, tell
the story of the large and dramatic
migrations over the five
continents.
Scuderie Papali
✉ *Via XXIV Maggio 16*
☎ *06/678–6648*

Art in Italy: The Test of Modernity
November 2000–January 2001
A critical assessment of modernity
in art, captured between the end of
the 19th century and the early
years of the 20th century.
Galleria Nazionale d'Arte Moderna
e Contemporanea
✉ *Viale delle Belle Arti 131*
☎ *06/322–981*

The Light of the Spirit in 20th-Century Art
July–October 2000
The concept of the sacred in
modern art viewed through the
works of the main artistic figures
of the century, from Picasso to
Matisse, Malevich, Mondrian,
Brancusi, and Boccioni, as well as
contemporary artists such as
Kounellis, Serra, Judd, and others.
Palazzo delle Esposizioni
✉ *Via Nazionale 194*
☎ *06/474–5903*

Botticelli and The Divine Comedy
September–December 2000
Drawings on parchment by Sandro
Botticelli illustrating the cantos of
the *Divine Comedy*. The works are
preserved at the Vatican's Apostolic
Library and in the collections of
the Staatliche Museen Preussischer
Kulturbesitz in Berlin.
Scuderie Papali
✉ *Via XXIV Maggio 16*
☎ *06/678–6648*

St. Caecilia: The Myth of Music Between the Sacred and the Profane
October 2000–January 2001
Palazzo Barberini (Cardinal
Francesco Library)
✉ *Via delle Quattro Fontane 13*
☎ *06/481–4591*

Cleopatra
October 2000
Organized in collaboration with
the British Museum and the
National Gallery in Washington.
The first complete exhibition on
the historical figure of Cleopatra,
queen of Egypt, enemy of the
Romans, and arbiter of the destiny
of the ancient world.
Palazzo Ruspoli
✉ *Via del Corso 418*
☎ *06/687–4704.*

The Hidden God
October–December 2000
Collection of 17th-century French
religious masterpieces by Poussin,
Champagne, Le Nain, and others,
accompanied by a conference and
musical events.
Villa Medici
✉ *Viale Trinità dei Monti 1/A*
☎ *06/676–11*

Christian Rome
October 2000
The closing archaeological exhibit
of the year 2000, tracing the
transition from classical Roman art
under the influence of Christian
Rome from the 3rd century to the
end of the 4th century. The show
provides complete documentation
of all forms of art in Rome:
painting, sculpture, minor arts,
and monuments. The exhibit will
feature special itineraries.
Palazzo delle Esposizioni
✉ *Via Nazionale 194*
☎ *06/474–5903*

Jerico: Ten Thousands Years of History in Palestine

November 2000
Museo Nazionale di Castel Sant'Angelo
✉ *Lungotevere Castello 1*
☎ *06/681–911*

The 20th Century

December 2000
An exhibit of some 180 paintings and sculptures from the most important schools of 20th-century Italian art.
Scuderie Papali
✉ *Via XXIV Maggio 16*
☎ *06/678–6648*

The Beaux-Arts Tradition

Dates to be determined
An exploration of American artistic circles at the close of the nineteenth century, assessing the impact of classical culture on artists such as Augustus St. Gaudens, John La Farge, Charles Follen McKim and many others.
American Academy in Rome
✉ *Via A. Masina 5*
☎ *06/584–6425*

Music and Theater

The start of the musical season of the Jubilee year is dominated by two major events: Mozart's *Coronation Mass,* directed by Riccardo Muti in S. Pietro on Christmas Eve 1999, and the inauguration of the Città della Musica with a concert directed by Myung-Whun Chung. The soloists are Cecilia Bartoli, Natalie Dessay, Martha Argerich, and Maximilian Vengerov.

Throughout the year the entire city and much of the region of Lazio will host a continous series of musical events, both in traditional settings for music and in churches, squares, abbeys, and archaeological sites that fill the area.

The **Accademia di Santa Cecilia** has dedicated a special concert season to the Holy Year, distinguished by the rediscovery of the great Italian tradition of sacred music.

The Easter Festival will be a special occasion for sacred music, with the revival of the ancient tradition of music in churches and oratories as accompaniment for all the rites of Easter week.

In *Orfeo ed Euridice* by Gluck, *Mosè* by Rossini (in the original French edition), and *Parsifal* by Wagner, the three composers tackle the themes of rebirth and redemption. This is the poetic motif that runs through the program of the **Teatro dell'Opera di Roma** in the year 2000, offering a musical reflection on the theme of the sacred without neglecting the traditional repertory, which will highlight Puccini's *Tosca* and Bellini's *Norma.*

A multitude of other musical and theatrical events has been planned. The most important include the twice daily concerts in the Benedictine church of S. Anselmo all'Aventino and the Festival of the Sacred, organized by the Fondazione Romaeuropa, with music and dance from around the world.

The **Teatro di Roma** has organized a series of productions for the Jubilee to addresses the spiritual and social issues facing us in the new millennium. The special Jubilee season opens in January with the Raffaello Sanzio group's production of *Genesi, from the Museum of Sleep* by Romeo Castellucci, with an original score by Scott Gibbons. It continues in the spring with *La seconda vita di Francesco d'Assisi* by José Saramango, directed by Marco Baliani.

The year 2000 will also see a new itinerant production of Luca Ronconi's *Laudari medioevali,* Raffaele Viviani's *I Dieci Comandamenti,* Giorgio Barberio Corsetti's *Graal,* and many other events, including Pina Bausch's special Jubilee production, *Ein Stück.*

During the summer, Teatro Argentina will put on *Sette Spettacoli per un Nuovo Teatro Italiano e per il 2000,* seven new productions selected in a public competition that seek to create a new theatrical idiom.

The calendar of events is not devoted solely to sacred music, but also includes many other initiatives ranging from modern music to theater and dance: from the Festa Italiana with traditional dance and music at the Teatro Sistina, to the European Music Festival in all the piazzas of the city, to the Autumn Festival, organized by ETI (the Italian Theater Council), with concerts and international avant-garde theater productions.

This section of the guide has been prepared by the Agenzia Romana per la Preparazione del Giubileo (Rome Agency for Jubilee Preparations). The Agency is a publicly owned limited company. Its task is to provide technical and organizational support to the government bodies in charge of

supplying the services needed by visitors during the Jubilee. Its shareholders are the City of Rome, the Province of Rome, Lazio Region, the Rome Chamber of Commerce, the Ministry of the Treasury (through the Deposits and Loans Fund), the City of Florence, and the City of Naples.

Piazza Adriana 12, 00193 Rome
Phone ++39/06/681–671
Web site: www.romagiubileo.it
e-mail: agenzia@romagiubileo.it

Artists in Rome
Index
Rome Atlas

The Contarelli Chapel, in the church of S. Luigi dei Francesi, with St. Matthew and the Angel *and the* Calling of Matthew, *by Caravaggio*

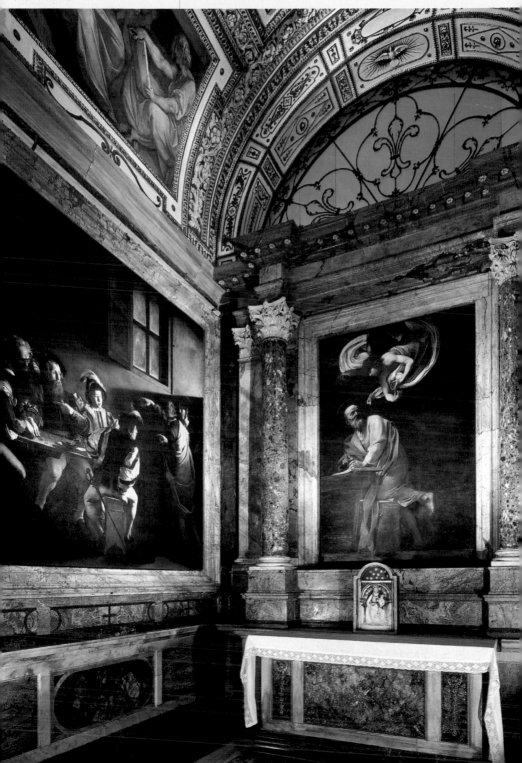

Artists in Rome

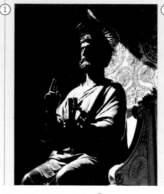

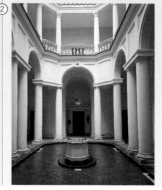

From time immemorial, Rome, the capital of Christianity, has been the center of artistic activity, more than any other city in Europe. Artists of extraordinary talent and fame created works that punctuate the landscape of the Eternal City. The pages that follow present some of the most celebrated architects, painters, and sculptors in Rome, who gave most to the city and are mentioned most frequently in the pages of Holy Rome. A series of concise biographies will acquaint readers with the artists who have shaped the face of Rome over the centuries.

Alessandro Algardi
Sculptor (1595–1654)
Algardi's apprenticeship with Ludovico Carracci in Bologna and his restoration work of ancient stuccos for Cardinal Ludovisi in Rome (1625) were fundamental parts of his training. While sensitive to the poetics of Bernini and the paintings of Pietro da Cortona, he was inspired by classical ideals of composure and compositional balance. Significant works include his stucco statues of *St. John the Evangelist* and the *Magdalen* for S. Silvestro al Quirinale (1628–1629); *St. Philip and the Angel*, for S. Maria in Vallicella (1640); and the monumental projects undertaken during the papcy of Innocent X Pamphilj (*Monument to Leo XI* and a marble altarpiece depicting *The Meeting of Attila and Pope Leo*, both in S. Pietro). He also executed numerous significant portraits: *Olimpia Pamphilj*, now in the Galleria Doria Pamphilj, and *Garzia Mellini*, in S. Maria del Popolo.

Arnolfo di Cambio ①
Sculptor and architect (1245–1302)
Influenced by the Gothic style, Arnolfo di Cambio harmoniously merged three-dimensional decoration and architecture. After working as an assistant to Nicola Pisano in Siena, he went to Rome in 1277 to work for Charles of Anjou. There he came under new influences, including classical and late antique sculpture and the French Gothic style, with its elegant linear quality. In two large baldachins, in S. Paolo Fuori le Mura (1285) and S. Cecilia in Trastevere (1293), he created original architectural schemes that merge with the sculpted portions. Although his works in Rome are signed (a votive chapel of S. Boniface VIII in the old S. Pietro in the Vatican, 1301; a bronze statue of St. Peter in the Vatican basilica, ☞*photograph above*), they are most likely from his workshop. It is probable that he also participated in the alterations to S. Maria in Aracoeli (1280–1285).

Gian Lorenzo Bernini ③
Architect, sculptor, and set designer (1598–1680)
Bernini was the dominant figure in Baroque Rome. His career as an architect began with the election of Pope Urban VIII (1623) and reached its apex during the papacy of Alexander VII. In the basilica of S. Pietro he created the bronze baldachin with spiral columns (☞*photograph at right*), the throne of St. Peter (1657–1666), the Scala Regia, and the final layout of the elliptical piazza (beginning in 1656). He designed fountains (the Fontana del Tritone in Piazza Barberini, the Fontana dei Fiumi in Piazza Navona), churches (S. Andrea al Quirinale), and palaces (Palazzo Montecitorio and Palazzo Barberini). His most memorable sculptures include *The Ecstasy of St. Teresa* in S. Maria della Vittoria

(1644–1652), *Blessed Ludovica Albertoni* in S. Francesco a Ripa, and the marble groups of *Apollo and Daphne, Aeneas and Anchises,* and *David* in the Galleria Borghese.

Francesco Borromini ②
(Francesco Castelli) Architect (1599–1667)
A brilliant figure in the architectural world of Baroque Rome, Borromini spent some years in Milan before going, at the end of 1619, to the capital, where he remained for the rest of his life. He began his activity working as a stonecutter in S. Pietro. He then went to work for Bernini and became his principal assistant. His first independent project was the construction of the cloister (☞*photograph above*), monastery, and church for S. Carlo alle Quattro Fontane (1638–1641). Here, as in his later works in Rome (the oratory and monastery of the Filippini, S. Ivo alla Sapienza, the renovation of the interior of S. Giovanni in Laterano, S. Agnese, the facade of the Collegio di Propaganda Fide), he experimented with novel spatial inventions (elliptical plans, undulating surfaces, theatrical arrangement of light sources, decorative abundance).

Bramante
(Donato di Pascuccio di Antonio) Architect and painter (1444–1514)
Bramante arrived in Rome after the fall of the Sforza family in Milan (1499). In the Eternal City, he designed the cloister of S. Maria della Pace (1500) and the circular tempietto of S. Pietro in Montorio (begun in 1502). The latter was the first great mid-Renaissance monument, and its elements, taken from ancient architecture, make it a symbol of universal harmony. When Julius II ascended to the papacy (1503), Bramante found an ideal client. He was involved in the

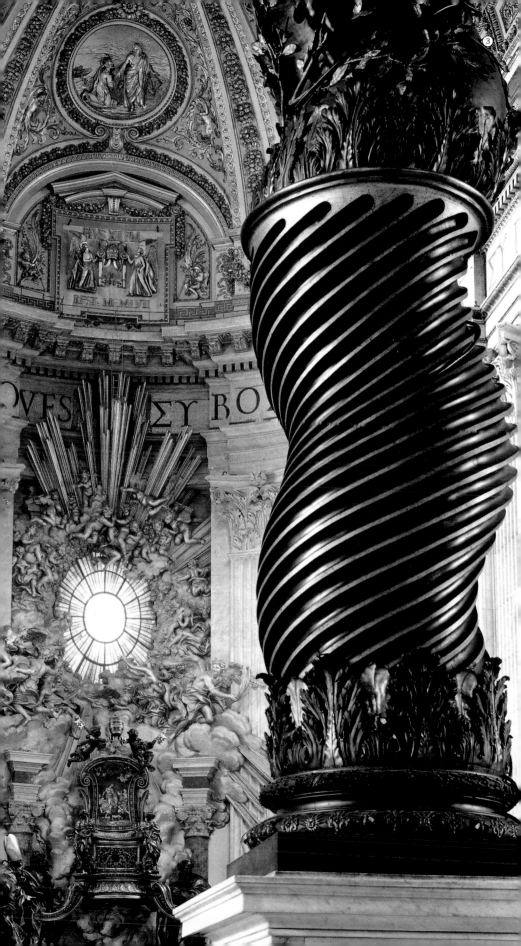

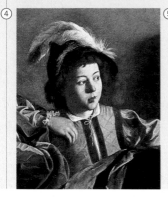

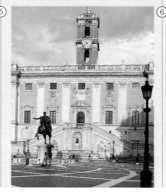

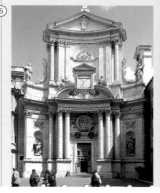

renovation projects for the Holy See, where he designed the Belvedere courtyard, which links the palace and villa of Innocent VIII. It is articulated on three levels and culminates in a large semicircular piazza. He proposed a central plan for S. Pietro surmounted by a vast dome, a scheme favored by humanist culture. The building was begun, but the death of the pope put an end to the project.

Caravaggio ④
(Michelangelo Merisi) Painter
(1571–1610)
Caravaggio grew up in Lombardy, and during his early years in Rome (1592–1593), he painted predominantly still lifes. Cardinal Francesco Maria del Monte, his first powerful patron in Rome, gave him lodgings in his palace and entrusted him with the fresco decoration of his laboratory (Casino Ludovisi). His genre scenes (*The Card Players*, 1595) and his early religious subjects for private use (*Rest on the Flight into Egypt*, 1595) date from this period. Thanks to the cardinal's patronage, he decorated the Contarelli Chapel in S. Luigi dei Francesi (1599–1602, ☞ 151). There, in *The Calling of Matthew* (☞ *see detail above*) and *The Martyrdom of Matthew*, everyday reality invades a grand sacred scene for the first time. The dramatic use of light and the somewhat unseemly realism of the subjects is accentuated in works such as the *Conversion of Paul* (S. Maria del Popolo), the *Deposition* (Vatican Pinacoteca), and the *Madonna of the Pilgrims* (S. Agostino).

Annibale and Agostino Carracci
Painters
(1560–1609 and 1557–1602)
In 1582 brothers Agostino and Annibale Carracci founded the Accademia dei Desiderosi in Bologna (later renamed Accademia

degli Incamminati), where the art of the Renaissance was evoked in works with simple tones and figures with faces and stances that were both natural and idealized. From 1595 onward, Annibale was in Rome, working for Odoardo Farnese. Agostino asked his brother to decorate the Farnese Gallery (1597), but disagreements between the two led Agostino to leave the city. In his work, Annibale returned to Renaissance forms and proposed a new concept of landscape, which became the central element of his compositions (*Flight into Egypt*, c. 1604, in the chapel of the Palazzo Aldobrandini).

Giacomo della Porta ⑤
Architect and sculptor (1533–1602)
A student of Vignola and follower of Michelangelo, Giacomo della Porta created a substantial body of work that helped to solidify those great Renaissance architects' concepts (the two-story church facade, the palazzo) into definitive building types. He continued Michelangelo's Campidoglio project (Palazzo dei Conservatori; Palazzo Senatorio, ☞ *see photograph above*), and he succeeded Vignola as architect of the Chiesa del Gesù in Rome, designing its facade (1573–1584). He became the architect of S. Pietro, where he completed Michelangelo's facade overlooking the garden and constructed the smaller domes and the great dome. He also designed the Oratory of the Crucifix (1568) and the nave of S. Giovanni dei Fiorentini (1582–1592).

Domenichino ⑦
(Domenico Zampieri) Painter
(1581–1641)
A student of Ludovico Carracci in Bologna, Domenichino arrived in Rome and entered the circle of Annibale Carracci, collaborating with him on the Farnese Gallery. Using Carracci as a model, he

developed a formula for classicism that is characterized by precision of drawing and compositional balance. The classical ideal did not prevent him from looking at reality, which he maintained as an essential point of reference. In S. Luigi dei Francesi, his *Scenes from the Life of St. Caecilia* (1614, ☞ *see detail at right*) represent the culmination of his style. He painted his *Last Communion of St. Jerome* (1614, Vatican Pinacoteca) and *Diana and Nymphs Hunting* (Galleria Borghese) during the second decade of the century. His frescoes for S. Andrea della Valle are noteworthy, although they fail to achieve the triumphant Baroque vision expressed in the dome by Lanfranco, his contemporary.

Carlo Fontana ⑥
Architect (1634–1714)
Carlo Fontana settled in Rome in 1655. He began his activity as an assistant to Pietro da Cortona, Rainaldi, and Bernini, for whom he worked for 10 years. He executed numerous projects, including S. Margherita in Trastevere, S. Biagio in Campitelli, the concave facade of S. Marcello al Corso (1683, ☞ *see photograph above*), and the Ospizio Apostolico in S. Michele a Ripa Grande, in collaboration with Ferdinando Fuga. He designed numerous chapels for churches in Rome, including the Cybo Chapel in S. Maria del Popolo (1683–1687), as well as the baptismal font in S. Pietro (1692–1698). He restored and in large part rebuilt the church of SS. Apostoli (1702) and completed Palazzo Montecitorio by Bernini, from whom he had inherited the position of papal architect. Over time he became the undisputed leading architect in Rome and was considered the person most responsible for the classicizing academic style into which the Baroque declined.

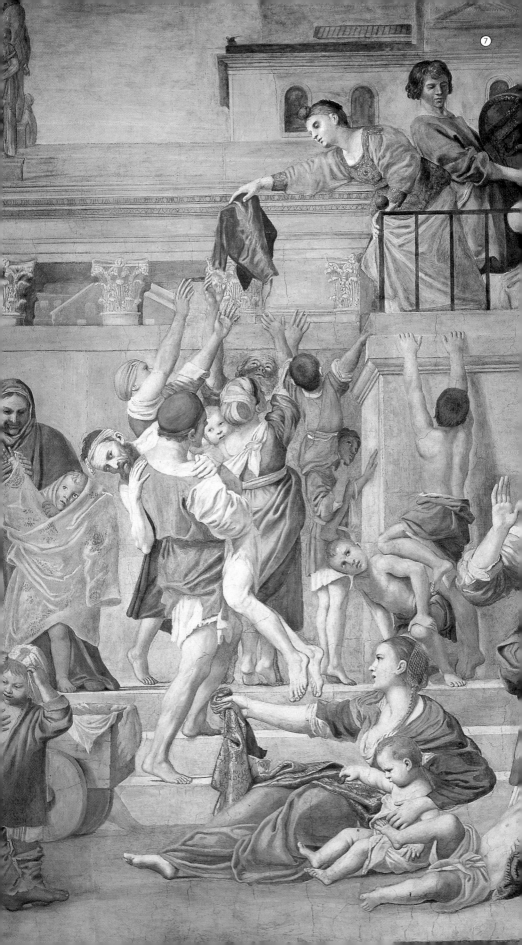

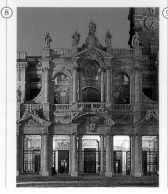

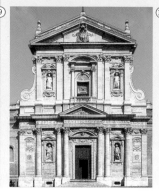

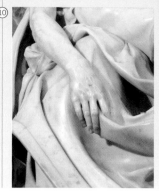

Domenico Fontana
Architect (1543–1607)

Architect to Sixtus V, he designed and saw to completion the urban redesign of Rome, with the opening of the Via Sistina and the streets that run from S. Maria Maggiore to S. Giovanni in Laterano, S. Croce in Gerusalemme, and S. Lorenzo. Fontana is also known for the erection of the obelisk in Piazza S. Pietro and for various engineering and hydraulic projects. His masterpiece is the Palazzo Lateranense (1586), followed by the SS. Sacramento Chapel in S. Maria Maggiore, which has a central plan. Little remains of his Ospizio dei Cento Preti, a building commissioned by the pope in 1587. He designed the original Salone Sistino in the Vatican Library (1587–1589), which contains opulent late-16th-century frescoes.

Ferdinando Fuga ⑧
Architect (1699–1782)

A Florentine by birth, Fuga created all his principal projects in Rome. Chosen by Clement XII and then by Benedict XIV to be architect of the papal palaces, he completed the Quirinal Palace, adding the Segretario delle Cifre building and a new wing, the "manica lunga." His works in Rome reveal a passage from a personal vocabulary adhering to Baroque parameters to forms more closely tied to classicism. These projects include the Palazzo della Consulta (1732–1737), the facade for S. Maria Maggiore (1741–1743, ☞ see photograph above), and alterations to the Palazzo Corsini, formerly the Riario (1736). In the latter project, his sophisticated late-Baroque language achieves its most elegant results. His other works include the churches of S. Maria dell'Orazione e Morte (1733–1737) and S. Apollinare.

Carlo Maderno ⑨
Architect (1556–1629)

In 1588 Maderno settled in Rome and became an assistant to his uncle, Domenico Fontana. In 1603 he was appointed architect of S. Pietro; that same year he completed the facade for the church of S. Susanna (☞ see photograph above), a revolutionary design that broke with the then current Mannerist style and announced the Baroque. S. Susanna and the majestic dome of S. Andrea della Valle are considered his masterpieces, although he is better known for his work on S. Pietro. During the papacy of Paul V, he won a competition to complete the basilica. He elongated Michelangelo's centralized plan and built the facade (1612). Other noteworthy projects include the remarkable dome for S. Giovanni dei Fiorentini (1519), the Palazzo Mattei, and the Palazzo Barberini (built almost entirely after his death, by Bernini).

Michelangelo Buonarroti ⑩
Architect, sculptor, painter, and poet (1475–1564)

Michelangelo left his indelible mark during each of his sojourns in Rome. He sculpted the Pietà (☞ see detail atbove) and, for the tomb of Julius II, the Rebel Slave, the Dying Slave, and the Moses (1513–1516). Between 1508 and 1512 he painted a magnificent fresco cycle for the Sistine Chapel, with powerful figures of Prophets, Sybils, and Nudes and scenes from Genesis. Clement VII commissioned him to add a fresco of the Last Judgment (1537–1541), which would become a turning point in the artistic development of the Western world. He is responsible for the urban plan of the Piazza del Campidoglio (1546–1547) and the church of S. Maria degli Angeli, and the construction of the apse portion of S. Pietro (1547), with its majestic dome.

Pietro da Cortona
(Pietro Berrettini) Painter and architect (1596–1669)

The official artist of the papal court, Pietro da Cortona is second only to Bernini in the history of the Roman Baroque. He arrived in Rome in 1613 and was a follower of both the classicism of Annibale Carracci and the pictorial freedom of Rubens. The warm, gilded images of his large-scale frescoes convey his great inventiveness and talent: Triumph of Divine Providence (1633–1639) on the ceiling of the great hall of the Palazzo Barberini, Story of Aeneas (1647) in the Palazzo Pamphilj, frescoes for the dome and nave of the Chiesa Nuova. His first important building, the church of Ss. Luca e Martina, is considered the first great Baroque church; his use of concave and convex forms in the facade of S. Maria della Pace can also be classified as Baroque. His facade for S. Maria in Via Lata exhibits a gradual elimination of Mannerist elements and an acceptance of those elements typical of Roman monumentality.

Pinturicchio ⑪
(Bernardino di Betto) Painter (1454–1513)

Pinturicchio worked in close proximity to Verrocchio's circle. He later worked autonomously in Rome, Perugia, Spoleto and Orvieto. In Rome, he collaborated with Perugino on the decoration of the Sistine Chapel (1481–1483) for Sixtus IV. His most challenging undertaking was the decoration of the Borgia Apartment (1492–1494, ☞ see detail of Resurrection at right)). His other projects in Rome are the Bufalini Chapel in the church of the Aracoeli and S. Maria del Popolo (Chapel of S. Girolamo, 1488; Chapel of S. Caterina, 1489; Cybo Chapel).

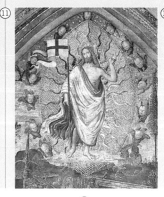

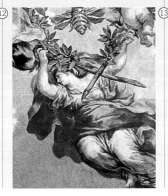

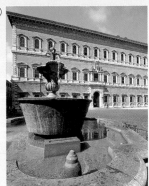

Raphael Sanzio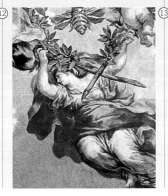
Painter and architect (1483–1520)
Raphael was brought to Rome by
Julius II in 1508, to work with
Perugino, Sodoma, Bramantino,
and others on the decoration of
the Vatican *Stanze* (1509–1514).
During this period, he painted the
Triumph of Galatea fresco for
Agostino Chigi, in the loggia of the
Farnesina (☞ *see detail above*), and
the Sybil frescoes for the Chigi
Chapel in S. Maria della Pace. He
also devoted his energies to architecture. His first building was S.
Eligio degli Orefici (1509, rebuilt
in the early 17th century). In 1517,
as Superintendent of Antiquities, he
demonstrated his interests in his
design for the Villa Madama,
which had a circular courtyard and
numerous rooms with apses and
niches, inspired by Roman baths.
He was named papal architect in
1514, a post previously held by
Bramante; in this capacity he
designed a variation on Bramante's
plan for S. Pietro. Raphael's Chigi
Chapel in S. Maria del Popolo
(1512–1513), on a central plan,
was finished by Bernini.

Carlo Rainaldi
Architect (1611–1691)
A dominant figure in Rome's late
17th-century architecture, Rainaldi
developed his own majestic manner, notable for its theatrical qualities and for the mix of Mannerist
and Baroque elements employed
by his great contemporaries (particularly Bernini). With his father,
he began S. Agnese in Agone, on a
Greek cross plan, but the project
was taken away from him the
following year and turned over to
Borromini. Carlo Rainaldi's
principal projects are all in Rome:
S. Maria in Campitelli; the facade
of S. Andrea della Valle; the exteri-
or of the apse and tribune of S. Maria
Maggiore; S. Maria in Montesanto
and S. Maria dei Miracoli, the twin
churches in Piazza del Popolo that
connect Via del Babuino, Via del
Corso, and Via Ripetta, the three
principal streets that radiate out
toward the center of the city.

Guido Reni
Painter (1575–1642)
Bolognese painter Guido Reni was
a champion of classicism. A student
of Ludovico Carracci, he often
worked in the papal city, where he
was influenced by the work of both
Raphael and Caravaggio. His
Crucifixion of St. Peter (1604),
painted for the church of S. Paolo
alle Tre Fontane and now in the
Vatican Pinacoteca, follows
Caravaggio's style. Fulfilling presti-
gious commissions, he frescoed the
Sala delle Nozze Aldobrandini, the
Sala delle Dame in the Vatican
(1608–1609), and S. Gregorio al
Celio. He also decorated the
Chapel of the Annunciata on the
Quirinale. His greatest work in
Rome is the fresco *Aurora*, in the
Casino of the Palazzo Pallavicini
Rospigliosi (c. 1612–1614).

Jacopo Sansovino
(Jacopo d'Antonio Tatti) Sculptor
and architect (1486–1570)
A Florentine who worked predominantly as a sculptor, Sansovino
arrived in Rome in 1506. His first
works in the city bear the sign of
competition with Michelangelo,
and after a bitter conflict with him,
he drew upon classical precursors
to an even greater degree. In 1519
he won a competition for the
design of the church of S. Giovanni
dei Fiorentini, but his initial design
with a central plan was soon abandoned. During the 1527 sack of
Rome he fled to Venice, where he
remained until his death. His
works in Rome include a statue of
St. James in S. Maria Monserrato
and the *Madonna and Child* (1521)
in S. Agostino, a much-loved devotional effigy. The church of
S. Marcello al Corso also bears
signs of his contribution.

Sangallo the Younger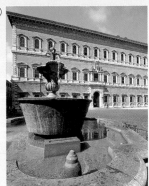
(Antonio Giamberti da Sangallo)
Architect (1484–1546)
From 1503 onward, Sangallo the
Younger worked in Rome, where,
after the death of Raphael, he
became the principal architect of
the high Renaissance for two
decades. He trained with his uncles
(he was the nephew of Antonio da
Sangallo the Elder and Giuliano da
Sangallo) and worked as a designer
for the architects Bramante and
Peruzzi. In 1516 he assisted
Raphael, who was working in
S. Pietro reinforcing Bramante's
walls. Various palazzi have been
attributed to him, particularly the
Palazzo Baldassini (1520) and the
Palazzo del Banco di S. Spirito
(1521–1524). His masterpiece is
the Palazzo Farnese (begun in
1534, completed by Michelangelo
in 1546), the most monumental of
the Renaissance palaces (☞ *see
photograph above*).

Vignola
(Jacopo Barozzi) Architect and
author (1507–1573)
In the mid-16th century this
Bolognese artist moved to Rome,
where he became the favored
architect of the Farnese family. He
worked within civil architecture
circles, both in the capital and in
various towns in Lazio (the suburban residence of Julius II, the Villa
Giulia, and the Palazzo Farnese in
Caprarola), but his religious buildings are his most successful. The
tempietto of S. Andrea was the first
example of sacred architecture on
an oval plan, a scheme that was
widely taken up by Baroque architects. He repeated this plan in his
design for S. Anna dei Palafrenieri
(1555). In his Chiesa del Gesù, he
conceived an architectural model
that became the prototype for
Counter-Reformation churches.

Index

Rome
Atlas

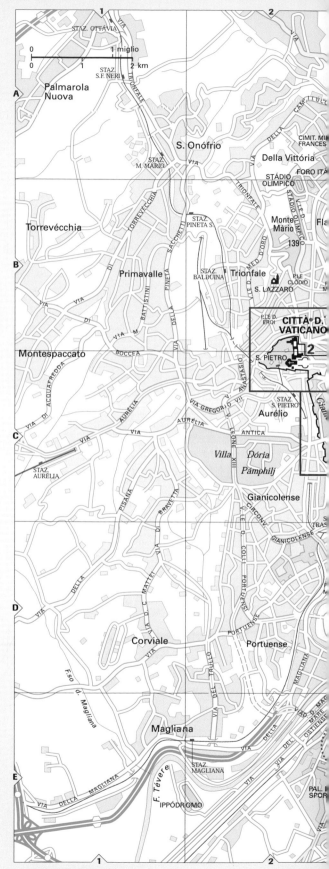

Main thoroughfare.

Street with steps and arcade.

Railway.

Ⓜ **COLOSSEO**

Subway/Underground stop.

Walls and archeological sites.

Important landmark.

Palace or public building;
hospital; developed area.

Church. Synagogue.

Park or garden.

Cemetery.

Scale 1:7500 (1 cm = 75 m)

164

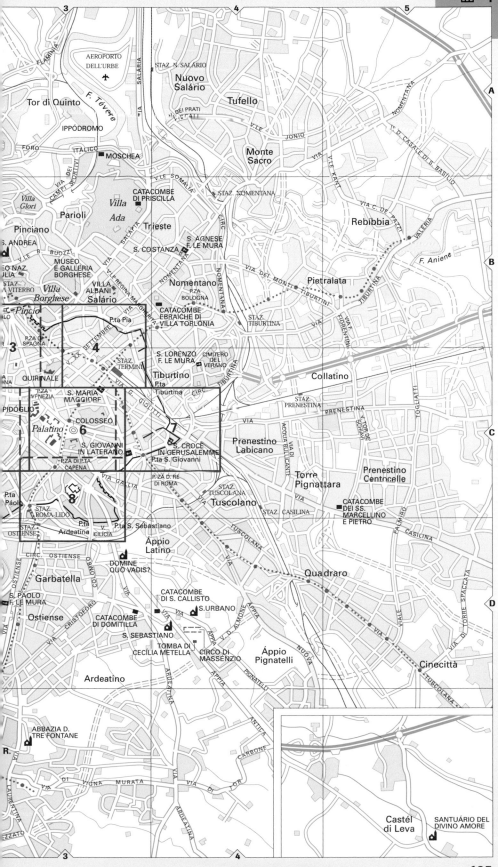

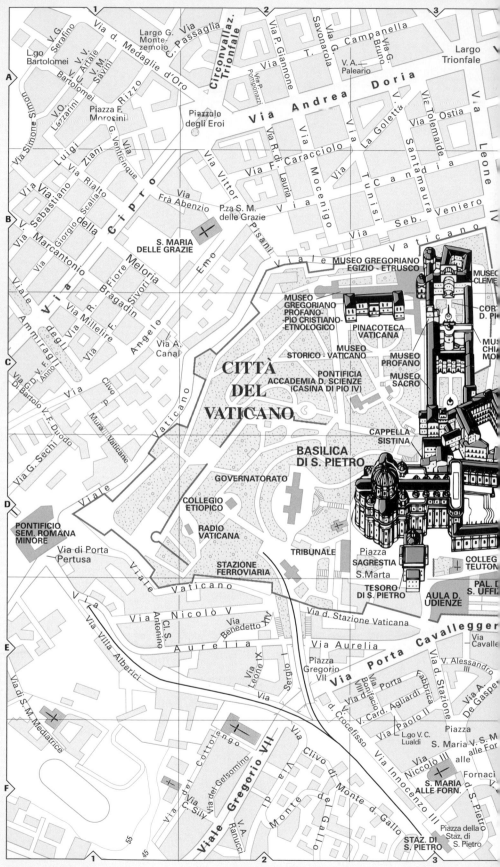

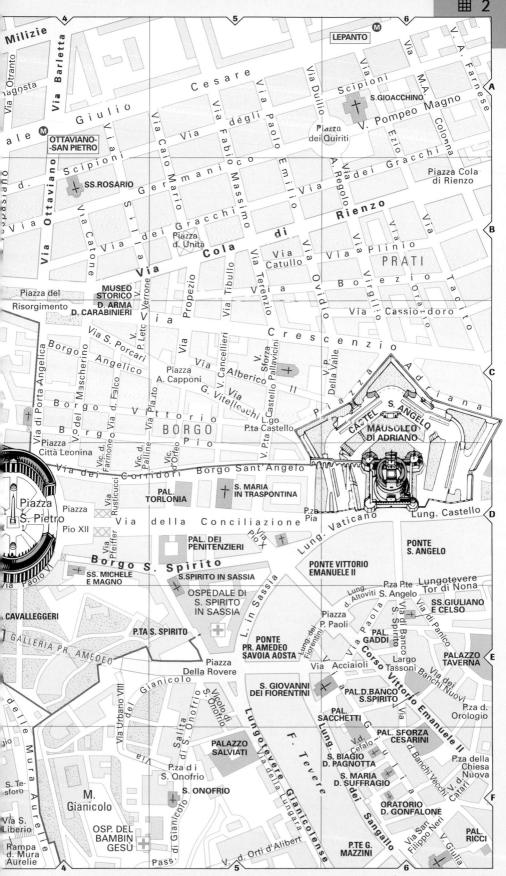

Milizie

V. A. Farnese

LEPANTO Ⓜ

Via Barletta

Via Otranto

agosta

Cesare

Via Duilio

Via

Scipioni

S.GIOACCHINO

Ⓐ

Giulio

Via degli

Via Paolo

M.A.

Piazza
dei Quiriti

V. Pompeo Magno

Colonna

 ⓂOTTAVIANO
-SAN PIETRO

Via Fabio

Via

Ezio

Via Caio Mario

Via Germanico

Via Calo

Emilio

A. Regolo

Via dei Gracchi

Piazza Cola
di Rienzo

Scipioni

Via Massimo

Silla

SS.ROSARIO

Via Catone

Via dei Gracchi

Via Cola

Via Catullo

Via Terenzio

Via Plinio

di

Rienzo

PRATI Ⓑ

Via Ovidio

Via

Via Tibullo

Via Propezio

Via Verrone

P. Leto

Via Cassiodoro

Virgilio

B o r g o

Orazio

Vezio

Tacito

Piazza del
Risorgimento

MUSEO
STORICO
D. ARMA
D. CARABINIERI

Via S. Porcari

Via Cancellieri

V. Sforza
Pallavicini

V.P.
Della Valle

Piazza Adriana

Ⓒ

Borgo

Angelico

Via Alberico

V.P. di Castello

L.go
P.ta Castello

C r e s c e n z i o

Via

Via di Porta Angelica

Borgo Mascherino

Via d. Falco

Piazza
A. Capponi

G. Vitelleschi

II

V i t t o r i o

CASTEL S. ANGELO

MAUSOLEO
DI ADRIANO

Borgo

Via del Pianto

BORGO

P i o

Piazza
Città Leonina

Vic. d.
Farinone

Vic. d.
Palline

Vic.
d'Orfeo

Borgo Sant'Angelo

Via dei Corridori

P.zza
Pia

Lung. Castello Ⓓ

Piazza
S. Pietro

Piazza
Pio XII

Via Rusticucci

PAL.
TORLONIA

S. MARIA
IN TRASPONTINA

Via della Conciliazione

Lung. Vaticano

PONTE
S. ANGELO

Borgo S. Spirito

Via Pfeiffer

Via
Pio X

PAL. DEI
PENITENZIERI

PONTE VITTORIO
EMANUELE II

Via
Paolo

SS. MICHELE
E MAGNO

S.SPIRITO IN SASSIA

L. in Sassia

Lung.
d. Altoviti S. Angelo

P.za Pte
Tor di Nona

SS.GIULIANO
E CELSO

Ⓔ

CAVALLEGGERI

OSPEDALE DI
S. SPIRITO
IN SASSIA

Piazza
P. Paoli

Via di Panico

GALLERIA PR. AMEDEO

P.TA S. SPIRITO

PONTE
PR. AMEDEO
SAVOIA AOSTA

Lung. dei
Fiorentini

Via di Banco

PAL.
GADDI

Corso Vittorio Emanuele II

PALAZZO
TAVERNA

Piazza
Della Rovere

Via Acciaioli

Largo
Tassoni

Via dei
Banchi Nuovi

Via S. Spirito

P.za di
Orologio

delle Mura Aurelie

Via Urbano VIII

del Gianicolo

Salita di S. Onofrio

Vicolo di
S. Onofrio

S. GIOVANNI
DEI FIORENTINI

PAL.D.BANCO
S.SPIRITO

P.za della
Chiesa
Nuova

Via
Urbano VIII

PAL.
SACCHETTI

PAL. SFORZA
CESARINI

d. Banchi Vecchi

V. d.
Catari

S. Tesforo

M.
Gianicolo

P.za di
S. Onofrio

PALAZZO
SALVIATI

Lungotevere Gianicolense

F. Tevere

Lung. dei Sangallo

V.d.
Cefalo

S. BIAGIO
D. PAGNOTTA

S. MARIA
D. SUFFRAGIO

ORATORIO
D. GONFALONE

Via San
Filippo Neri

V. Giulia

PAL.
RICCI

Ⓕ

Via S.
Liberio

Rampa
d. Mura
Aurelie

OSP. DEL
BAMBIN
GESÙ

S. ONOFRIO

Via di Gianicolo

Via della Lungara

V. d. Orti d'Alibert

P.TE G.
MAZZINI

Pass.

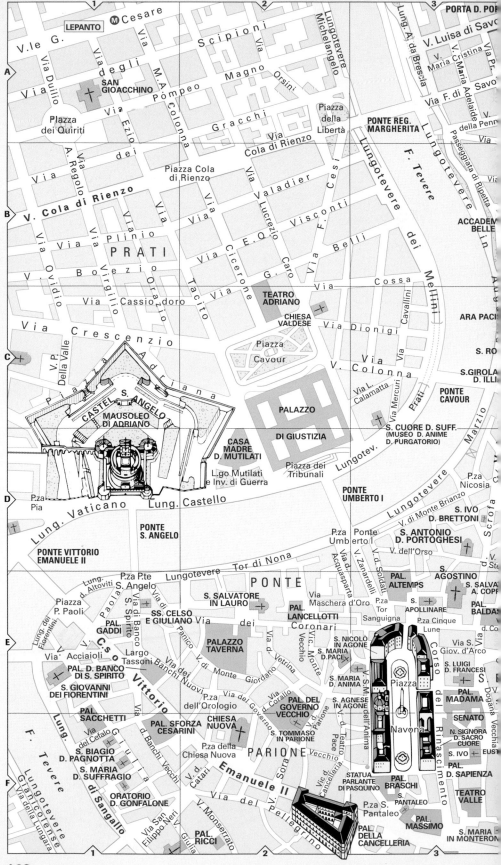

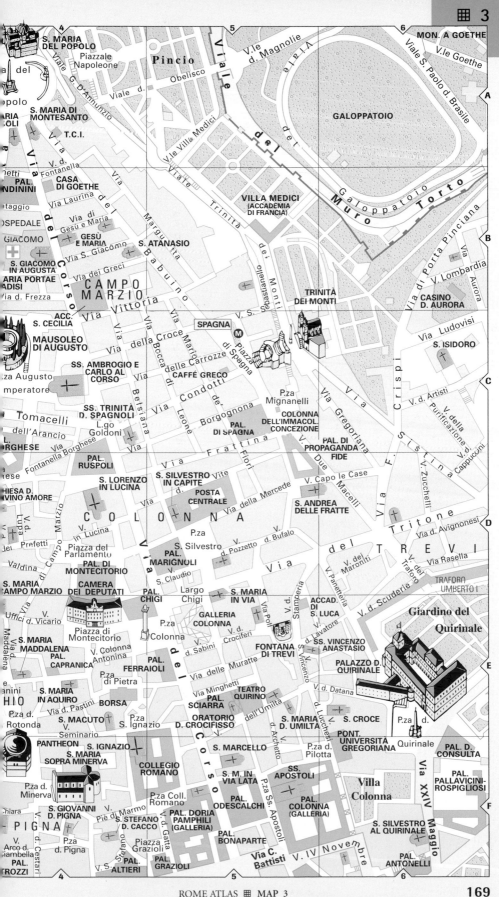

MON. A GOETHE

V.le Goethe

Viale S. Paolo d. Brasile

S. MARIA
DEL POPOLO

Piazzale
Napoleone

Pincio

Viale d. G. D'Annunzio

Viale d.

Obelisco

V.le d. Magnolie

Viale

Viale

del

GALOPPATOIO

A

opolo
del

ARIA
OLI

S. MARIA DI
MONTESANTO

T.C.I.

Fontanella

CASA
DI GOETHE

Via Laurina

Via di
Gesù e Maria

Via

Margutta

Muro

Torto

Galoppatoio

Via di Porta Pinciana

V. Lombardia

Aurora

B

etti
NDININI

PAL.

ottaggio

OSPEDALE

GIACOMO

S. GIACOMO
IN AUGUSTA

ARIA PORTAE
ADISI

Via d. Frezza

GESÙ
E MARIA

Via S. Giacomo

S. ATANASIO

Via dei Greci

CAMPO
MARZIO

Via Vittoria

Babuino

V.le Villa Medici

Viale

Trinità

dei

Monti

V.le Villa Medici

VILLA MEDICI
(ACCADEMIA
DI FRANCIA)

TRINITÀ
DEI MONTI

Via di Porta Pinciana

CASINO
D. AURORA

Via Ludovisi

S. ISIDORO

Crispi

V. della Purificazione

V. d. Artisti

V. d. Cappuccini

ACC.
S. CECILIA

MAUSOLEO
DI AUGUSTO

za Augusto
mperatore

SS. AMBROGIO E
CARLO AL
CORSO

Via della Croce

Via

delle Carrozze

Belsiana

CAFFÈ GRECO

SPAGNA
Ⓜ

Via S.

P.za
di Spagna

Via

S.

Via

Gregoriana

Sistina

Via F.

V. Zucchelli

C

Tomacelli

dell'Arancio

RGHESE

ese

SS. TRINITÀ
D. SPAGNOLI

L.go
Goldoni

Fontanella Borghese

PAL.
RUSPOLI

Via

Condotti

Leone

de

Borgognona

Via

Frattina

Fiori

PAL.
DI SPAGNA

P.za
Mignanelli

COLONNA
DELL'IMMACOL.
CONCEZIONE

PAL. DI
PROPAGANDA
FIDE

Due

Macelli

V. Capo le Case

V. d. Avignonesi

D

CHIESA D.
VINO AMORE

S. LORENZO
IN LUCINA

S. SILVESTRO
IN CAPITE

POSTA
CENTRALE

Via della Mercede

S. ANDREA
DELLE FRATTE

del

Tritone

TREVI

Via Rasella

V. d.

in Lucina

V. d.
Lupa

Via di Campo Marzio

COLONNA

P.za
S. Silvestro

d. Pozzetto d. Bufalo

Via

V. dei
Maroniti

Via d. Traforo

TRAFORO
UMBERTO I

el Prefetti

Valdina

Piazza del
Parlamento

PAL. DI
MONTECITORIO

PAL.
MARIGNOLI

S. Claudio

Largo
Chigi

S. MARIA
IN VIA

A. Panetteria

ACCAD.
DI
S. LUCA

V. d. Scuderie

Giardino del

Quirinale

E

S. MARIA
CAMPO MARZIO

Uffici d. Vicario

S. MARIA
MADDALENA

CAMERA
DEI DEPUTATI

Piazza di
Montecitorio

V.
Uffici d. Vicario

PAL.
CHIGI

P.za
Colonna

GALLERIA
COLONNA

V. d.
Crociferi

d. Sabini

FONTANA
DI TREVI

SS. VINCENZO
ANASTASIO

V. d. Lavatore

V. S. Vincenzo

PALAZZO D.
QUIRINALE

PAL. D.
QUIRINALE

V. d. Datana

PAL.
FERRAIOLI

V. Colonna
Antonina

PAL.
CAPRANICA

P.za
di Pietra

Via delle Murate

TEATRO
QUIRINO

PAL.
SCIARRA

dell'Umiltà

V. d. Lucchesi

S. CROCE

P.za d.

anini

HIO

S. MARIA
IN AQUIRO

V. d.
Maddalena

BORSA

Via d. Pastini

P.za
S. Ignazio

S. MARIA
D. UMILTA

PONT.
UNIVERSITÀ
GREGORIANA

Quirinale

PAL. D.
CONSULTA

F

P.za d.
Rotonda

PANTHEON

S. MACUTO

V.
Seminario

S. IGNAZIO

S. MARIA
SOPRA MINERVA

ORATORIO
D. CROCIFISSO

d'Archetto

S. MARCELLO

P.za d.
Pilotta

Villa

Colonna

PAL.
PALLAVICINI-
ROSPIGLIOSI

Chiara

P.za d.
Minerva

S. GIOVANNI
D. PIGNA

COLLEGIO
ROMANO

P.za Coll.
Romano

S. M. IN
VIA LATA

SS.
APOSTOLI

P.za Ss. Apostoli

Via XXIV

Maggio

S. SILVESTRO
AL QUIRINALE

PIGNA

V.
Arco d.
iambella

P.za
d. Pigna

Piè di Marmo

S. STEFANO
D. CACCO

PAL. DORIA
PAMPHILI
(GALLERIA)

PAL.
ODESCALCHI

PAL.
COLONNA
(GALLERIA)

PAL.
TROZZI

PAL.
ALTIERI

PAL.
GRAZIOLI

Piazza
Grazioli

PAL.
BONAPARTE

Via C.
Battisti

V. IV Novembre

PAL.
ANTONELLI

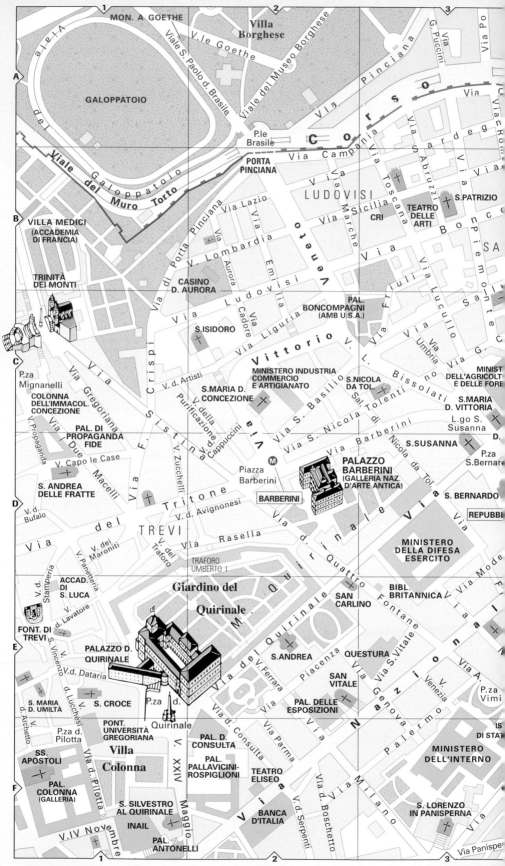

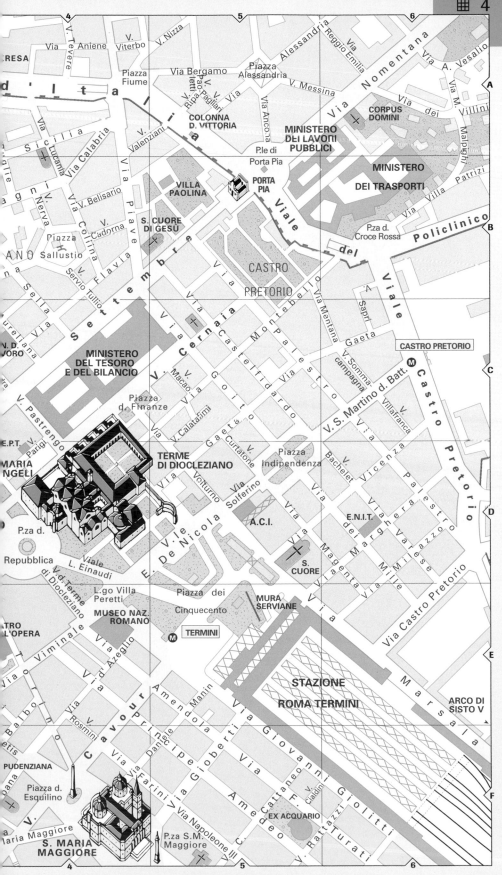

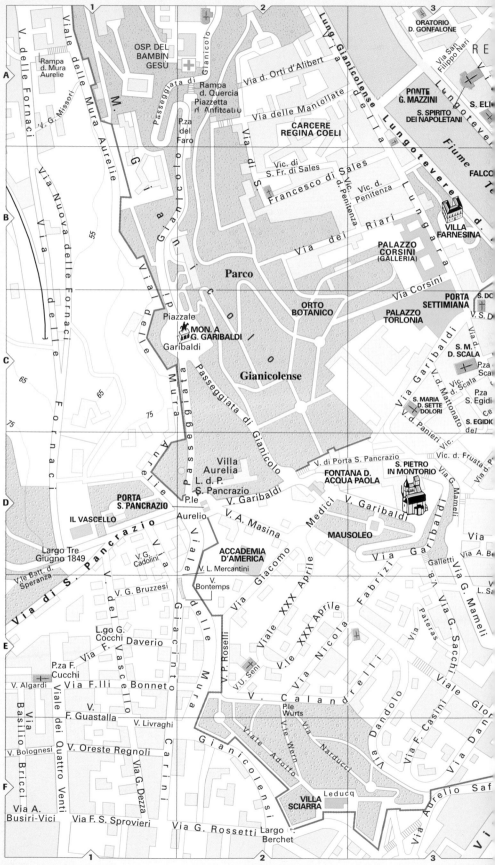

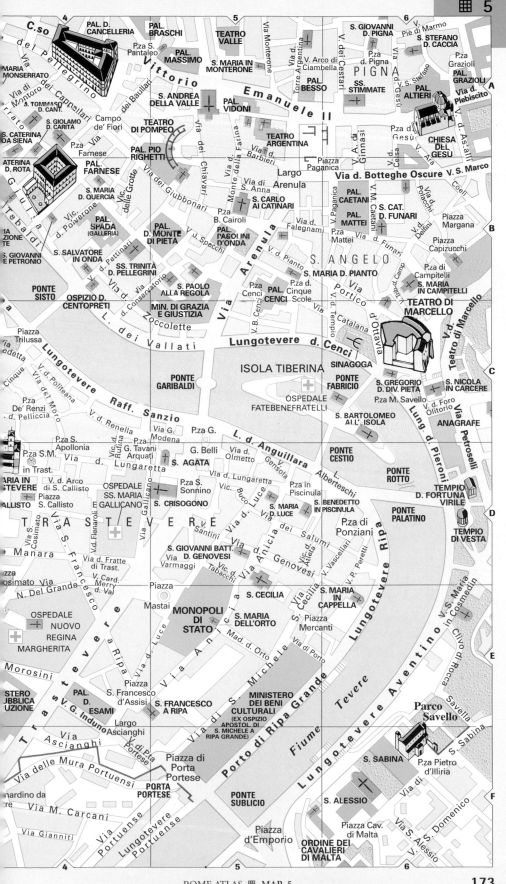

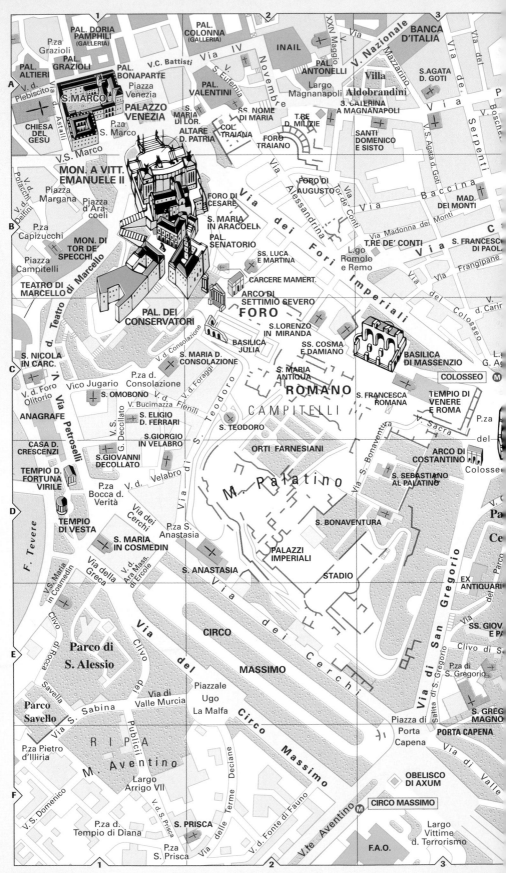

174

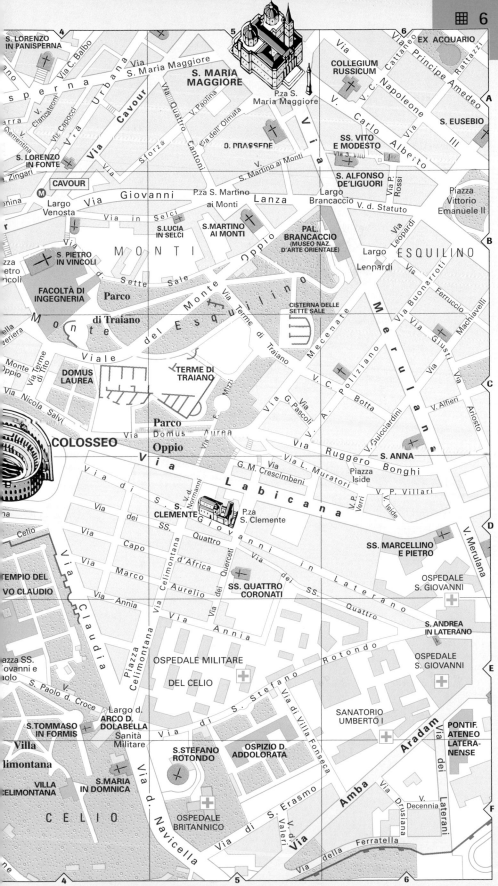

S. LORENZO
IN PANISPERNA

Via C. Balbo

Via Urbana

Via Cavour

S. Maria Maggiore

S. MARIA
MAGGIORE

P.za S.
Maria Maggiore

COLLEGIUM
RUSSICUM

Via

Via Principe Amedeo

Via Cattaneo

Via Rattazzi

EX ACQUARIO

V. C. Napoleone

Via Carlo Alberto

S. EUSEBIO

III

V. Ciancaleoni

V. Capocci

V. Paolina

Quattro Cantoni

Via dell' Olmata

O. PRASSEDE

SS. VITO
E MODESTO

V. Clementina

Via Zingari

S. LORENZO
IN FONTE

Sforza

V. Martino ai Monti

V. S. Vito

S. ALFONSO
DE'LIGUORI

Via P. Rossi

Piazza
Vittorio
Emanuele II

CAVOUR

Via Giovanni

Largo
Venosta

Via in Selci

P.za S. Martino
ai Monti

Lanza

Largo
Brancaccio

V. d. Statuto

Via Leopardi

S. LUCIA
IN SELCI

S.MARTINO
AI MONTI

PAL.
BRANCACCIO
(MUSEO NAZ.
D'ARTE ORIENTALE)

Largo
Leopardi

ESQUILINO

S. PIETRO
IN VINCOLI

M O N T I

Oppio

Via Buonarroti

Via Giusti

Via Machiavelli

FACOLTÀ DI
INGEGNERIA

Parco

Sette Sale

del Esquilino

CISTERNA DELLE
SETTE SALE

Via Ferruccio

di Traiano

Monte

Monte

Via Terme di Traiano

Mecenate

V. C. Poliziano

Via Alfieri

Ariosto

Viale

Via Terme
di Tito

DOMUS
LAUREA

Monte
Oppio

TERME DI
TRAIANO

A. Mizzi

V. C. Botta

V. Guicciardini

Via Nicola Salvi

Parco

Domus

Aurea

Via G. Pascoli

S. ANNA

Ruggero Bonghi

COLOSSEO

Oppio

V i a

Domus Aurea

G. M. Crescimbeni

Labicana

Via L. Muratori

Piazza
Iside

V. P. Villari

V. Iside

V.P. Verri

S. S.

CLEMENTE

V. d. Normanni

P.za
S. Clemente

Giovanni

in

Laterano

SS. MARCELLINO
E PIETRO

V. Merulana

Via di

Via

Via dei

Via dei SS.

Quattro

OSPEDALE
S. GIOVANNI

TEMPIO DEL
VO CLAUDIO

Via dei

Capo

Celimontana

d'Africa

Quattro

Querceti

SS. QUATTRO
CORONATI

Quattro

S. ANDREA
IN LATERANO

Via

Claudia

Via Marco

Aurelio

Via Annia

Via Annia

Rotondo

OSPEDALE
S. GIOVANNI

azza SS.
ovanni e
aolo

S. Paolo d. Croce

Piazza
Celimontana

OSPEDALE MILITARE

DEL CELIO

Via di S. Stefano

Via di Villa Fonseca

SANATORIO
UMBERTO I

Aradam

PONTIF.
ATENEO
LATERA-
NENSE

S.TOMMASO
IN FORMIS

Largo d.
ARCO D.
DOLABELLA

Sanità
Militare

Via dei

Villa
limontana

VILLA
CELIMONTANA

S.MARIA
IN DOMNICA

S.STEFANO
ROTONDO

OSPIZIO D.
ADDOLORATA

Via di S. Erasmo

Amba

Via Drusiana

V.
Decennia

Laterani

C E L I O

Via d. Navicella

OSPEDALE
BRITANNICO

V. d.
Valeri

Via

della

Ferratella

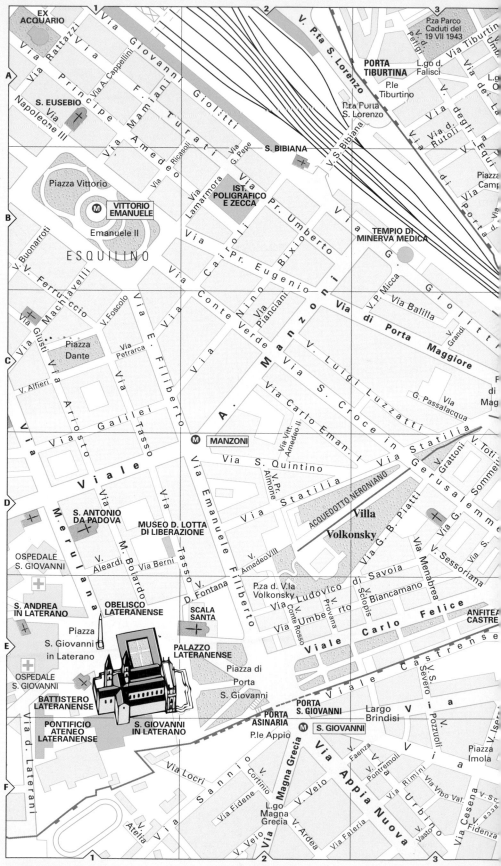

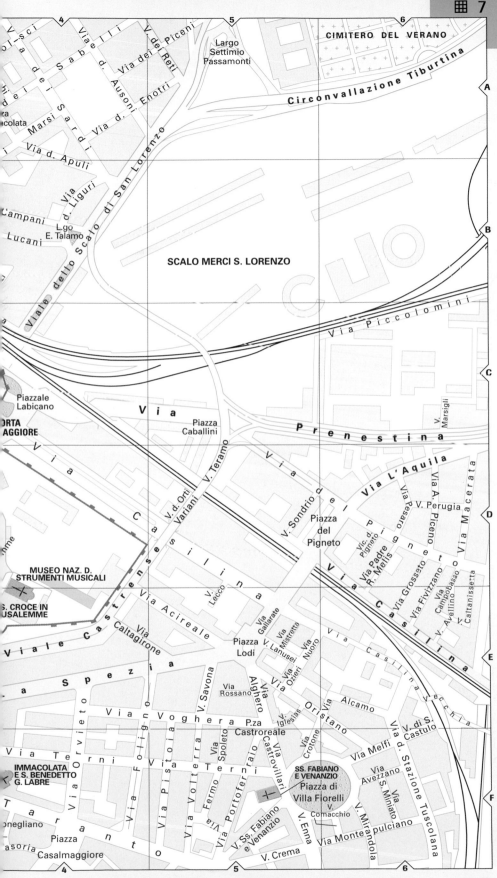

CIMITERO DEL VERANO

Largo
Settimio
Passamonti

Circonvallazione Tiburtina

A

Via d. Piceni
Via d. Reti
Via dei Reti
Via dei Sabelli
Via d. Ausoni
Via d. Enotri
Via dei Sardi
Via dei Marsi
Via d. Apuli
Via d. Liguri
Via dello Scalo di San Lorenzo
Campani
Via d. Marsi
L.go
E. Talamo
Lucani

B

SCALO MERCI S. LORENZO

Via Piccolomini

C

Piazzale
Labicano

Via
Prenestina

Piazza
Caballini

ORTA
AGGIORE

Piazza
Caballini

Via
Marsigli

V i a

Via L'Aquila

Via A. Piceno
V. Perugia
V. Pesaro
Via Macerata

D

V. d. Orti
Variani
V. Teramo
V. Sondrio del
Piazza
del
Pigneto
Vic. d.
Pigneto
Via
padre
R. Melis

MUSEO NAZ. D.
STRUMENTI MUSICALI

Via Grossato
Via Fivizzano
Via Campobasso
Via Avellino
Caltanissetta

S. CROCE IN
USALEMME

Via Acireale
V.
Lecco
Via
Galarate
V i a
C a s i l i n a

Via
Caltagirone

Via Casilina Vecchia

E

V i a l e   C a s t r e n s e

Via
Savona
V.
Algero
Via
Mistretta
V. Lanusei
Piazza
Lodi
V. Ozieri
V. Nuoro

L a   S p e z i a

Via
Rossano

Via
Voghera
V. di S.
Castulo

Alcamo

V i a   T e r n i
Via Orvieto
Via Foligno
Via Pistoia
Via Voltera
Via
Spoleto
P.za
Castroreale
V.
Iglesias
Via Oristano
Via Crotone
Via Melfi
V. di S.
Castulo
Via
Avezzano
Via
S. Miniato
Via
Stazione Tuscolana

IMMACOLATA
E S. BENEDETTO
G. LABRE

Via Fermo
Via Terni
Via Portoferaio
Via Castrovillari
SS. FABIANO
E VENANZIO
Piazza di
Villa Fiorelli
V.
Comacchio
Via Mirandola

F

onegliano
V. SS. Fabiano
e Venanzio
V. Enna
Via Montepulciano

Piazza
Casalmaggiore
asoria
V. Crema

4   5   6

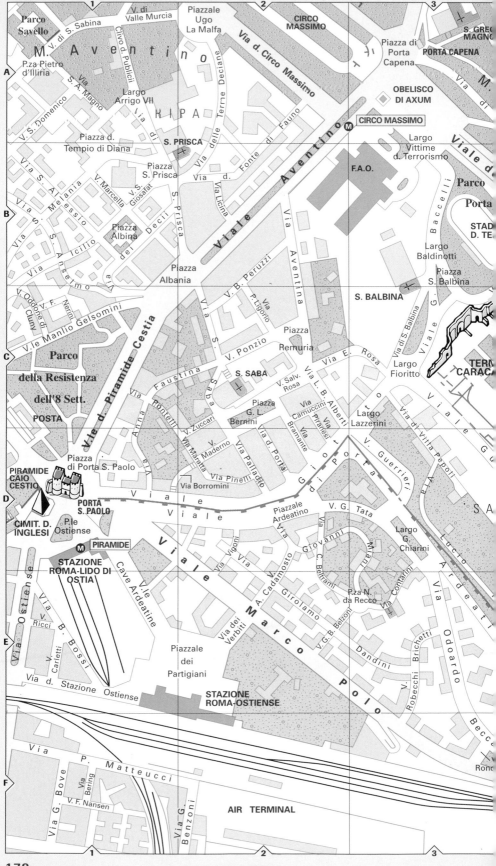

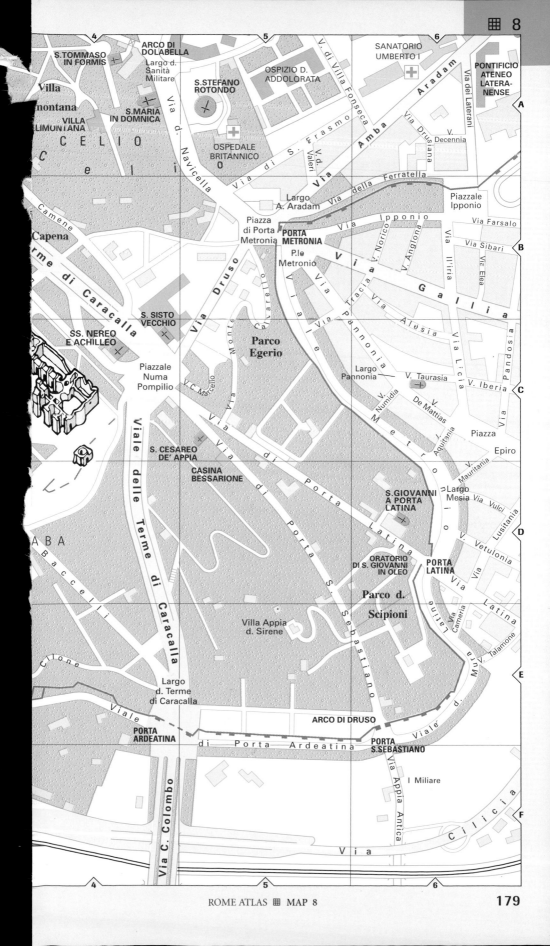

PHOTO CREDITS

The churches of S. Andrea al Quirinale, S. Ignazio, S. Maria sopra Minerva, S. Maria della Scala, S. Prassede, S. Pudenziana, S. Sabina, S. Silvestro in Capite, Ss. Cosma e Damiano, Ss. Giovanni e Paolo are owned by the Fondo Edifici di Culto, which is administered by the Department of Interior's Central Office for Religious Affairs. We thank the F.E.C. for providing the necessary permits.

Rome Agency for Jubilee Preparations: 136, 137, 146 right, 148 left (by kind permission of the magazine *Capitolium*)

Marco Anelli (by kind permission of Fabbrica di San Pietro in Vaticano): 145 left

Photographic Archive of the Touring Club Italino: 12, 24 d, 26 top, 30, 32 bottom left, 36 left, 43 top, 43 center, 46–47, 58 left, 58 right, 80 right

Olivo Barbieri from *San Pietro in Vaticano. Emozioni nel tempo*, TCI 1998 (by kind permission of Fabbrica di San Pietro in Vaticano): 5, 22, 28 bottom, 152 left, 153, 156 right

Giancarlo Costa: 34 top, 35 top, 37 top, 38 top, 39 top, 42 bottom, 44 center, 45 top

Aralodo De Luca: 26 bottom left, 26 bottom right, 95, 128, 129, 157 center

Double's: 40, 43 bottom left, 46, 47 bottom

Fototeca Storica Nazionale: 44 right

Il Dagherrotipo: Stefano Chieppa 23 bottom, 35 bottom; Stefano Occhibelli 68 left, 68 right; Giovanni Rinaldi 18 top, 146 left

Marka: Vito Arcomanno 19 bottom, 48; U.P.P.A. 48

Scala: 13, 14 left, 15 top, 16 left, 17, 20 top, 20 bottom, 21 right, 21 bottom, 24 left, 27, 28 left, 33 top, 33 bottom, 41 top, 41 bottom left, 41 bottom right, 42 left, 43 bottom right, 44 left, 45 bottom, 47 top, 57 left, 57 right, 63 right, 64, 85 right, 92 left, 127 right, 130 left, 131, 154 left, 155, 157 left, 157 right

Antonio Sferlazzo: 12 bottom, 38 bottom left, 38 bottom right, 39 bottom, 49, 54 left, 71 left, 72 left

Sime: Johanna Huber 15 bottom, 31, 53, 54 right, 55, 56, 67 right, 74, 92 right, 108 left, 130 right, 132, 133, 134 right; Giovanni Simeone 2–3, 52, 70 left, 70 right, 94, 110, 111, 121 left, 123, 144

Luca Sorrentino (by kind permission of the magazine *Capitolium*): 145 right